REMAKING THE HUMAN

Politics of Repair

Series Editors:
Francisco Martínez, University of Leicester
Patrick Laviolette, Masaryk University

Politics materializes in buildings lacking maintenance, disrepair infrastructures, and potholes on the road. But what kind of politics, precisely? The volumes in this series put an emphasis on repair and maintenance as an analytical means for studying how we think about and imagine social relations. Politics of Repair is set up to study the social efficacy of fixing and mending as well as the link between the negligence of built forms and the visibility of power. The series welcomes comparative anthropological studies addressing how repair practices and perceptions of brokenness vary culturally and the resulting consequences for how we think about politics.

Volume 2
Remaking the Human: Cosmetic Technologies of Body Repair, Reshaping, and Replacement
Edited by Alvao Jarrín and Chiara Pussetti

Volume 1
Repair, Brokenness, Breakthrough: Ethnographic Responses
Edited by Francisco Martínez and Patrick Laviolette

Remaking the Human
Cosmetic Technologies of Body Repair, Reshaping, and Replacement

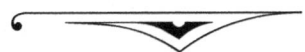

Edited by
ALVARO JARRÍN AND CHIARA PUSSETTI

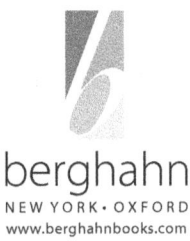

berghahn
NEW YORK • OXFORD
www.berghahnbooks.com

First published in 2021 by
Berghahn Books
www.berghahnbooks.com

© 2021, 2024 Alvaro Jarrín and Chiara Pussetti
First paperback edition published in 2024

All rights reserved. Except for the quotation of short passages
for the purposes of criticism and review, no part of this book
may be reproduced in any form or by any means, electronic or
mechanical, including photocopying, recording, or any information
storage and retrieval system now known or to be invented,
without written permission of the publisher.

Library of Congress Cataloging-in-Publication Data

Names: Jarrín, Alvaro, editor. | Pussetti, Chiara, editor.
Title: Remaking the Human: Cosmetic Technologies of Body Repair,
    Reshaping, and Replacement / edited by Alvaro Jarrín and Chiara Pussetti.
Description: New York: Berghahn Books, 2021. | Series: Politics of Repair;
    volume 2 | Includes bibliographical references and index.
Identifiers: LCCN 2021004787 (print) | LCCN 2021004788 (ebook) |
    ISBN 9781800730311 (Hardback) | ISBN 9781800730328 (eBook)
Subjects: LCSH: Material culture—Cross-cultural studies. | Repairing—Social
    aspects—Cross-cultural studies. | Applied anthropology—Cross-cultural
    studies.
Classification: LCC GN406 .R436 2021 (print) | LCC GN406 (ebook) |
    DDC 306—dc23
LC record available at https://lccn.loc.gov/2021004787
LC ebook record available at https://lccn.loc.gov/2021004788

British Library Cataloguing in Publication Data

A catalogue record for this book is available from the British Library

ISBN 978-1-80073-031-1 hardback
ISBN 978-1-80539-337-5 paperback
ISBN 978-1-80539-446-4 epub
ISBN 978-1-80073-032-8 web pdf

https://doi.org/10.3167/9781800730311

CONTENTS

List of Illustrations	vii
Acknowledgments	ix
Introduction. The Uncanny Aesthetics of Repairing, Reshaping, and Replacing Human Bodies *Alvaro Jarrín and Chiara Pussetti*	1

Part I. REPAIR

Chapter 1. Ideologies of Repair in Erectile Dysfunction Treatment and "Men's Health" Medicine *Emily Wentzell*	17
Chapter 2. Repairing Sexual Aging: Italian GPs' Discourses in the Viagra Era *Raffaella Ferrero Camoletto*	35
Chapter 3. Repairing the Body and Improving the Nation: Corrective Plastic Surgeries for Protruding Ears in Brazil *Marcelle Schimitt*	52
Chapter 4. The Itinerant Beauty Brigade: Repairing Social Fractures through the *Apapacho Estético* *Eva Carpigo*	67

Part II. RESHAPING

Chapter 5. Shaping the European Body: The Cosmetic Construction of Whiteness *Chiara Pussetti*	93

Chapter 6. Reshaping Masculinities and the Beauty Industry
   in Colombia   123
   Alejandro Arango-Londoño

Chapter 7. Reshaping and Hacking Gendered Bodies: Gay Bears
   and Pro-Independence Catalan Militants   141
   Begonya Enguix Grau

Chapter 8. Remaking (Post-)Human Bodies in the Anthropocene
   through Bioart Practices   165
   Christine Beaudoin

Part III. REPLACEMENT

Chapter 9. Can You See the Real Me? Cyborg, Supercrip,
   or Simply a Lover of Sport?   189
   P. David Howe and Carla Filomena Silva

Chapter 10. Unfixing Blindness: Retinal Implants and
   Negotiations of Ability in Postsocialist Russia   207
   Svetlana Borodina

Chapter 11. Learning through Apps: The Replacement of
   Offline Cis-Female Bodies with Digital Pregnancies
   and Menstruations   224
   Daniela Tonelli Manica, Marina Fisher Nucci, and
   Gabriela Cabral Paletta

Chapter 12. Remaking Desires and Femininities: Testosterone
   "Replacement" for Treating Women's Sexuality in Brazil   240
   Fabíola Rohden

Afterword. Beyond the Flesh   256
   Lenore Manderson

Index   268

ILLUSTRATIONS

Figures

4.1. Diego Sexto, the founder of the Itinerant Beauty Brigade, is an itinerant hairdresser. He works in a park in Mexico City. Mexico, 2017. Photo by the author. 70

4.2. Itinerant Beauty Brigade at Casa Xochiquetzal, a refuge for elderly sex workers. Venues are refitted, and little areas (for makeup, nails, face masks, haircuts, image consulting) are created in the courtyard. Mexico City, 2016. Photo by the author. 72

4.3. Women from Casa Xochiquetzal, elderly sex workers, participants at a Beauty Brigade. Mexico City, 2016. Photo by the author. 74

4.4. A session of self-care for Itinerant Beauty Brigade's volunteers. Mexico City, 2016. Photo by the author. 77

4.5. Lula and Berenice animate the encounter between volunteers of the Beauty Brigade and people with scleroderma. Mexico City, 2017. Photo by the author. 78

4.6. Volunteers of the Itinerant Beauty Brigade are doing a scalp massage for women with scleroderma. Mexico City, 2017. Photo by the author. 80

4.7. Albert, hairstylist volunteer of the Itinerant Beauty Brigade, is receiving the symbolic "gift" from a Casa Xochiquetzal resident: hand massage and benediction. Mexico City, 2016. Photo by the author. 82

4.8. Closing picture of a Beauty Brigade in Casa Xochiquetzal (house for elderly sex workers in Mexico City). Mexico City, 2016. Photo by Francisco Cano Z.   83

5.1. Skin-lightening products available at a beauty store in Rua dos Anjos, Lisbon. Photo by the author.   102

5.2. Products available at an African beauty salon in the Almirante Reis Avenue, Lisbon. Photo by the author.   105

5.3. Skin-lightening product with corticosteroids in a small Pakistani market in Avenida Almirante Reis, Lisbon. Photo by the author.   109

7.1. Madrid LGBT Pride State Demonstration, 2008. Photo by the author.   152

7.2. A poster on the streets of Barcelona. Photo by the author.   154

7.3. Barcelona: demonstration for Catalonia's National Day, 11 September 2018. Photo by the author.   156

7.4. Militants in black bloc. Barcelona, 11 September 2019. Photo by the author.   157

8.1. Setup for mammalian tissue culture in a biosafety cabinet at SymbioticA, 2016. Photo by the author.   170

8.2. Guy Ben-Ary's vials to make the biochemical soup that allows his external brain to grow. At SymbioticA, 2016. Photo by the author.   173

8.3. Following the recipe shared by Tarsh Bates to make agar plates that support growth of yeast, bacteria, and fungi. At the microbiology lab where she worked on her art at the University of Western Australia, 2016. Photo by the author.   175

Tables

5.1 List of products found in the main perfumeries of the city center of Lisbon.   112

7.1. Gay Body types. Source: John Hollywood, "Gay Men: Are You a Jock, Otter, Bear or Wolf?," *Paired Life* (blog), 17 June 2019, retrieved 18 July 2019 from https://pairedlife.com/dating/Gay-Men-Are-you-a-Jock-Otter-Bear-or-Wolf.   150

ACKNOWLEDGMENTS

This work is supported by the project EXCEL: The Pursuit of Excellence; Biotechnologies, Enhancement and Body Capital in Portugal, which has received funding from the Portuguese Foundation for Science and Technology (FCT), under the grant agreement PTDC/SOC-ANT/30572/2017. The grant is coordinated by the Institute of Social Sciences at the University of Lisbon by principal investigator Chiara Pussetti.

We are grateful for the opportunity to collaborate, learn about each other, build friendship, and travel together. We believe it has been a successful journey, and this book marks the beginning of new adventures together.

In the process of book editing we have benefited from the support of many people, but we are particularly thankful to Lenore Manderson, who not only wrote the afterword but provided each author additional individual feedback. We are thankful for her intellectual generosity. We also want to thank our editor at Berghahn Books, Tom Bonnington, and the series editor who encouraged us to submit a book proposal, Francisco Martínez. Thanks as well to the three anonymous reviewers of the volume.

Through all the layers of research and writing, family members have warmed our hearts. Chiara wants to thank her daughter, Sole, who teaches her every day the courage to be free, to unmake and remake our identity, as a project always in progress. Much thanks to Sole for her uncanny and poetic view of the world. Alvaro wants to thank his husband, Fox Jarrín, for his unwavering support, for introducing him to Ray Kurzweil, and for cheering him up during a difficult 2020. Here's to a better cyborg future that is less unequal and more hopeful!

INTRODUCTION

The Uncanny Aesthetics of Repairing, Reshaping, and Replacing Human Bodies

ALVARO JARRÍN AND CHIARA PUSSETTI

A portrait from the photography series "Beauty Warriors," by the Latvian artist Evija Laivina, graces the cover of this book. In the photograph, a woman is wearing a "face slimmer," a pink plastic mouthpiece shaped like oversized lips, available for five dollars on Amazon and advertised as a "simple solution to the timeless problem of how to give sagging facial skin and muscles that much-needed daily lift." The mouthpiece forces the mouth open, and the person wearing it is supposed to sound out the five vowels over and over again, for three minutes every day, in order to strengthen her facial muscles and gain both youth and a slimmer face. We know the mouthpiece is gendered female due to its pink color, and although a picture of a white woman is used to advertise the product on Amazon, the makers claim that the product is very popular in Japan, evoking some transnational appeal. What is fascinating about the image created by Evija Laivina, however, is the way the model wearing the "face slimmer" stares off into space, while the oversized plastic lips frame her open mouth in a grotesque manner. We cannot but help wonder what is in her mind as she wears this uncomfortable contraption and why consumers of this item go through the pain of wearing it. Without context, we are unaware of how the plastic mouthpiece works and whether it has become a permanent part of the model's body. The portrait is meant to denaturalize our global pursuit of better and more beautiful bodies, hinting at more invasive procedures like plastic surgery, and thus render uncanny the process by which we produce human beauty.

We would like to propose the concept of "uncanny aesthetics" to think through the ways in which we are remaking the human in the contemporary moment. The "uncanny valley" is a popular concept in robotics and graphic animation, which describes the feeling of unease caused by robots or digital creations that resemble humans too closely, startling us when they reveal their nonhuman nature to us. Masahiro Mori (2012), an authority within the field of robotics, posits that this feeling of eeriness is probably instinctual, developing from our need to fear unhealthy humans and corpses, of which nonliving robots remind us. Jennifer Rhee critiques Mori for this assumption and points out the unstable nature of the human in the first place, against which nonhuman others are supposed to be measured. The uncanny valley, Rhee (2013) argues, is the product of a long history that orients us toward specific definitions and demarcations of the human, and thus the discomfort that we feel toward the almost human reveals not our instincts but rather our entanglement with what lies beyond the human. Our emphasis in this volume on uncanny aesthetics is a call to deploy our productive unease as scholars regarding the permeable limits of the human. In a similar way to how Evija Laivina's art denaturalizes the bodily modification products available online, our work seeks to render the familiar strange and the strange familiar and analyze the power dynamics behind our global rush to repair bodies, reshape bodies, and replace body parts.

Allow us to unpack the notion of uncanny aesthetics a bit further. First, why the focus on aesthetics? All of the essays in this volume are concerned with bodily aesthetics or with the impulse to normalize bodies in one way or another, which in some ways presumes an aesthetic or physical ideal against which non-normative bodies are measured. When the objectively "healthy" or "beautiful" body is uncritically assumed to exist, a wide array of bodies are immediately labeled as wanting or as lacking in comparison—disabled bodies, queer bodies, racialized bodies, (de)sexualized bodies, unfit bodies, aging bodies, and/or poor bodies become the mirror opposite of what is desirable. Very frequently, there is a biopolitical impulse behind the labeling of bodies as beautiful and desirable, insofar as these bodily norms become linked to what Lauren Berlant (1997) calls the "National Symbolic"—the body of the nation is equated with the body of the ideal citizen. Biopolitics—the politics of fostering life—defines the healthy and normative body as necessary for the nation to prosper (Foucault 1990), and we would add that this body also has to be aesthetically appealing, engendering a "biopolitics of beauty" (Jarrín 2017). Medical, racial, and political discourses have long reinforced this biopolitical norm, violently excluding those deemed outside the norm or at the very least devaluing their existence (Garland 2009). Globalization, however, allows these biopolitical norms to transcend national borders, as transnational brands and global media transmit these messages about beauty across the globe. As Marcia Ochoa (2014) argues, national bodily ideals have become transnationalized through mediatized events like beauty pageants, where nations compete against one another for recognition within a global beauty economy. Even the work of empire, Mimi Thi Nguyen (2011, 2016) reminds us, can benefit from the "biopower of beauty," as beautification regimes in Afghanistan and Cambodia get deployed by Americans as symbols of renewed female agency and the supposed benevolence of US militarism.

As the contributions to this volume demonstrate, the body is increasingly understood as something to be consumed, enhanced, and perfected under neoliberal capitalism. The global beauty economy provides the tools and technologies for beautification, but it does not necessarily impose a singular and hegemonic beauty standard, as Claudia Liebelt (2018) points out. Instead, aesthetic norms circulate in ways that produce unexpected, uncanny effects on the populations they encounter. Global notions of beauty intersect with local aesthetic hierarchies, producing new norms (Jafar and Casanova 2013). Those who possess non-normative bodies sometimes submit their bodies to these biopolitical norms, avidly consuming the plastic surgeries, hormones, pharmaceuticals, prosthetics, skin-lightening creams, or other bodily enhancements that promise them social inclusion, upward mobility, citizenship, and well-being. At other times, however, people resist those biopolitical norms and craft their own aesthetic, affective, and/or political responses that denaturalize, queer, or hack bodily ideals and the very idea of a model citizen. Frequently, it is difficult to distinguish compliance from resistance, because both structure and agency are folded into one another, like a moebius strip. As Begonya Enguix Grau argues in this volume, "bodies are a battleground and a playground." The personal is always already political as we all strive to remake the human through the myriad technologies at our disposal.

It is important to resist the impulse to romanticize unaltered bodies, as if we could return to a time when our biology was not irrevocably intertwined with technology. As Lenore Manderson points out, our science fiction narratives demonstrate that we are simultaneously eager and fearful of what our cyborg future will bring, yet we miss the fact that cyborgs are already here. It is almost impossible nowadays to grow old without submitting one's body to any number of medical interventions that insert technology into our body: countless numbers of people live their daily lives thanks to pacemakers, hip and knee replacements, intraocular lenses, heart stents, prosthetics, and dental implants (Manderson 2011). Most women know intimately how technology helps regulate their reproduction, and almost everyone with the means or the insurance coverage will make use of common medical technologies like X-rays, MRIs, blood tests, echocardiograms, and other diagnostic technologies. To quote Katherine Hayles (1999), we "became posthuman" without even noticing it, and the everyday ubiquity of technologies that remake the human is what renders them so commonplace, normalized, and desirable. We are less interested, therefore, in hypothetical discussions about "designer babies" (Green 2007), "human enhancement" (Agar 2004), "the singularity" (Kurzweil 1999), or other cyborg technologies that only exist in theory at the moment and want to focus instead on practices that are already widely available, but which potently reshape our relationship to our gendered, racialized, sexualized, classed, differently abled, and aging bodies. Insights regarding what is already in place should shape bioethical discussions of what will or should occur in the future.

We believe ethnography is particularly well positioned as a methodology to examine these ubiquitous technologies, because it gives insight into the intimate and visceral ways that people imagine their subjectivities in relation to technologies that repair, reshape, and replace their bodies. Technologies are not embraced or rejected according to abstract ethical standards—they are lived in ambivalent ways by people within particular sociocultural, economic, and political contexts that give meaning to those technologies. We propose uncanny aesthetics as a concept that helps preserve the complexity revealed by the field, because to reside in the uncanny valley is to question what is human in the first place, before deciding how the human is being remade. Some practices like skin lightening are often exoticized as something that only "other" cultures engage in, while other practices like laser hair removal are so normalized that we do not critically examine why they are desirable. There is a productive unease that arises from sitting with the uncanny feeling one gets when strange practices become familiar and beckon to us or when a familiar practice is rendered strange by the context it occurs in—an insight long familiar to anthropologists, but which becomes even more crucial when the question is how the human is being remade. As Donna Haraway argues, the "ubiquity and invisibility of cyborgs" is why we need to sit with the discomfort of not knowing what the human is in today's world, and part of the progressive political work we can do in our scholarship is to remain attentive to the "transgressed boundaries, potent fusions, and dangerous possibilities" emerging from these new ways of being human (Haraway 2016: 13–14).

Human Malleability and Its Limits

What are the limits of the human, today, if any? Futurists like Ray Kurzweil (1999) predict the onset of an era where the human body is utterly transformed or made irrelevant—our organic bodies constantly repaired by nanobots or replaced by prostheses, and our minds uploaded into cybernetic networks. Ian Wilmut, the creator of the first cloned sheep, promised an "age of biological control" that would transform not only our reproductive future, but all of life's processes (Wilmut, Campbell, and Tudge 2000). These grand predictions not only play into the speculative forms of capital that seek to create surplus value from life itself (Cooper 2008), but they seem to forget the very materiality of the body and imagine our biology as infinitely "plastic, flexible, and partible" despite evidence to the contrary (Franklin 2007: 33). As Katherine Hayles (1999) has argued, these disembodied versions of the post-human are problematic because they reaffirm the liberal humanist subject—self-contained, masterful, rational—rather than recognize our finitude, our vulnerability, and our embeddedness within complex material worlds that contain other beings aside from ourselves.

Nonetheless, it is undeniable that humanity is malleable in ways that undermine any notion of a universal and undeviating human nature. Many authors share the idea that the only sensible thing to say about human nature is that it exceeds the natural through sociocultural means and that it is "in" that nature for humanity to continuously reconstruct itself and its own history. The Italian cultural anthropologist Francesco Remotti (2006, 2013) proposed the term *anthropo-poiesis*—from the classic Greek *poiein*—to identify the specific human capacity to "making," "creating," or "shaping" particular, culturally specific, and socially negotiated forms of humanness. In Remotti's terms, "humanity is not given ... but has to be constructed and molded" (1999: 111). We are constantly engaged in processes of "human making," and this "making" (*poiein*) is first and foremost a "shaping" (*plassein*) (2013: 40) on the basis of specific ideals, values, models, or "forms of humanity" (Remotti 1999)—which can be hegemonic, non-hegemonic, or counter-hegemonic.

The theory of humanity as demiurge, "*homo faber sui*," "*homo creator*," or "*homo technicus*" (Ihde and Malafouris 2019) is based on a long tradition of thought that includes philosophers such as Giovanni Pico della Mirandola, Michel de Montaigne, Blaise Pascal, Giambattista Vico, Johann Gottfried Herder, Friedrich Nietzsche, Arnold Gehlen, Jean-Paul Sartre, the anthropologist Clifford Geertz, the evolutionary geneticist Richard Lewontin, the neurobiologist Steven Rose, and the psychologist Leon Kamin, among others. According to all these authors, the human condition is defined by indeterminateness, incompleteness, and indefiniteness and consequently by the unlimited possibility of being and of building ourselves. If human nature is "not in our genes" (Lewontin, Rose, and Kamin 1984) and not even in the hands of some god, human beings are "poetic" (Leach 1976: 5): they possess the "divine capacity" (Leach 1969: 90) to create, reshape, transform, and replace themselves and their physical, social, and cultural environment (Leach 1969: 26). Human beings are left to their own devices, without pre-defined models or archetypes, and therefore condemned, as Jean-Paul Sartre (1965: 543) has argued, to construct the reference models from which they themselves will be built.

Anthropo-poiesis and *anthropo-plassein* have always been our deepest nature: not a "post"-human, but an ever-present condition, which defines us as human beings. Human beings are—using Pico della Mirandola's expression—"*plastes et factor* [shapers]" (Picco della Mirandola [1486] 1998: 5) of themselves, and this shaping intervention is an artistic, cosmetic (from the Greek root *kosmein*, "to create an order, to organize, to produce, to design"), and technical (from the Greek root word *techne*, "art," linked to the idea of *poiesis*) activity. *Techne*—the material (objects, tools, artifacts) techniques and the cultural and discursive technologies of the self—and *soma*—our phenomenological corporeality—have always been intimately integrated and inextricably connected. According to Ihde and Malafouris, "We are *Homo faber* not just because we make things but also because we are made by them" (2019: 209). This relational human-technology ontology, in which people and things are inseparably intertwined and co-constituted, is an embodied and processual relation. This essential and foundational interconnection implies also that there is no "core" or "essential" humanity (biological or otherwise) that pre-exists our subjectivation, but only a process of continuous becoming in which humanity is incessantly remade, reshaped, altered, enhanced, or extended by technological interventions.

An implication of this "becoming" dimension is that "technological change is not always progressive, linear or in any sense controlled and pre-planned" (Ihde and Malafouris 2019: 204). Humans may believe they control their destiny through technology, but technology always co-constitutes humanity in return, in ways that are unpredictable and bely our mastery over our own bodies and subjectivities. Additionally, pre-existing power dynamics inevitably shape how new technologies are implemented in different contexts. Elizabeth Roberts (2012), for example, provides compelling evidence of how Ecuador's racial hierarchies shaped the ways in which in vitro fertilization was implemented in that country, employing it as a technology that could whiten the nation by favoring lighter-skinned egg and sperm donors. Thus, while some authors like Nikolas Rose (2006) see the potential for "active biological citizens" who take ownership of biopower and transform it into an individualized project of self-improvement, others are more skeptical and warn us of the ways in which neoliberal forms of biopower can produce a "flexible eugenics" that pressures individuals into eliminating certain human characteristics, like disability, from the general population (Taussig, Rapp and Heath 2003). This volume provides both optimistic and pessimistic viewpoints into the effects of technology on pre-existing inequalities around the world.

Structural inequalities and new forms of governmentality also shape how technologies are differentially deployed onto some populations and not others, creating different forms of risk. Emilia Sanabria (2016), for example, notes how low-income patients in Brazilian public hospitals are disciplined by state actors to submit their bodies to hormonal medical treatments, in contrast to the choices provided to consumer-citizens within private medical practices. The authors of this introduction have seen similar issues within our own research, either in the ways that low-income Brazilians are asked to assume the risks of experimental plastic surgeries, before these procedures are marketed more widely for profit (Jarrín 2017), or in the ways that skin lighteners remain unregulated by Portuguese medical authorities, because most of those who consume those products are immigrants from former Portuguese colonies (Pussetti, chapter 5 in this volume). In both these cases, the risks of unproven technologies are externalized onto more vulnerable populations (most of them women), either purposely or due to neglect, and those populations suffer the grave consequences of botched plastic surgeries and exposure to toxic chemicals like mercury and hydroquinone. The huge profits of the plastic surgery industry and of the transnational corporations that produce skin lighteners demonstrates that "biocapital" (Cooper 2008; Sunder Rajan 2006) is still dependent on a biopolitical hierarchy where some bodies matter more than others. The human body may be conceived as infinitely malleable by futurists and trans-humanists, but the truth is that there are biological limits to the bodily transformations we subject the body to, and these limits, not surprisingly, traverse old fault lines of race, class, gender, and colonial power.

Outline of the Book

In the age of the explosion and spread of "wish-fulfilling" biotechnologies destined to repair, reshape, and replace human characteristics and functions, the human being has been radically reconceptualized. Moreover, these procedures are booming and becoming increasingly common, more affordable, and minimally invasive. We sought contributions to the volume that addressed the complex imbrications between humans and widely available technologies and sought to cover a wide variety of topics and geographic areas within the region of the world that Paul Gilroy calls "the Black Atlantic" (1993). Although not every author in the collection tackles race, we found that notions of beauty, health, and bodily improvement traverse familiar circuits between Europe, Africa, Latin America, and North

America—borrowing from one another and influenced by a common history of the transatlantic slave trade. As Sharon Patricia Holland argues, "The transatlantic slave trade altered the very shape of sexuality" for everyone in the Black Atlantic, not only for those of African descent, because it inaugurated racialized and gendered hierarchies, tied to specific forms of erotic desire, that exist until today (2012: 56). We want to push the argument even further and argue that how people desire to remake themselves and others today is also shaped by these violent histories and the biopolitical trends they inaugurated.

We also sought contributions that were very thoughtful about the intersections between race, class, gender, sexuality, age, disability, and nationality. As useful as the concept of "intersectionality" has been to any type of scholarship that tackles human embodiment (Crenshaw 1990), intersectional analysis can sometimes fall short when it is simply additive, doing analysis of a single category and then complementing it with a few details about how other categories factor within that master narrative. Intersectionality, in that instance, is treated like a traffic intersection in a road, barely slowing down the chosen path, and it can produce two-dimensional characterizations of complex forms of embodiment. The authors included in this collection take seriously how categories of embodiment are coproduced, emerging simultaneously during any process of subjectivation. As Jasbir Puar (2007) points out, embodiment is a multifaceted, messy, and fluid affair that feels less like intersecting identities and more like an ongoing assemblage, perpetually in motion. The human cyborgs that come into being in the interface between the human, the animal, and the technological are not only blurring the boundaries between nature and culture, but they also make evident the gendered aspects of race, the class dimensions of gender performances, the racialization of sexuality and age, the national and transnational concerns tied to sexuality and disability, and a myriad other human assemblages.

We organized this collection into three distinct sections, focused on the subjects of repairing, reshaping, and replacing the human. Each of these themes overlaps with one another, but they do indicate different developments within the rush to remake the human. Repair implies a return to some original, restoring the body to a former or ideal version of itself. Repair can be experienced as a form of self-care, but it can also impose aesthetic ideals of youth, normative gender, or normative appearance on bodies that would otherwise be considered ordinary but have been deemed abnormal in view of the existing norms. Reshaping goes a step further and implies a transformation of the human into something new. Reshaping the body can mean intervening on human biology, through surgery and pharmaceuticals, to comply with existing norms, but it can also mean that people celebrate the malleability of their bodies and pursue unique ways of being human. Finally, replacement understands the body as a machine made of interchangeable parts and claims that a certain bodily part or bodily function can be replaced with a specific technology. The promise of replacement is that the body can exceed its biological limits, but the peril of replacement is that an enhanced body becomes more desirable than a differently abled body, thus endangering disability rights. Repairing, reshaping, and replacing the human body are not necessarily normalizing procedures, because there are opportunities to redefine the human as we transform the body, but the norm always lurks in the background, as an example to follow or as a pattern that people seek to disrupt.

In the first section on repair, the authors reflect on how the ideologies and practices of repair are implicated in bodily transformations. Emily Wentzell and Raffaella Ferrero Camoletto investigate the treatment of erectile dysfunction, and the initiative to "repair" masculinity, in three different countries: Mexico, the United States, and Italy. Wentzell demonstrates that aging working-class men in Mexico reject erectile dysfunction drugs and resist the medical discourses that seek to medicalize their biology, focusing instead on repairing problematic forms of masculinity like machismo. Within the United States, Wentzell shows that the reception of erectile dysfunction marketing is more varied, with some practitioners embracing the focus on "men's health," while others were critical of biological essentialism and sought to undermine the gender and racial stereotypes that might shape the care men receive. Camoletto sees a similar diversity in the approaches of Italian practitioners, who either avoid the topic of sexual dysfunction with their patients or embrace the management of "healthy sexual aging" through drugs like Viagra. Masculinity, given the evidence provided by Wentzell and Camoletto, seems somewhat resistant to medicalization depending on the context, but men's gendered bodies are still interpellated by erectile dysfunction drugs in ways that require the active rejection of these drugs or embracing them as a way to delay an effect of aging.

In their chapters, Marcelle Schimitt and Eva Carpigo tackle efforts to beautify low-income individuals in Brazil and Mexico; they offer contrasting examples of repair, either as a way to improve the nation or as a conduit for self-care and the creation of community. Schimitt argues that corrective plastic surgeries for protruding ears in Brazilian children are labeled as "reparative," even though they do not repair any biological function, because they are perceived by plastic surgeons as producing social normalcy. These medical discourses by surgeons are eerily similar to older eugenic discourses, which tied the individual repair of young bodies to the collective improvement of the nation, demonstrating continuities between eugenic aims and contemporary plastic surgery. Carpigo provides a more optimistic view of repair in her analysis of the Beauty Brigade in Mexico City, a bottom-up initiative of mutual aid that provides beauty makeovers free of charge to those in need and allows for real human connections to flourish. In the space generated by the Beauty Brigades, the vulnerability of those giving and receiving beauty makeovers is acknowledged, and human dignity and diversity are valued rather than undermined. Schimitt's and Carpigo's chapters show that beauty can be a normalizing force or an affirming force for those involved in beautifying practices.

The next section of the book, focusing on reshaping the human, also begins with two chapters on beauty: Chiara Pussetti describes the use of skin-lightening products in Portugal; Alejandro Arango-Londoño examines men's plastic surgeries in Colombia. The chapter by Pussetti analyzes how Afro-Portuguese women and immigrants to Portugal who use skin lighteners emphasize that the use of these creams is simply an aesthetic choice, yet they also understand that skin-lightening products can provide upward mobility by bringing their bodies closer to a European bodily ideal. Whiteness, Pussetti argues, becomes an aesthetic marker of Europeanness that dates back to the colonial era and that also associates white women with a classic, refined femininity, in contrast to the more animalistic and sensual femininity associated with women of color. Arango-Londoño similarly emphasizes gendered beauty as men's plastic surgeries gain popularity and reshape the masculinities available for consumption in neoliberal Colombia. The plastic surgeries and aesthetic procedures that are acceptable among men, however, are those that reinforce the gender binary and produce an athletic, hyper-virile, and cosmopolitan masculinity, generating a new economic niche that markets specialized procedures intended to increase a men's value and biocapital. Both Pussetti and Arango-Londoño consider that beautification technologies are deeply entangled with class and racial markers, in ways that become very alluring for consumers.

In contrast, Begonya Enguix Grau and by Christine Beaudoin provide more hopeful instances of body reshaping in Catalunya, Canada, and Australia. Enguix Grau offers two case studies of collectives in Catalunya that "hack" normative gender relations—the "bear" subculture of gay men that revalues fat and hairy bodies, and the feminist independence activists who subvert gender norms by adopting outfits and attitudes that reject traditional femininity. Enguix Grau makes the case that these two groups demonstrate that bodies can become political weapons in the struggle to change relationships between nations and its subjects, producing new, non-normative assemblages. Beaudoin describes how biohackers and bioartists from Australia and Canada create tissue cultures and other artworks from mammals or from their own bodies, thus blurring the boundaries between our bodies and others, between humans and machines, even between species. This blurriness, Beaudoin argues, is particularly relevant in our effort to rethink the human during the Anthropocene, because it allows us to think how our post-human futures can provide new ways of confronting our global environmental crisis. Enguix Grau and Beaudoin, therefore, state that "hacking" the human is a way to positively transform it and open it up for new possibilities.

The final section, on replacement, begins with two chapters on disability. David Howe and Carla Filomena Silva address the image of the cyborg athlete within the Paralympics, and Svetlana Borodina focuses on retinal implants in Russia. Howe and Silva assert that the media attention given to prosthetic technologies in the Paralympics has led to the celebration of "supercrips"—athletes are recognized according to the extent of their "cyborgization." This leads to the marginalization of athletes who make less use of technologies, either because they come from developing countries and cannot afford this technology or because they do not require prosthetics, due to conditions such as cerebral palsy and other neurological disabilities. Borodina argues that additional technology does not necessarily translate into additional agency or equality for those with disabilities. Her vision-impaired interlocutors perceive retinal implants as devaluing their unique sensory modes and as failing to solve the social and political exclusion they experience. Medical and state discourses are deeply invested in "fixing" blindness and promise fantastical futures, thus reinforcing the marginalization that blind Russians experience today. The disability movement has as much to lose as to gain from new technological developments that remake the human.

In the final two chapters, Daniela Tonelli Manica, Marina Fisher Nucci, and Gabriela Cabral Paletta focus on how Brazilian women use apps during pregnancy and menstruation to monitor their own bodies, and Fabíola Rohden describes how women make use of hormonal replacement therapies. Manica and colleagues argue that the use of digital apps during pregnancy helps women gather useful information about their bodily transformations but that this generates a "cyborg baby" that seems to remain alive digitally even after a woman suffers a miscarriage, thus causing further pain. Similarly, the ability to monitor one's own fertility cycles through apps allows women to replace other contraceptives with a digital version that allows them to circumvent Catholic disapproval. Fabíola Rohden discusses the use of testosterone to improve the loss of libido in Brazilian women, which is problematic not only because of the medical risks involved, but because it seems to frequently stem from complaints offered by the women's husbands rather than concerns of their own. Ultimately, the medical discourses espoused by doctors reinforce the idea that sexual desire is a masculine trait that women lose with age and needs to be replaced. The last two chapters, therefore, demonstrate that technology (digital software and hormones) can replace gendered experiences and thus reinforce and reshape gender norms.

Repairing, reshaping, and replacing the human with technology cannot be reduced to a positive or negative development in human history. The complexities of particular situations are hugely important to determine if remaking the human has opened opportunities or closed possibilities for those involved and whether the promises of a given technology outweigh the perils or risks it entails. To better understand these questions, it is very important to continue having these discussions and to draw on ethnographic data to understand how people's motivations, aspirations, and practices regarding particular technologies are entangled with larger negotiations over class, race, gender, age, and nationality. Abstract bioethical discussions that are not grounded in local realities miss how these new technologies are lived in practice and what we can expect when new technologies are implemented in different contexts.

Alvaro Jarrín received his PhD from Duke University and is an associate professor of anthropology at College of the Holy Cross. His research explores the imbrication of medicine, the body and inequality in Brazil, with foci on plastic surgery, genomics, and gender nonconforming activism. He is the author of *The Biopolitics of Beauty: Cosmetic Citizenship and Affective Capital in Brazil* (University of California Press), which explores the eugenic underpinnings of racio-logical thought among plastic surgeons and the aesthetic hierarchies of beauty that reinforce racial inequality in Brazil.

Chiara Pussetti is currently auxiliar researcher at the Institute of Social Sciences at the University of Lisbon. Over the last eighteen years, she has lectured at graduate and postgraduate levels in Italy, Portugal, and Brazil and has researched and published extensively on the subjects of migration, healthcare, gender, body and emotions, social inequality, suffering, and well-being in urban contexts. She is also principal investigator of the project EXCEL: The Pursuit of Excellence; Biotechnologies, Enhancement and Body Capital in Portugal (PTDC/SOC-ANT/30572/2017).

References

Agar, Nicholas. 2004. *Liberal Eugenics: In Defence of Human Enhancement.* Hoboken: Blackwell.
Berlant, Lauren. 1997. *The Queen of America Goes to Washington: Essays on Sex and Citizenship.* Durham, NC: Duke University Press.

Cooper, Melinda. 2008. *Life as Surplus: Biotechnology & Capitalism in the Neoliberal Era.* Seattle: University of Washington Press.
Crenshaw, Kimberle. 1990. "Mapping the Margins: Intersectionality, Identity Politics, and Violence against Women of Color." *Stanford Law Review* 43: 1241–99.
Foucault, Michel. 1990. *The History of Sexuality.* Vol. 1, *An Introduction.* New York: Vintage.
Franklin, Sarah. 2007. *Dolly Mixtures: The Remaking of a Genealogy.* Durham, NC: Duke University Press.
Garland-Thomson, Rosemarie. 2009. *Staring: How We Look.* Oxford: Oxford University Press.
Gilroy, Paul. 1993. *The Black Atlantic: Modernity and Double-Consciousness.* Cambridge, MA: Harvard University Press.
Green, Ronald. 2007. *Babies by Design: The Ethics of Genetic Choice.* New Haven, CT: Yale University Press.
Haraway, Donna. 2016. "A Cyborg Manifesto: Science, Technology, and Socialist Feminism in the Late Twentieth Century." In *Manifestly Haraway.* Minneapolis: University of Minnesota Press, pp. 3–90.
Hayles, Katherine N. 1999. *How We Became Posthuman: Virtual Bodies in Cybernetics, Literature, and Informatics.* Chicago: University of Chicago Press.
Holland, Sharon Patricia. 2012. *The Erotic Life of Racism.* Durham, NC: Duke University Press.
Ihde, D., and L. Malafouris. 2019. "*Homo faber* Revisited: Postphenomenology and Material Engagement Theory." *Philosophy & Technology* 32(2): 195–214.
Jafar, Afshan, and Erynn Masi de Casanova. 2013. "Bodies, Beauty and Location: An Introduction." In Afshan Jafar and Erynn Masi de Casanova (eds.), *Global Beauty, Local Bodies.* New York: Palgrave Macmillan, pp. xi–xxv.
Jarrín, Alvaro. 2017. *The Biopolitics of Beauty: Cosmetic Citizenship and Affective Capital in Brazil.* Berkeley: University of California Press.
Kurzweil, Ray. 1999. *The Age of Spiritual Machines: When Computers Exceed Human Intelligence.* New York: Penguin Books.
Leach, Edmund. 1969. *A Runaway World? The 1967 Reith Lectures.* London: Oxford University Press.
———. 1976. *Culture and Communication.* Cambridge: Cambridge University Press.
Lewontin, Richard, Steven Rose, and Leon Kamin. 1984. *Not in Our Genes: Biology, Ideology and Human Nature.* New York: Pantheon.
Liebelt, Claudia. 2018. "Beauty and the Norm: An Introduction." In Claudia Liebelt, Sarah Bollinger, and Ulf Vierke (eds.), *Beauty and the Norm.* London: Palgrave and Macmillan, pp. 1–19.
Manderson, Lenore. 2011. *Surface Tensions: Surgery, Bodily Boundaries, and the Social Self.* London: Routledge.
Mori, Masahiro. 2012. "The Uncanny Valley." Translated by Karl F. MacDorman and Norri Kageki. *IEEE Robotics & Automation Magazine* 19(2): 98–100.
Nguyen, Mimi Thi. 2011. "The Biopower of Beauty: Humanitarian Imperialisms and Global Feminisms in an Age of Terror." *Signs* 36(2): 359–83.
———. 2016. "The Right to Be Beautiful." *The Account: A Journal of Poetry, Prose and Thought.* Retrieved 4 December 2020 from theaccountmagazine.com.
Ochoa, Marcia. 2014. *Queen for a Day: Transformistas, Beauty Queens and the Performance of Femininity in Venezuela.* Durham, NC: Duke University Press.

Picco della Mirandola, Giovanni. (1486) 1998. *Oration on the Dignity of Man*. Indianapolis/Cambridge: Hackett Publishing Classics.
Puar, Jasbir K. 2007. *Terrorist Assemblages: Homonationalism in Queer Times*. Durham, NC: Duke University Press.
Remotti, Francesco. 1999. *Forme di Umanità. Progetti incompleti e cantieri sempre aperti*. Torino: Paravia Scriptorium.
——. 2006. *Prima Lezione di Antropologia*. Bari: Laterza, 2006.
——. 2013. *Fare Umanitá. I Drammi dell'Antropo-poiesi*. Bari: Laterza.
Rhee, Jennifer. 2013. "Beyond the Uncanny Valley: Masahiro Mori and Phillip K. Dick's *Do Androids Dream of Electric Sheep?*" *Configurations* 21(3): 301–29.
Roberts, Elizabeth. 2012. *God's Laboratory: Assisted Reproduction in the Andes*. Berkeley: University of California Press.
Rose, Nikolas. 2006. *The Politics of Life Itself: Biomedicine, Power, and Subjectivity in the Twenty-First Century*. Princeton, NJ: Princeton University Press.
Sanabria, Emilia. 2016. *Plastic Bodies: Sex Hormones and Menstrual Suppression in Brazil*. Durham: Duke University Press.
Sartre, Jean-Paul. 1965. *L'Être et le Néant*. Paris: Gallimard.
Sunder Rajan, Kaushik. 2006. *Biocapital: The Constitution of Post-genomic Life*. Durham, NC: Duke University Press.
Taussig, Karen-Sue, Rayna Rapp, and Deborah Heath. 2003. "Flexible Eugenics: Technologies of the Self in the Age of Genetics." In Alan H. Goodman, Deborah Heath, and M. Susan Lindee (eds.), *Genetic Nature/Culture: Anthropology and Science Beyond the Two-Culture Divide*. Berkeley: University of California Press, pp. 58–76.
Wilmut, Ian, Keith Campbell, and Colin Tudge. 2000. *The Second Creation: The Age of Biological Control by the Scientists Who Cloned Dolly*. London: Headline.

PART I
REPAIR

CHAPTER 1

Ideologies of Repair in Erectile Dysfunction Treatment and "Men's Health" Medicine

EMILY WENTZELL

Medical treatment requires health-care providers to identify bodily parts or processes that are functioning abnormally. Doing so requires working from baseline definitions of normal bodies and embodied behaviors. While such definitions are key for health intervention, they are also based on culturally specific understandings of what constitute normal, ideal, and pathological functions (Canguilhem 1989). This situation only becomes problematic when the cultural nature of these norms is denied or left unexamined. In such cases, common in the world of Western biomedicine, medical intervention and marketing can normalize and perpetuate cultural ideologies that worsen inequalities and cause other forms of suffering. It is thus necessary to critically analyze the ideologies at play behind the ways professionals and patients define pathology in order to heal without doing social harm.

This is especially clear in the case of health interventions related to sex and gender. The biological fact of wide human variation in the traits we define as physical sex and the range of ways that different cultures have defined the numbers and types of sexes, genders (forms of behavior understood to be related to sex characteristics), and sexualities (people's sexual practices and identities) demonstrate that there is no universal norm for any of these categories (Fausto-Sterling 1985; Ross and Rapp 1983). Instead, individual sex, gender, and sexuality emerge from the intersection of biosocial factors including genetics and epigenetics, material environment, and cultural context (Niewöhner and Lock 2018). Medical treatment that overlooks this diversity and takes culturally specific understandings of "normal" sex, gender, and sexuality as natural and universal can thus impose narrow norms that cause patients harm. This is exemplified by interventions like intersex "normalization" surgery and conversion therapy, which were identified as damaging only after activists exposed the problematic and prejudiced ideas of normal on which these practices are based (Karkazis 2008; Drescher et al. 2016).

In this chapter, I analyze interview data to investigate differences among patients' and providers' understandings of what the objects of repair should be in medical treatments targeted at men. I first focus on the experiences of one set of patients, discussing the divergences between older Mexican men's understandings of decreased erectile function and the medical concept of erectile dysfunction (ED), which has been globalized through the marketing and prescription of drugs like Viagra. I then focus on the institutional level, in the emergent medical subspecialty of "men's health medicine," which has developed in part from the blockbuster success of ED drugs. I examine the significant differences in understandings of what to target for repair among different types of US-based health professionals working in or adjacent to the men's health field. In all cases, I analyze how people's cultural ideologies about masculinity influence what they define as pathological rather than normal variation. These ideologies vary widely, from the notion that an essential male biology dictates a normative masculinity, to understandings of both those categories as context dependent. The ways that people define "men" determine what issues they believe require medical repair and what they see as the purview of medicine itself.

Viagra: Repairing Erections and Maintaining Masculinities

ED Drugs as "Masculinity Pills"

People have understood decreasing erectile function diversely in different times and places, including as normal aging, a sign of emotional distress, and a consequence of witchcraft (Wentzell 2008; McLaren 2007). Since the 1990s, understandings of this bodily change as the medical pathology "erectile dysfunction" have become prevalent worldwide, largely due to the introduction, marketing, and media coverage of ED drugs like Viagra (Tiefer 2006). While such drugs have aided men distressed by decreasing erectile function, they have also had wide-ranging cultural consequences for people's ideologies of masculinity and health. Framing decreasing erection as pathology requires implicit acceptance of a specific idea about what kind of sexuality is normal and healthy for men: unceasing erection and penetrative sexuality across the life course, regardless of one's age or social interactions with partners (Wentzell 2017). This is not an objective scientific fact, but a culturally specific understanding of who men are and should be; this understanding can itself perpetuate social suffering.

By enabling men to align their bodies with this specific ideal of gendered sexuality, ED drugs serve as "masculinity pills" (Loe 2006: 31; Both 2015). ED drug treatment naturalizes specifically Western cultural notions of men's sexuality as mechanistic and homogenously focused on penetrative heterosexual sex rather than on other kinds of acts, partners, or more relational desires (Grace et al. 2006; Mamo and Fishman 2001). This ideology also naturalizes ideas of aging as inherently pathological (Katz and Marshall 2002; Marshall 2008). From this perspective, any bodily deviation from stereotypically youthful and penetration-oriented sexuality is a medical problem in need of repair, rather than normal human variation between people or across one's life course.

Yet not everyone uncritically accepts either this normative idea of male sexuality or the idea that decreasing erectile function is a problem or pathology. In many cultural contexts, living out respectable aging by decreasing or ceasing one's sexual practice is highly valued (e.g., van der Geest 2001). Even in settings where youthfulness and unceasing penetrative sexuality are commonly valorized, some people might embrace these norms while others understand appropriate male aging as shifting away from emphasis on sexuality to other forms of social interaction (Potts et al. 2004; Sandberg 2013). It is also common for people, even spouses, to disagree about what counts as normal, positive, or desirable sexuality for men in later life (e.g., Moore 2010).

A Mexican Case Study

People draw on culturally specific ideologies regarding male biology and "good" masculinities as they decide whether decreasing erectile function should be a target of medical repair. I found this in my research on the topic in urban, central Mexico. Ideas about who Mexican men are and should be have long been a key topic of debate in Mexican popular culture. These discussions draw on a locally specific racial ideology, which has been promoted by public intellectuals and government interventions since the revolution in the early twentieth century. This ideology states that there is a discrete Mexican populace, formed from the ongoing intermixing of people of Indigenous and Spanish heritage, that would eventually homogenize into a unique *mestizo* (mixed) race ideally suited for modernity (Vasconcelos [1925] 1997; cf. Alonso 2004). This discourse of *mestizaje* (mixing) also included quite negative notions about Mexican men: the idea that as the progeny of forced reproduction between Conquistador forefathers and Indigenous foremothers, they inherited problematic traits of patriarchal womanizing and emotional closure known as machismo (cf. Paz [1961] 1985). These ideas are not biological truths; the notion of race itself is not biologically valid, although it carries powerful social significance that affects people's lives and bodies (Fuentes et al. 2019). Nevertheless, these understandings of Mexican maleness and masculinity had powerful consequences.

While the idea that Mexican men are inherently predisposed to machismo is prevalent in popular culture, this form of masculinity has been critiqued for several decades. People frame machismo as problematically regressive, amid calls for more egalitarian gender roles and the emerging valorization of marriage based on love, intimacy, and fidelity rather than economic support and reproduction (e.g., Amuchástegui and Szasz 2007). Yet the way people tend to criticize machismo keeps the idea of it alive; rather than dismissing it, people often discuss it as a biocultural inheritance against which good Mexican men must struggle (Gutmann 1996; Ramirez 2009; Amuchástegui Herrera 2008).

These ideas and social changes influenced people's interpretations of decreasing erectile function. In 2007–8 I interviewed over 250 men, about 50 together with their wives, who were seeking urology treatment at a government-run clinic in the city of Cuernavaca. As part of a federal system offering free care to all formally employed workers and their families, the clinic offers good treatment but long waits that encourage those with greater means to seek private care. The clinic consequently served mostly working-class patients. Staff urologists invited any patient they thought might be experiencing decreased erectile function, due to aging or conditions like type 2 diabetes, to join my study. Most were pleased with the opportunity to discuss their experiences with an engaged listener from outside their social worlds (for details, see Wentzell 2013). Here, I discuss the ways that many participants drew on local understandings of Mexican men's natures as they made sense of changing sexual function.

The vast majority of study participants had experienced decreased erectile function and knew how and where to access ED drugs, yet rejected the idea that their bodily changes were a medical pathology. Instead, they understood the kind of masculinity that ED drugs might support as the problem in need of repair. Participants often described macho sexuality as biologically innate to Mexican men, as one man explained: "Here in Mexico, [infidelity is] something normal. They say the Mexican is passionate. They say the man is polygamous by nature." However, they also discussed the ways that ideals of "good" masculinity had changed around them over the courses of their lives. For instance, one man said that while men of his generation were taught that "the woman needs to be behind," they needed to learn that "the wife isn't a thing—she's a person, she's a comrade." Many who had once focused on extramarital sexuality as a source of masculine pride framed themselves as "*ex-machista[s]*," as one man termed it; they had learned over time to value faithful, domestically oriented masculinities.

This shift enabled men to keep up with cultural changes in gender ideologies and to live out masculinities seen as appropriate and respectable in later life. Rejecting the idea of aging as pathology, men overwhelmingly embraced changing their embodiments of masculinity as they aged. In a life trajectory so common that one man glossed it "the Mexican classic," men often understood decreasing erectile function as a signal that they should shift from youthful forms of virility to more mature forms of manliness focused on the domestic sphere. They thus framed sexual function change as "normal" and "natural." As one man explained, decreasing erectile function is "nature, I'm diminishing, and I take that as something normal." Men also tended to cast this change as a normal consequence of hard work in their youths, as another man noted: "My work is a little rough, heavy. I carry a lot, so I feel a little tiredness. Now, I can't have as much sex as before. This is normal. Now it's not the same—when I was young, more potency. Now with my age, not anymore." Thus, meeting the manly obligation to provide for one's family led naturally to bodily changes in later life that included decreased sexual function.

Many men understood such physical change as support for a shift away from innate but socially problematic and age-inappropriate sexual desires. Many saw the sexual behavior that had marked them as manly in their youths as problematic now. For instance, one man said he had been "a womanizer," but "now I don't have the same capacity. I'm fifty-five, I know what I am. I don't want problems with my wife. Like I deserve respect from her, she deserves it from me as well." For such participants, who sometimes commented that "the macho comes out of us [Mexican men]" when seeing an attractive woman, following what they saw as youthfully innate impulses led to the expression of a male sexuality that was no longer seen as socially desirable and was frankly "silly" in older men. Men's "changing capacity" enabled them to treat women in ways seen as respectful, guided by their new values rather than what some perceived to be the dictates of their youthful biologies. Wives often advocated for such changes, including by characterizing their husband's decreasing erectile function as "natural" and discussing their desires for emotional closeness, fidelity, and respect rather than frequent penetrative sex.

These perspectives led participants to be suspicious of the healthfulness of ED drugs. Since most saw decreasing erectile function as normal rather than pathological, they tended to frame ED drug use as the abnormal condition. One man explained his disinterest in ED treatment by explaining, "I don't like to use things that aren't normal. I don't like to force my body."

Many feared that forcing one's body to perform "youthful" sexual behavior in older age would do harm. Participants frequently mused that ED drugs would inappropriately "accelerate" their bodies, as one man explained, possibly "to your death. Many friends have told me, they will accelerate you a lot, then you'll collapse, that stuff will kill you." While men often engaged in a process of accepting decreased erectile function over time, by using the narratives presented above, even those who were initially unhappy about physiological changes overwhelmingly sought gentler interventions like vitamins or healthy lifestyle changes to encourage erection without "unbalancing" or otherwise harming their system.

There were some exceptions to these trends; a few men did seek ED treatment. Some had never felt they had performed masculinity successfully and were thus engaged in a lifelong quest to embody ideal manliness. Others expressed ideas similar to those above but did not yet see themselves as old enough to age out of youthful sexuality. Nevertheless, despite the global prevalence of ED drugs and the norms of masculinity they perpetuate, study participants overwhelmingly understood macho sexuality rather than decreasing erectile function to be the pathology in need of repair.

Providers' ideologies of masculinity and health also influenced patients' understandings. The urologists who treated these men shared their views of decreased erectile function not as pathological but, as one remarked, as "normal, because of the stress people have" and because of the bodily experiences of aging and chronic illness. Even when men were distressed by this change, the IMSS urologists tended to define it as a transient emotional problem rather than a cue to diagnose ED. One doctor articulated this while asking me to help the patient cope with this difficulty when I interviewed him: "This patient does not feel confident in himself; he had problems with his wife and his self-esteem decreased. He thinks he needs pills but what he needs is to feel better about himself, so you should talk to him about that."

The urologists held this ideology while also prescribing ED drugs for younger and wealthier patients in their own private practices. This demonstrates that physicians can hold multiple, seemingly conflicting understandings of bodily change, applying them variously to different kinds of patients in ways mediated by structural context. The mostly working-class IMSS patients generally felt "older" by their fifties, after lifetimes of hard work and, often, long-standing experiences of chronic disease such as type 2 diabetes. Their physicians thus interpreted these men as ready to make a life course shift away from a focus on penetrative sex. This assessment was encouraged by structural deterrents against diagnosing ED in the IMSS. These included time pressures that made it unattractive to diagnose new conditions beyond those for which patients sought treatment. They also included economic constraints. The IMSS hospital pharmacy could not afford to stock the ED drugs on the list of medications that were supposed to be available to patients, so physicians knew that low-income patients would have to pay out of pocket for the drugs. In contrast, the urologists told me that private practice patients wanted and could afford ED treatment. The doctors thus saw private patients as able to embody youthful sexuality at numerically older ages than IMSS patients.

Men's Health Medicine: Varied Targets of Repair in an Emerging Field

I now shift from discussing the ways patients define erectile function change as normal versus pathological to examining the ways that medicine as an institution develops its ideologies of repair. To do so, I turn my lens from the users to the developers of men's health offerings. I present data from a research project on the development of the emerging medical field of men's health in order to discuss how medical providers' specific ideologies of gender and sexuality influence the normative assumptions that come to underlay their specialty's definitions of which bodily changes and experiences are unhealthy or abnormal. Specifically, I argue that in the emerging field of men's health, currently a heterogenous mix of providers from different specialties, practitioners' different philosophies of gender and health determine whether they define key targets of repair as men's bodies or men's gender ideologies.

The medical subfield of men's health was inspired by events ranging from the success of ED drugs to gay men's activism around urogenital cancers. It has also emerged in response to longer histories of gender-specific medicine in women's health. Specific instantiations of men's health can reflect any of these trajectories, as the field is defined quite varyingly by the multidisciplinary health professionals and organizations seeking to formalize it. Works seeking to define men's health thus range from calls for social scientifically grounded understandings of gender and health as complexly interrelated phenomena (e.g., Courtenay 2002) to men's health medical texts that focus on the technical treatment of and doctor-patient communication regarding testosterone and male genital pathologies (e.g., Lim 2013).

Here I draw on early findings from interviews with US-based men's health professionals to discuss how varied understandings of the natures of men and masculinities are influencing the emergence, content, and biosocial consequences of this nascent medical field. I analyze interviews with seventeen US-based health-care professionals who either define themselves as men's health practitioners or do activist work promoting health access for men. These professionals, identified via snowball sampling, largely from contacts I made at an international men's health conference, include urologists and cardiologists (the specialties most represented in US men's health programming), family medicine providers, public health practitioners, and an ob-gyn and nurse-midwives who sought to expand their scope of practice to cis- and transgender men. About a third of interviewees were female, a third were people of color, and about a fourth were born and/or raised outside the United States. While not comprehensive or representative, these data provide an instructive first look at the great variation within US-based men's health medicine in terms of professionals' understandings of men, their problems, and appropriate targets of repair for addressing these problems.

Defining Men's Needs Defines the Targets of Repair

Participants saw men as under- or poorly served within medicine, but what this meant to them varied according to their ideas of men's natures and needs. Several physicians saw men and women as two discrete biological groups and thus believed men were in need of specialized health services like those offered to women. For instance, one urologist who has been foundational in developing men's health professional associations defined men as "underserved" and said that men's lower life expectancy compared with women demonstrated the need "to get men into medical care more efficiently," and to this end he also argued the need to fund men's health programs. Similarly, a cardiologist noted that while heart disease was more prevalent in women, it seemed to make men sicker; given this, he called for research behind his observation that "when you go to a hospital you see that there are more men who look severely ill." Another cardiologist, who had been instrumental in bringing medical attention to women's unique physiological experiences of heart disease, noted that "everybody thinks we've neglected women, but we've also neglected men—why do men die six years before women?"

Physicians who foregrounded understandings of men as a biologically defined group also tended to attribute shared psychological traits to "men" that influenced their health-care behavior (and also implicitly based their understandings of men on research with white, middle-class men). The urologist quoted above stated that "men in general [exhibit a] universal avoidance of health care—that's certainly the case throughout Europe and mirrors what's true in the US." He noted that this reflected "male psychology of considering himself bulletproof" rather than access issues, since men in the United Kingdom had universal health care. Another voiced this common idea by explaining that "men are historically a lot worse at seeking help," meaning that men's health could be defined as addressing both men's biological needs and social barriers, or "helping men with male specific problems and letting them know that . . . it's not that embarrassing."

These physicians did identify differences within the category of men when asked about patients' different understandings of masculinity. The urologist just quoted responded by noting generational differences in men such as older men's stricter adherence to traditional gender roles. He then suggested that his work in his institution's LGBTQ clinic was more relevant for discussing gender. This comment suggested that he saw heterosexual and cisgender men's experiences of gender as less significant to their health care as that of men who diverged from implicit norms, mirroring a cultural history of gender studies and activism in which women have been seen as "having gender" and men were viewed as a normative, default category. Several physicians similarly identified gender as primarily significant for patients who were nonheterosexual or transgender, fusing awareness of difference with a core identification of one group of men with a common psychology as the default object of "men's health."

While many physicians primarily discussed men as a group defined by shared biology and psychology, they challenged some male stereotypes, such as the ideas that men are unemotional or focused on individualism. Instead, these doctors discussed the need for communication with patients that accounted for emotional and social needs they perceived as common to men as a group. For instance, a urologist who specialized in vasectomy said he always allotted thirty minutes for conversation at his pre-surgery consults to allay patients' fears, since "there is a lot to talk about in addition to the technical aspects of the procedure, in terms of: 'Will this affect my sexual function in the future?' 'Will this affect me as a man?'" These physicians also noted the relationality of men's lives. For some, this included talking to men's spouses, while others saw wives as drivers of men's health behavior. One urologist explained, "It's well known that 60–80 percent of health seeking in the family is driven by women." He then noted that "men's health is family health," since men were key contributors to their families' economic well-being.

Some providers (most but not all of whom were immigrants to the United States and people of color) further complicated this picture of "men" by discussing the ways that different ethnic, racial, or national backgrounds shaped men's experiences with health problems and care. For instance, the urologist discussing vasectomy communication above, himself a migrant to the United States, mused about regional differences in patient concerns. A urologist specializing in male infertility presented an analysis of cultural difference that contrasted with uniform ideas of "male psychology" and stereotypes of masculinity associated with ideas of ethnicity and race. He told me that for his patients of Asian, Middle Eastern, and African origin, it was "taboo" not to have children, and so experiences of infertility caused them great pain and shame, at a familial, couple, and individual level. He noted that this influenced their desires for fertility treatment but also noted that such desires did not conform to stereotypes of patriarchal masculinity. He recounted the story of an Indian man crying in his office because he blamed himself for his and his wife's infertility. They had had a child through in vitro fertilization but felt pressure from relatives to have more children. The physician noted that despite the stereotype that men from this culture (also the doctor's familial culture) wanted sons, this patient focused on wanting his family and wife to be happy.

Physicians who emphasized a universal male biology as key to men's health treatment tended to define the medical targets of repair based on the perspectives discussed above. Many voiced the idea that men avoided health care but would seek treatment for a few issues that they found particularly problematic, which one urologist called the "five s's: sex, streams, steroids, sperm, and sleep." These physicians advocated for a men's health approach that would use these as gateway conditions, enabling providers to connect men presenting with these problems to multidisciplinary care for the chronic illnesses that often caused them. For instance, a urologist said that a patient with ED could be given Viagra or a penile prosthetic instead of treatment for underlying chronic disease, but "if we were to approach that problem from a multidisciplinary approach, we may provide better outcomes and give that person a better chance of improving their life. . . . So, a men's health clinic ideally would be that all these physicians would come and approach that patient's problem from different perspectives." Such physicians sometimes noted that women were required to see physicians for reproductive issues throughout their whole lives but that men lacked such an impetus; they hoped to use the few concerns they believed drew in male patients as gateways to more comprehensive care and earlier intervention.

Some urologists sought to address structural targets of repair to facilitate appropriate care for men. Several defined "men's health" as simply a "marketing term" that might entice reticent men to see them. While all discussed strategies for making their practices or clinics welcoming to male patients, some worked to create dedicated men's health clinics, which would both be inviting for men and provide multidisciplinary medical care. Many discussed clinics that had focused on interior design as a major tool for attracting male patients. For example, a urologist described the "men's health clinics, especially in bigger cities like Chicago or New York" as "a place for the men to walk into and they're like, ah this is mahogany wood, there's a pool table in the back. . . . It's branding, and walking in and feeling like you're in a space that's unique for men." This approach made sense to those who focused on male psychology as a unified whole. Though none of the interviewees worked in such a clinic and many criticized the use of marketing by profit-driven testosterone and ED clinics, many understood them to be appealing to men.

Given the interviewees' emphasis on men as relational beings, it was more common for them to emphasize the health benefits that clinics attractive to men could create. This was true for the urologist who was a founder of key US men's health organizations and who was also creating a "male-focused clinic" at his home institution. He described this clinic as needing to appeal to men on a superficial level, including "decorating that looks male," but more importantly needing to meet men's lifestyle needs in order to attract patients and connect them with treatments from varied medical disciplines. For example, he prioritized offering "schedules and times that can appeal to men" likely to want early, late, or weekend appointments that fit around their work schedules, as well as easy parking and access from the highway. While such accommodations would certainly benefit all patients, he characterized these inconveniences as barriers that men were unwilling to overcome.

Two physicians, however, ran somewhat different kinds of men's health clinics, reflecting their different definitions of men. These doctors, who described themselves as having humanistic or social scientific bents and interests, defined men's health problems as what a social scientist would call fundamentally biopsychosocial. They understood the targets of repair they treated in their clinics—one focused on male pelvic pain and the other on male sexual dysfunction—as mind-body issues to be assessed and treated with methods from medicine as well as fields attuned to the social aspects of health, including masculinities understood as expressions of social experience rather than of a universal male biology.

Neither physician adopted the "mahogany and pool table" design approach. Instead, they structured their clinics to facilitate communication between patients and providers. This included material surroundings. One physician decorated his office with memorabilia and art that were meaningful to him and could put patients at ease and spark conversation. Both emphasized the structure of patient appointments, including extended time for conversation as most significant to providing good men's health care. For instance, the pelvic pain specialist had decided not to accept insurance because the reimbursement model emphasized procedures over communication. She said communication and medical thoroughness, rather than particularistic focus on procedures, is "what we believe so that's what we stand by. Ninety-minute appointments and a comprehensive physical exam from head to toe."

These doctors also included tools from beyond medicine into their practices. For instance, the pelvic pain specialist included genograms in each initial workup. These are a tool adapted from the field of family therapy to map the simultaneously biological and social inheritances from one's family. She explained, "You create a family tree, and you use at least three generations, and you are not only looking at past medical history or family history of medical diseases, but you also do dynamics. Like what kind of relationships were going on, were they abusive. . . . It goes beyond doing a family history for medicine." Similarly, the physician running the sexual-dysfunction-focused clinic noted that "most men I see suffer not only from the organic issues . . . but they also suffer from performance anxiety from the largest sex organ in the body, which is the brain." He often taught patients sensate focus techniques to treat the mental aspect of this mind/body condition, for example, encouraging them to do nonsexual massage with their partners to restore confidence and intimacy.

Using techniques from diverse disciplines and emphasizing communication enabled these providers to treat what they understood as biological problems with important social components. This approach was grounded in more diverse understandings of masculinities than that of some other men's health practitioners. For instance, the pelvic pain specialist critiqued the idea that "men are seen as so simple," as promoted in car-themed men's health materials that encouraged men to see their doctor for a "tune-up." She saw patients' biological problems and the gendered distress they caused—which would vary among men—both as objects of repair. She explained that "to me, taking care of men isn't like, 'oh did you get an STD or not, or your culture is negative or not.' It's like, why did this happen, what could we do maybe to prevent this from happening again? Because . . . it's not just your symptoms that are bothering you. You know you feel really scared and bad."

The physician who ran the sexual dysfunction clinic saw high-income patients but also worked in the public health service and in clinics largely attended by low-income patients. He thus incorporated assessment of the social effects of structural inequalities into his understanding of his patients as responding in individual ways to shared social and structural factors. For example, he noted that for a male patient who is "disabled, it's likely that they're going to feel disenfranchised and struggle, albeit not all [disabled] men. You can't generalize that for all men. Whether they're partnered or not, how many partners they have and how many children they might have with all the different partners, whether they're involved in their lives or not."

Medical providers who trained in women's health had still more socially focused ideas about their targets of repair. They employed social scientific understandings of gender as a context-specific construct in their men's health work and saw gender norms (expressed on both individual and structural levels) and biological pathologies as fundamentally interlinked objects of treatment. This was the case for an ob-gyn who saw women clinically but focused his research program on male contraception. He understood masculinity ideologies as key potential barriers to reproductive health care: "No matter what [male contraception] method you make ... no one's going to touch it unless the culture of men changes." In tandem with developing new contraceptive technologies, he undertook social-scientifically informed research on masculinities "to really debunk some of the stereotypes that currently exist about men and to expose a lot of our implicit biases." He saw gender-specific health as useful in that it provided "a safe, dedicated space" for women. But he also believed that providing care jointly to partners rather than "siloing" men and women would enhance patients' health, given the relational nature of sexual and reproductive issues. He defined such care as a site for intervening into the behaviors of "perpetrators" of gender-based violence and inequality in female-male relationships.

The two certified nurse-midwives (CNMs) I interviewed were deeply involved in structural work to reduce such siloing. Both had commenced their careers by treating women but incorporated men into their practices when they discovered unmet need. One midwife had been providing STI education and walk-in screening for women, when men kept asking for care. She said she "just added men to the [clinic's] web page and that was it!" Within a year 40 percent of her patients were men. She treated men successfully until she changed clinics and thus malpractice insurance providers. She then discovered that a change in her national association's scope of practice wording, defining patients as "women" and limiting treatment of men to women's STI-infected partners, meant she could no longer be insured to treat men.

These CNMs were fighting to change their association's language so that they could treat "men," while also employing feminist theory and social constructionist analyses of gender to argue that defining patients as "men" or "women" denied the sex and gender diversity of people, including those who might be transgender, nonbinary, or intersex. As one said, there are "so many people who are not binary identified and where do they fit in and who do they go to? ... I think what we need to do is move away from making a binary out of reproductive health." For them, reductive gendering of health care created another key kind of unmet need, and this too was a crucial target of repair. While they engaged with the world of men's health and sought to be identified as able to practice it, they both ultimately saw gendered care as exclusionary. The other CNM noted, "I'm interested in understanding the men's health perspective, particularly heterosexual men, to make the point that when you gender care, you're in fact excluding people who also need care. The ultimate goal is to work toward less gendering of care." They also resisted gendering good care; one noted that "one of the things that has been interesting to me looking at the literature—there is a thing about young men not being willing to wait. Guys are less patient, or less willing to put up with that? ... Why would women's time be any less valuable?" They also defined quality care as both inclusive and as centering relationality: "Really when you think about sexuality and reproduction it often, not always, often involves two people of different genders. And it really makes more sense for them to get care together."

The public health professionals I interviewed shared these providers' constructionist takes on gender, their attention to structural inequalities, and their understandings of their own disciplines as well as mainstream medical men's health as targets of repair. These researchers, both men of color dedicated to improving the health of other men of color through community and structural-level intervention, described themselves as outliers in a public health world of men's health that one glossed as "old, white, [and] clinical." Both understood typical public health understandings of men as homogenous, implicitly white and middle-class, suffering from health problems largely related to their own performance of toxic masculinities. The researchers identified a lack of theoretical sophistication in this approach, which left no room for the diversity of masculinities men lived out, nor for the complexly gendered, racial/ethnic, and class stigmas and forms of structural violence harming many men's health. One explained that the chorus of "men suck, men suck" based on homogenizing ideas of "men" led to the assumption that "brown and black men must suck" too, thus perpetuating health-demoting racism.

They extended this critique to the most common forms of the medical practice of men's health in the United States. For instance, one public health researcher noted that the clinics with interior design tailored to "men" with mahogany were not only built on a profit model centering white, well-off, and stereotypically masculine men, but reproduced inequalities by "cater[ing] to men's assumptions" about masculinity, "rather than challenging them." The other critiqued the field's narrow focus on sexual and reproductive health. While several physicians understood that approach to be "comprehensive" if it included multiple medical specialties, he thought that defining men's health around sexual and reproductive issues precluded a truly "comprehensive" approach that would include more sophisticated thinking about gender. He noted that "the idea that masculinities is a plural notion hasn't really taken hold. ... In men's health in the US, we kind of default back to 'yeah there's masculinities but we're going to talk about mostly hegemonic masculinities, we're going to treat all men the same, we're going to talk about . . . 'men don't go to the doctor, men don't do this, men don't like to ask for directions.'"

Both public health professionals addressed multiple targets of repair in their work. While their professional goals were to improve individual men's health, they understood it to be fundamentally shaped by raced, gendered, and classed systems that perpetuated health-demoting inequalities. As they ran community-based projects to assess and address men's specific health needs and barriers, they also sought to change medical and public health knowledge systems from within. Both were involved in creating quantitative scales of masculinity for men assigned to specific racial or ethnic categories, which would assess the diverse realities of those men's lived experience rather than employing pathologizing stereotypes.

Conclusion

Both examples presented here—men's sexual health in Mexico, and health professionals' perceptions of men's health in the United States—demonstrate how people's definitions of men dictate what they view as health problems and take on as medical targets of repair. The Mexican case study reveals divergence between the understandings of men embedded in ED drug marketing and those that emerge from Mexican cultural discourses about the nature of *mestizo* men and the persistence yet problematic nature of machismo. Both these discourses link men's sexuality and masculinity closely to an idea of male biology, but those definitions of male biology are quite different. They thus led study participants to define healthy and appropriate later-life male sexuality in ways that contradicted the promotion of lifelong virility assumed within the medical understanding of decreased erectile function as a biological pathology. The idea that their biologies encouraged socially negative forms of masculinity led older, working-class men seeking IMSS urologic treatment to see problematic forms of masculinity, rather than decreasing erectile function, as a target of repair. Instead of seeking ED treatment, most of these men and their partners understood the bio-cultural inheritance of macho male sexuality to be the problem and understood decreased erectile function in older age not as a medical pathology but as an aid and opportunity to resist problematic tendencies.

Similarly, what US professionals involved with "men's health" defined as problems in need of repair and what they defined as the scope and objects of their emergent medical field depended on their understandings of the nature of men and masculinity. Two different concepts and groups of practitioners appear to operate: some men's health practitioners base their work in ideas of gender and sex as social constructs, and others understand "men" to be a natural category defined by a shared biology and psychology that influence male behavior. Individual providers demonstrated great variability in whether they saw men most significantly as a single group or understand men to be variably affected by race, class, and other statuses that structure inequalities that affect health. These different intellectual starting points led providers to characterize men and their health needs differently and to seek out different primary targets for repair: namely, masculinity ideologies versus men's bodies. These foci then led providers to offer very different kinds of therapies and strive to create different kinds of clinics, with different consequences for patients. These differences also led providers to identify diverse structural targets of repair, from a lack of dedicated men's health medicine to be cured with new clinics to de-gendering medical practice.

These two cases demonstrate that people's culturally influenced understandings of men's natures shape "men's health" interactions from both the patient and provider sides. Locally specific ideologies of masculinity and health, which vary by factors ranging from nationality to one's form of medical training, shape what various actors view as health problems and solutions for male patients. People draw on such ideas—including beliefs about whether masculinity is a social construct or biological essence—in order to determine what problems are and how to fix them. In order to define and offer better care for men, it is thus imperative to first identify the ways that cultural assumptions about masculinity figure into our definitions of normal and ideal biology and our efforts to repair deviations from it.

Emily Wentzell is an associate professor of anthropology and director of the International Studies Program at the University of Iowa. Her research focuses on the relationships between changing gender norms and emerging sexual health interventions targeted at men and draws on ideas from medical anthropology, gender/sexuality studies, and science and technology studies. She has long focused on Mexican men's and families' experiences with these topics, using a life course perspective, and is currently researching the ways that varied local ideologies of masculinity, aging, and health are being incorporated into the emerging global field of men's health medicine.

References

Alonso, Ana María. 2004. "Conforming Disconformity: "Mestizaje," Hybridity, and the Aesthetics of Mexican Nationalism." *Cultural Anthropology* 19(4): 459–90. https://doi.org/10.1525/can.2004.19.4.459.
Amuchástegui, Ana, and Ivonne Szasz, eds. 2007. *Sucede que me canso de ser hombre*. Mexico City: El Colegio de Mexico.

Amuchástegui Herrera, Ana. 2008. "La masculinidad como culpa esencial: subjetivación, género y tecnología de sí en un programa de reeducación para hombres violentos." II Congreso Nacional Los Estudios de Género de los Hombres en México: Caminos Andados y Nuevos Retos en Investigación y Acción, Mexico City, 14 February.

Both, Rosalijn. 2015. "A Matter of Sexual Confidence: Young Men's Non-prescription Use of Viagra in Addis Ababa, Ethiopia." *Culture, Health & Sexuality* 18(5): 1–14.

Canguilhem, Georges. (1943) 1989. *The Normal and the Pathological.* Translated by Carolyn R. Fawcett. New York: Zone Books.

Courtenay, Will. 2002. "A Global Perspective on the Field of Men's Health: An Editorial." *International Journal of Men's Health* 1: 1–14.

Drescher, Jack, Alan Schwartz, Flávio Casoy, Christopher A. McIntosh, Brian Hurley, Kenneth Ashley, Mary Barber, David Goldenberg, Sarah E. Herbert, and Lorraine E. Lothwell. 2016. "The Growing Regulation of Conversion Therapy." *Journal of Medical Regulation* 102(2): 7.

Fausto-Sterling, Anne. 1985. *Myths of Gender: Biological Theories about Women and Men.* New York: Basic Books.

Fuentes, Agustín, Rebecca Rogers Ackermann, Sheela Athreya, Deborah Bolnick, Tina Lasisi, SangHee Lee, ShayAkil McLean, and Robin Nelson. 2019. "AAPA statement on race and racism." *American Journal of Physical Anthropology* 169(3): 400–402.

Grace, Victoria, Annie Potts, Nicola Gavey, and Tiina Vares. 2006. "The Discursive Condition of Viagra." *Sexualities* 9(3): 295–314.

Gutmann, Matthew C. 1996. *The Meanings of Macho: Being a Man in Mexico City.* Berkeley: University of California Press.

Karkazis, Katrina. 2008. *Fixing Sex: Intersex, Medical Authority, and Lived Experience.* Durham, NC: Duke University Press.

Katz, Stephen, and Barbara Marshall. 2002. "New Sex for Old: Lifestyle, Consumerism, and the Ethics of Aging Well." *Journal of Aging Studies* 17(1): 3–16.

Lim, Peter H. C. (ed.). 2013. *Men's Health.* London: Springer-Verlag.

Loe, Meika. 2006. "The Viagra Blues: Embracing or Resisting the Viagra Body." In Dana Rosenfeld and Christopher A. Faircloth (eds.), *Medicalized Masculinities.* Philadelphia: Temple University Press, pp. 21–44.

Mamo, L., and J. Fishman. 2001. "Potency in All the Right Places: Viagra as a Technology of the Gendered Body." *Body & Society* 7(4): 13–35.

Marshall, Barbara. 2008. "Older Men and Sexual Health: Post-Viagra Views of Changes in Function." *Generations* 32(1): 21–27.

McLaren, Angus. 2007. *Impotence: A Cultural History.* Chicago: University of Chicago Press.

Moore, Katrina L. 2010. "Sexuality and Sense of Self in Later Life: Japanese Men's and Women's Reflections on Sex and Aging." *Journal of Cross-Cultural Gerontology* 25(2): 149–63.

Niewöhner, Jörg, and Margaret Lock. 2018. "Situating Local Biologies: Anthropological Perspectives on Environment/Human Entanglements." *BioSocieties* 13(4): 681–97.

Paz, Octavio. (1961) 1985. *The Labyrinth of Solitude and Other Writings.* Translated by Lysander Kemp. New York: Grove Weidenfeld.

Potts, Annie, Victoria Grace, Nicola Gavey, and Tiina Vares. 2004. "'Viagra Stories': Challenging 'Erectile Dysfunction.'" *Social Science & Medicine* 59: 489–99.

Ramirez, Josué. 2009. *Against Machismo: Young Adult Voices in Mexico City*. New York: Berghahn Books.

Ross, Ellen, and Rayna Rapp. 1983. "Sex and Society: A Research Note from Social History and Anthropology." In Ann Snitow, Christine Stansell, and Sharon Thompson (eds.), *Powers of Desire: The Politics of Sexuality*. New York: Monthly Review Press, pp. 51–73.

Sandberg, Linn. 2013. "Just Feeling a Naked Body Close to You: Men, Sexuality and Intimacy in Later Life." *Sexualities* 16(3–4): 261–82.

Tiefer, Leonore. 2006. "The Viagra Phenomenon." *Sexualities* 9(3): 273–94.

van der Geest, Sjaak. 2001. "'No Strength': Sex and Old Age in A Rural Town in Ghana." *Social Science and Medicine* 53: 1383–96.

Vasconcelos, José. (1925) 1997. *The Cosmic Race: A Bilingual Edition*. Translated by Didier T. Jaén. Baltimore: Johns Hopkins University Press.

Wentzell, Emily. 2008. "Imagining Impotence in America: From Men's Deeds to Men's Minds to Viagra." *Michigan Discussions in Anthropology* 25: 153–78.

———. 2017. "How Did Erectile Dysfunction Become "Natural"? A Review of the Critical Social Scientific Literature on Medical Treatment for Male Sexual Dysfunction." *Journal of Sex Research* 54(4–5): 486–506. https://doi.org/10.1080/00224499.2016.1259386.

Wentzell, Emily A. 2013. *Maturing Masculinities: Aging, Chronic Illness, and Viagra in Mexico*. Durham, NC: Duke University Press.

CHAPTER 2

Repairing Sexual Aging
Italian GPs' Discourses in the Viagra Era

RAFFAELLA FERRERO CAMOLETTO

Partly as a result of the European ban on direct-to-consumer prescription drug advertising, from the beginning of the twenty-first century, social campaigns have "problematized" aspects of male sexual lifestyles and life courses, and repaired them by treatment and pharmaceuticals. Professional associations of physicians (e.g., urologists, andrologists, and sexologists) are behind these campaigns, which are also backed by both institutional bodies (e.g., the Ministry of Health) and pharmaceutical companies. Their objective is to spread information among people about various male sexual dysfunctions and available medical treatments. Thus they propagate the idea of male sexual health as a new public health and medical issue and in so doing convey a view of masculinity that needs to be "repaired." This in turn promotes new forms of medical expertise suitable for treating it (for a previous analysis of these campaigns, see Ferrero Camoletto and Bertone 2012).

This chapter[1] outlines the positions of Italian general practitioners in the panorama of multiple expert perspectives of sexual medicine, particularly how they handle the sexual aging process in dealing with their male patients' sexual health problems. I shall demonstrate that socially available representations and cultural norms defining sexual aging are embodied, conveyed, and sometimes questioned by medical discourses.

The arrival on the scene of Viagra and equivalent sexuopharmaceuticals[2] and the spreading rhetoric of "positive aging" in its various permutations ("active," "successful," and/or "healthy") are key components of medical experts' cultural environment. The intersection of these two cultural phenomena impacts upon the way people, men in particular, perceive and experience age-related sexual changes: from old age seen as characterized by a process of desexualization and "sexual retirement" to seeing aging people as "sexy oldies" (Gott 2005) or "sexy seniors" (Marshall 2010).

This clinical and cultural revolution calls into question accepted medical (and commonsensical) views of sexual aging; as a result, medical experts are forced to address a heated debate about conflicting perceptions and definitions of normalcy in sexual aging. Previous research (Andrews and Piterman 2007; Bauer, McAuliffe, and Nay 2007; Gott and Hinchliff 2003; Gott, Galena, Hinchliff, and Elford 2004; Gott, Hinchliff, and Galena 2004; Taylor and Gosney 2011) has evidenced the uneasiness of general practitioners when dealing with sexual issues, especially with midlife and older patients.

I shall analyze GPs' adoption and questioning of socially available scripts of aging, gender, and sexuality, based on a recent Italian mixed-method qualitative research project. As a consequence, I shall show how GPs, in their clinical practice, have a tendency to combine the natural, the normal, and the normative (Jones and Higgs 2010) by reinterpreting "sexual health" medically in terms of their perceptions of what constitutes—for aging men and women—an age-appropriate "respectable sexuality" (Bertone and Ferrero Camoletto 2009; Wentzell 2013b). In so doing, medical discourses may convey a biomedicalized ideology of repair, reproducing an understanding of aging as a pathological process to be monitored and counteracted. Keeping older bodies sexually active, and thereby fixing the sex machine (Loe 2001), becomes a core issue for GPs to address and to cure and care for their patients' sexual health.

Positive Aging and Sexuopharmaceuticals: Re-sexualizing Later Life

Successful aging seems to have become one of the contemporary obsessions (Lamb 2017), focusing on individual agency and choice to maintain "busy bodies" (Katz 2000) and to withstand the cultural markers of old age (Gross and Blundo 2005; Katz and Calasanti 2015; Katz and Marshall 2004). As Twigg and Martin (2015: 355) pointed out, this opens up "new territory for empirical investigation in which the body is understood as a key site for the operation of new forms of governmentality. . . . The bodies of older people are disciplined and made subject to regimes of fitness and health in which responsibility for ageing well becomes a moral imperative."

Gerontologists have criticized these notions of "successful" and "active" aging because of their neoliberal focus on productivity and their consumeristic antiaging approach, both of which restrict the understanding of the aging process (Boudiny and Mortelmans 2011; Bülow and Soderqvist 2014; Katz and Calasanti 2015; Martinson and Berridge 2015; Rubinstein and de Medeiros 2014). Within this frame, a "lifelong sexual function" (Marshall and Katz 2002) becomes a primary aspect of healthy and successful ageing, imposing the new imperative of "sex for life" (Katz and Marshall 2003), envisaging a "virility surveillance" (Marshall 2010) by which "the floppy penis" (Calasanti and King 2005) in aging men is seen as a warning signal of a precariously abnormal condition, current or future, requiring medically assisted restoration (Loe 2001; Marshall 2009).

The so-called Viagra studies have emerged as one of the research streams investigating men's aging and sexuality within a medicalized frame (Ferrero Camoletto and Bertone 2012, 2017; Gurevich et al. 2018; Hinchliff, Gott, and Galena 2004; Humphery and Nazareth 2001; Johnson, Sjögren, and Åsberg 2016; Loe 2001; Low et al. 2004; Mamo and Fishman 2001; Marshall 2006, 2007, 2008, 2012; Potts 2005; Potts et al. 2004; Tiefer 1986, 2006; Wentzell 2013a, 2013b; Wentzell and Salmerón 2009). Thus, the advent of Viagra has triggered a radical transformation in the perception of age-related changes in male sexuality.

In their reconstruction of the Western cultural scenario in the pre-Viagra era, Potts and colleagues (2006) pointed out how the prevailing narrative about male aging was the notion of an inevitable sexual decline, associated with a physiological reduction of erectile ability. Other narratives were available, but less used and less acknowledged, for example, the so-called progressive narrative, interpreting the effects of decreased erectile ability as an opportunity to live a sexuality less centered on penetrative potency, but open to the experimentation of different sources and forms of sex. In the Viagra era, both these narratives have been replaced by that of the "sexy oldie," connecting healthy aging with lifelong sexual activity following a "forever functional" imperative (Marshall and Katz 2002). Progress then has been reinterpreted in terms of a restoration of youthful sexual skills and of the enhancement of never-attained sexual performances, constructing a new pharmacologically assisted virility (Marshall 2006, 2010) and a "cyborg masculinity" (Potts 2005). This notion of a forever functional sexuality reflects a critical node of recent medical development, the shift from a medicine focused on needs to a medicine addressing desires; in Italy, in particular, this is witnessed by the recent introduction, in the medical deontological code, of the term "enhancement medicine" (Giglio 2015). As a consequence, in the field of sexual aging, the boundaries between the purpose of care and that of optimization and enhancement, between the therapeutic uses and the extra-therapeutic and recreational uses of medical and pharmaceutical technologies are becoming increasingly blurred, paving the way for a techno-mediated aging sexuality always open to repair.

Research on aging men has outlined, however, the persistence of the narrative of decline. For instance, a study of Mexican men (Wentzell 2013b;

see also chapter 1) showed how ED medicines can endanger men's notion of a respectable sexuality and of a mature and responsible masculinity. Sexual difficulties can therefore be reinterpreted as natural sexual changes, rejecting the pathologizing label of sexual dysfunction and the risk of "getting viagraed" by an artificially produced pharma-mediated sexuality (Wentzell and Salmerón 2009). The research literature has also noted that some aging men may adopt the narrative of progress (Potts et al. 2006; Wentzell 2013b) as an alternative understanding of sexual aging; for instance, in her analysis of older Swedish people's accounts, Sandberg (2011, 2013) introduced the notion of an "intimacy narrative" to frame how her interviewees tended to interpret life-course-related sexual changes as an opportunity to experience different, richer forms of sexual expression.

GPs Facing the Viagra Revolution

While providing a multifaceted picture of patients and consumers, Viagra studies often assign to medical experts the role of transmission chains of a top-down process of medicalization of sexuality. In fact, few studies have investigated how physicians—either as sexual medicine professionals or as general practitioners—culturally define, and accordingly treat, life-course-related sexual changes. In what is depicted as medical experts' compliance with the new engine of "pharmaceuticalization," the possibility of their reflexivity and resistance seems to have been overlooked.[3]

A review of the literature provides a picture of scattered, mainly quantitative, research on this topic. In Europe,[4] the most investigated national case is the UK (Gott and Hinchliff 2003; Gott, Galena, Hinchliff, and Elford 2004; Gott, Hinchliff, and Galena 2004; Gott 2005; Humphrey and Nazareth 2001), while other national contexts are only partly covered: France (Giami 2010), Ireland (Byrne et al. 2010), Portugal (Alarcão et al. 2012; Ribeiro et al. 2011, 2014), and Switzerland (Platano et al. 2008a, 2008b). These studies outline different barriers to raising the subject of sex among both GPs and their (older and not-so-old) patients.

Physicians, on the one hand, describe their own difficulties in addressing sexual issues. The most common justification is the lack of time in everyday clinical practice (e.g., Ribeiro et al. 2014); however, this perception of a time constraint can be influenced by the cultural belief that sexual health is not a priority issue when dealing with older patients, therefore endorsing commonsensical notions of an asexual old age (Alarcão et al. 2012; Gott, Hinchliff, and Galena 2004). Another relevant, recurring barrier is GPs' admission of, and complaints about, a lack of training and education in their academic curricula on such a sensitive topic. For instance, in British qualitative studies, physicians describe their fear and discomfort in initiating a dialogue on sexual issues by adopting catchphrases like "opening a can of worms" (Gott, Galena, Hinchliff, and Elford 2004a) or "opening a floodgate" (Humphrey and Nazareth 2001).

Because of this combination of lack of time and lack of training, GPs often seem to consider sexual health as an inappropriate and non-legitimate topic to be proactively introduced into their professional interaction with older patients. As a consequence, many physicians adopt a reactive style, limiting themselves to responding to sexual concerns and problems brought to them by patients. However, some GPs acknowledge the importance of their role as gatekeepers of the definitions of healthy aging and therefore in their "permission granting role" of legitimizing normal and appropriate age-related sexualities (Gott 2005).

Giami (2010), in his qualitative study on French GPs, provides a useful typological summary of approaches to sexual issues. The first approach is evasion (*évitement*), involving selective exclusion of and resistance to tackling sexual issues due to the abovementioned excuses such as lack of time and pressure from other clinical priorities, irrelevance of the topic for older patients, and fear of violation of patients' privacy and intimacy. The second approach is called medical reappropriation, when the GP adopts a relative, partial avoidance by reframing sexual problems as a matter of physiology, infections, contraception, etc., and therefore acknowledging them as legitimate medical problems. The third approach is called holistic because it makes reference to GPs' adoption of a more comprehensive understanding of health issues, including sexual issues as a key dimension of well-being. The fourth approach is the quest for some sort of sexological specialization pointing out the importance of specialized training in sexual medicine for GPs' academic curricula and clinical practice.

In this fragmented review of the literature, Italy appears to be lagging behind; among the studies addressing Italian general practitioners' attitudes and behavior within their medical profession, the style of management of sexual health issues seems to be a neglected theme (for an exception among clinical studies, see De Berardis et al. 2009). This shortfall in research points to the need for exploring the complexity of GPs' accounts of their experience in dealing with their older patients' sexualities.

Current Study: Context and Methodology

In this chapter, I draw upon empirical material collected within a current multi-method qualitative follow-up research project (started in 2016) on the transformation of representations and experiences of aging and sexuality in Italy. Previous research (Ferrero Camoletto and Bertone 2012, 2017; Ferrero Camoletto, Bertone, and Salis 2015) carried out in Italy from 2010 to 2015 focused on social awareness campaigns about male sexual health. These campaigns aimed to inform the general population about the diversity of men's sexual problems and to promote obtaining medical advice, thereby constructing a definition of the problem to be solved, the patients to be cured, and the strategies for resolution, including treatments to be adopted. This research project included a thematic analysis of visual and textual documentary material produced by major national awareness campaigns on male sexual health websites and videos ("Amare senza pensieri," 2008–9; "Amico andrologo," since 2009; "Basta scuse," 2010; "Chiedi aiuto," 2012; "Uomo e salute," 2013); websites on male sexual health managed by medical experts (www.pianetauomo.eu, promoted by SIU, the Italian Urological Society; www.prevenzioneandrologica.it, promoted by SIA, the Italian Andrological Society); and websites by pharmaceutical companies (www.lillyuroandrologia.it, promoted by Lilly). Nineteen interviews were carried out, along with one roundtable of experts in the field of sexual medicine (urologists, endocrinologists, sexologists, sex counselors), recruited because of their involvement in these campaigns.[5] In addition, interviews with two groups of product-development and marketing managers from two major pharmaceutical companies' Italian subsidiaries (Lilly and Menarini) were conducted.

The project narrowed the field of investigation by focusing on the impact of the Viagra revolution and of the rhetoric of active aging on the representations and experiences of sexual aging and on the controversial notion of ageless sex. The project involved an analysis of media and medical documents on older people's sexual health, interviews with GPs (twenty-three), and focus groups and interviews with older people (four and seven, respectively) in order to explore their perceptions and experiences of sexual aging.

As an empirical basis, I focus on the in-depth interviews with general practitioners. The interviews, lasting from 30–40 to 90 minutes, have been fully transcribed and submitted to open, axial coding procedures with Atlas.ti software. Following a thematic analysis (Braun and Clarke 2014), I reconstructed how doctors debate the issue of sexual aging. To summarize how GPs differ in their views of older people's sexual health, I combined the two typologies of the abovementioned qualitative studies (Gott, Hinchliff, and Galena 2004b for the UK; Giami 2010 for France), identifying five styles of sexual health management:

(a) *Reactive evasion*, when sexual issues are not seen as a priority or are considered a risky topic to be dealt with only when patients introduce it

(b) *Reactive sexological specialization* (or *delegation*), when sexual issues are delegated to sexual-medicine experts
(c) *Proactive medical appropriation*, when sexual problems are reframed as medical problems relating to physiology, infections, contraception, etc.
(d) *Proactive holistic approach*, when sexual issues are framed within a more general view of well-being
(e) *Proactive sexological specialization*, when GP's training in sexual issues is demanded

In the following sections, some of the preliminary results are presented and discussed.

"Letting Sleeping Dogs Lie": Between Avoidance and Delegation

In Italy, as outlined in research into other national contexts (e.g., see above), GPs do not appear at ease in dealing with sexual issues in their everyday interactions with older people; sexuality is perceived as a buck to be passed on as often as possible and to be managed cautiously when unavoidable. Talking about sex, therefore, seems to be legitimate only if patients introduce the topic. GPs fear being accused of invading patients' private spheres and of their patients' unpredictable reactions when such a sensitive topic is mentioned.

> It means being available to help them in relation to this issue ... if they mention it. ... If they don't say anything, it's a bit more difficult for me to initiate the conversation about it because I don't know how the patient will react. (GP, female, 60)

> These are niche topics, speaking about male patients, since women absolutely don't talk about them because for women to stop having sex after the menopause is perfectly normal. For a man the problem is still present at an older age, but in my experience it is an issue I rarely deal with because I let sleeping dogs lie. (GP, male, 52)

Not only are sexual issues perceived as a sensitive, private matter, but some physicians refer to sexuality as an inappropriate topic beyond medical jurisdiction. Talking about sex appears to be a more mundane practice to be dealt with in a confessional by a spiritual guide or within psychological counseling, requiring a different kind of professional training and environment.

> Some patients reacted with "Mind your own business!" as if they didn't consider this query of professional interest, as if this issue were detached from general health ... as if it should not be investigated by someone wearing scrubs, but rather by someone wearing a cassock or a psychiatrist. (GP, male, 51)

Some GPs, on the contrary, acknowledge the relevance of sexual health and the importance of managing sexual problems, but they tend to delegate this task to specialists in sexual medicine.

> If a patient introduces the problem, I take it into account, I give the appropriate therapeutic indications. ... I always do a checkup, then I send him/her to a specialist. ... [Sexual issues] are very often related to other pathologies ... they are delegated to urologists or gynecologists. (GP, female, 51)

The risk in this approach seems to be that of reducing the GP's role to sorting patients or, as is often admitted, to solving sexual problems mainly or only by prescribing pharmaceuticals.

> It is a niche issue, not so often dealt with in general practice. I personally don't encourage the patients very much, that's true, but it's very rare for a patient to talk to me about sexual problems, or if he does it's because he knows there is a little pill, a little help requiring medical prescription, so in the end [my role] comes down to prescribing these drugs. (GP, male, 52)

Proactive Approaches: Sexual Issues as a Gateway to Older Patients' Health

For some GPs, managing their older patients' sexual impairment is perceived not only as legitimate clinical practice, but also as an opportunity to build stronger therapeutic compliance. Thus, some GPs claim a more proactive role. This can mean a medical reappropriation of the investigation of sexual issues, as in this long quotation from a GP for whom managing patients' sexual difficulties emerges as the most satisfying part of his job for two reasons: because it makes the patients happy and meets their real needs, and because it triggers a stronger doctor-patient relationship, empowering therapeutic alliance and reinforcing GPs' professional status.

> The best part of my work is the rare occasions when you have direct contact. When the patient comes, takes a seat, opens up, says: "Listen, doctor, I have a problem, things are not going well with my wife." He approaches it indirectly. So you ask: "What do you mean?" "Well, it isn't working properly." So you start to put your heads together, you explain which drugs are available, how they work, how to use them, you crack some jokes. ... It's different from prescribing an-

tibiotics against bronchitis; maybe it works but the following week the patient doesn't come to say "Thanks." The patient with erectile deficit, if the treatment is successful, comes back with a smile from ear to ear. (GP, male, 45)

The specificity of sexual issues within this approach is reinterpreted positively; no longer perceived as an inconvenient, delicate topic, it acquires the role of door opener to gain the patient's trust. Moreover, for a few GPs a proactive style of medical management also conveys a more comprehensive and holistic notion of health, including sexual issues as a core dimension; talking about sex is part of an "all-embracing" view of the patient's well-being.

Well, if we want to take into account the individual's well-being, we must necessarily manage it [sexual health] too. . . . Well-being is a completion of physical, psychological and—why not?—sexual dimensions. Therefore it is all-embracing, it is present in all our medical investigations. (GP, female, 56)

Within this perspective, GPs tend to consider sexual problems as an important sentinel and as predictors of a wider range of dysfunctions and pathologies, and therefore requiring careful, committed medical attention. The acknowledgment of sexual health as a legitimate topic for GPs leads some to admit their lack of an appropriate academic background and to ask for specific training in sexual medicine as a useful tool to deal better with their patients and solve their problems.

In my opinion, it [talking about sex] should be part of our . . . like when we ask, "Does it hurt when you urinate? What does it smell like?" . . . We should remember to ask it. . . . But first of all, we need scientific evidence . . . because I wasn't specifically trained for that. So, if we had had specific training, we could intervene more appropriately on certain problems, replacing the smile on our patients' faces. (GP, male, 45)

Unpacking Healthy Sexual Aging

In addition to the distinction between reactive and proactive approaches, GPs' narratives reveal some ambivalence about the definition of sexual aging and what is natural or normal in later-life sexuality. As pointed out at the beginning of the chapter, medical discourses are enmeshed with cultural beliefs, values, and representations of gender, aging, and sexualities.

The diverse styles of medical management of old people's sexual health problems also channel and express different ways of defining and understanding what is appropriate in sexual aging. Some GPs seem to introduce a normative dimension into their clinical approach, conveying the new "must" of lifelong active sexuality (Marshall and Katz 2002): older people are expected to continue an active sexual life as part of a healthy lifestyle. Therefore GPs "willingly" handle the request in order to support their patients' sexual "rebirth" and a lifestyle of "being fully aware of your body."

> It is clear that at 70 you cannot perform as you could at 30, but you can (and should) have an active physical—including sexual—life, naturally using different ways and means. . . . People at 65–70 have no sexual life, and I, in my 50s, think this is sad and tragic. (GP, female, 51)

> Let's open GPs' minds to sexuality, please! Because sometimes they are more bigoted than their patients. . . . The aim is to make patients more alive, respecting and promoting sexual activity as producing beneficial effects. . . . What could be better than living healthily, with this lifestyle, being fully aware of your body? (GP, female, 56)

In opposition to this enthusiastic view of later sexuality as a rebirth and reappropriation of an active sexual lifestyle, other GPs outspokenly make reference to an overlapping of natural/biological and social/moral standards in defining age-appropriate sexual conduct (Marshall and Katz 2012).

> To increase your performance is a current pipe dream, not only in sex. . . . But I believe, not only as a GP but also personally, that you pay for this. If you go against nature, against the opportunities nature provides, you can end up not being able to use what your age allows. I have some cases in mind . . . patients who resist my attempts to discourage them from seeking from drugs what nature hasn't given them. And they have lives which are ridiculous in my opinion. . . . What makes me laugh is that they believe they are successful because they perform extraordinarily well. The only evidence is that they have extraordinary brains [laughing], small ones. (GP, male, 51)

The quest for a pharma-assisted everlasting sexuality is reinterpreted as a consumeristic approach and as an artificial way of coping with the naturalness and inevitability of the aging process. Moreover, this obsession with sexual rejuvenation exposes patients to the risk of looking ridiculous and paying the price. However, in a few GPs' narratives I found some room for the acknowledgment of a wider range of options of age-related sexual expressions, providing, especially for men, the possibility of moving beyond the sex-machine script. In the following quote we can see a GP legitimizing different ways of managing sexual aging: a midlife man who is seeking to ensure his own and his partner's wider well-being, as well as an older man admitting that he is no longer interested in sex after losing his wife.

The point is everyone has the right to an appropriate healthy and pleasant sexual life at any stage of the life course, being aware of the different bodily options and pleasure available at different ages.

> It reminds me of a patient I had a few years ago, who told me, "You know, I have a new partner and I want to make her feel well, to feel well myself too, therefore ... do you think I should do something about it?" I think this is very healthy and positive.... Last week a 78-year-old patient told me, "Listen, since my wife [with whom he had lived for 50 years] died last year, I don't desire other women, I don't feel like it," and I replied, "I think it's physiological, because you are 80 and you have always lived with your wife," with whom he had an active sexual life. It's absolutely normal.... There should be more publicity about the right of a man, even at 70, to have a pleasant sexual life; about the right of a woman, at 15, 60, 70, 103, to have a pleasant sexual life, using different ways and means, which is evidently physiological. At 60 you don't run a marathon, you do a little jogging. (GP, female, 55)

The reference to a context-dependent understanding of aging and sexuality seems to create some space to question a reductionist naturalized notion of sexual functioning in order to recognize the influence of social and cultural dimensions shaping how older people make sense of their sexualities across their life course. However, as I'll discuss in the last section, GPs' accounts more frequently tend to endorse a "healthicization" of sexuality (Epstein and Mamo 2017), which, in defining what is a healthy sexual lifestyle in later life, merges the natural, the normal, and the normative.

Conclusion: Sexual Aging under Repair?

In this chapter I have examined the various impacts on GPs' narratives of discourses about active aging and ageless pharma-mediated sex. There is evidence of the aging process being normalized by the overlapping of moral and health debates (Jones and Higgs 2010). This process can be interpreted as an expression of neoliberal biopolitics concerning the responsibilities of bio-citizens to maintain and repair their own bodies (Rose 2007). As Marshall states, "The centering of sexual function as an indicator of overall health and/or a warning sign of disease in aging men signals a new regime of virility surveillance, and grounds the contemporary construction of the 'aging male' as a biomedical object" (2009: 262).

GPs are fully embedded in this biomedicalized discourse on sexual aging as a process to be carefully monitored, managed, and fixed; thus it is possible for GPs to risk affirming or reinforcing a (new?) normative model of a forever-functional sexuality, felt not only as a right but also as a duty for older people (Marshall 2012). Viagra triggered a new ageless virility; maintaining sexual potency, that is, penetrative capacity, is interpreted as a sign of good health and of positive/active/successful aging.

But there is a tension between the two points of view, according to GPs' accounts: on the one hand, accepting the right and expectation of new generations of sexually active seniors to continue a satisfying level of sexual activity as a result of pharmacological and mechanical devices; on the other hand, refusing a consumeristic attitude toward sex and conserving their social role as guardians of sexual health and respectable sexual aging. By defining "functional age" ambiguously, at the crossroads of biological and biographical trajectories, GPs endorse the "contradictions of 'post-ageist' discourses and practices that promise to liberate bodies from chronological age, while simultaneously re-naturalizing gender in sexed bodies" (Marshall and Katz 2012: 222).

In fact, the GPs' narratives convey a multidimensional understanding of normalcy, thereby merging its physiological, statistical, and social definitions. GPs determine the boundaries of age-appropriate sexual health by taking into account the gendered script of a "respectable sexuality" (Bertone and Ferrero Camoletto 2009; Wentzell 2013b), according to which men should balance the risk of maintaining their sexual activity without becoming "dirty old men" or "sugar-daddies" (Walz 2002), while women have to find equilibrium between continuing sexual desire/attractiveness and avoiding ridicule as "cougars" or "mutton dressed as lamb" (Fairhurst 1998).

In some cases, GPs seem to be helpful in deconstructing stereotypes and prejudices about older people's sexuality: more specifically, they adopt what Gott (2005) called a "permission-granting role," expanding concepts of normal, appropriate aging sexualities, thereby enabling older patients to define their sexualities in less restricted ways. Some accounts suggest making space for a "progressive narrative" by accepting a more varied range of age-related sexual expressions (Potts et al. 2006; Sandberg 2013) and thereby legitimating different ways—for both men and women—to come to terms with sexual changes during their life courses. This "minority report," in some GPs' discourses, allows also them to distance themselves from a notion of medicine focused on enhancement and to question an ideology of repair reducing the aging bodies to sex machines to be fixed or optimized.

Raffaella Ferrero Camoletto is associate professor in sociology of culture at the Department of Cultures, Politics and Society, University of Turin, Italy. She has been working on two topics: body, gender, and space in emerging urban sports, and critical perspectives on masculinities and (hetero) sexualities, with a specific focus on the social impact of Viagra.

Notes

1. A different version of this chapter can be found in Ferrero Camoletto 2020.
2. On the notion of sexuopharmaceuticals, see Cacchioni 2015.
3. For an investigation and introduction to a social debate on this issue in the Italian context, see Ferrero Camoletto and Bertone 2012, 2017, and Ferrero Camoletto, Bertone, and Salis 2015.
4. On Malaysia, for an interesting study adopting focus groups to explore GPs' attitudes toward sexual health outside Europe, see Low et al. 2004.
5. The key limitation of the study depends on the small scale of the sample, restricting the possibility of taking into account the influence of some structural dimensions, mainly gender and age cohorts of the medical experts interviewed.

References

Alarcão, Violeta, Sofia Ribeiro, Filipe Leão Miranda, Mario Dias Carreira, Teresa Dias, Joaquim Garcia e Costa, and Alberto GalvãoTeles. 2012. "General Practitioners' Knowledge, Attitudes, Beliefs, and Practices in the Management of Sexual Dysfunction—Results of the Portuguese Sexos Study." *Journal of Sexual Medicine* 9(10): 2508–15.

Andrews, Catherine N., and Leon Piterman. 2007. "Sex and the Older Man: GP Perceptions and Management." *Australian Family Physician* 36(10): 867–69.

Bauer, Michael, Linda McAuliffe, and Rhonda Nay. 2007. "Sexuality, Health Care and the Older Person: An Overview of the Literature." *International Journal of Older People Nursing* 2(1): 63–68.

Bertone, Chiara, and Raffaella Ferrero Camoletto. 2009. "Beyond the Sex Machine? Sexual Practices and Masculinity in Adult Men's Heterosexual Accounts." *Journal of Gender Studies* 18(4): 369–86.

Boudiny, Kim, and Dimitri Mortelmans. 2011. "A Critical Perspective: Towards a Broader Understanding of 'Active Ageing.'" *Electronic Journal of Applied Psychology* 7(1): 8–14.

Braun, Virginia, and Victoria Clarke. 2014. "What Can 'Thematic Analysis' Offer Health and Wellbeing Researchers?" *International Journal of Qualitative Studies on Health and Well-Being* 9: 26152.

Bülow, Morten Hillgaard, and Thomas Söderqvist. 2014. "Successful Ageing: A Historical Overview and Critical Analysis of a Successful Concept." *Journal of Aging Studies* 31: 139–49.

Byrne, Molly, Sally Doherty, Hannah M. McGee, and Andrew Murphy. 2010. "General Practitioner Views about Discussing Sexual Issues with Patients with Coronary Heart Disease: A National Survey in Ireland." *BMC Family Practice* 11(1): 40–47.

Cacchioni, Thea. 2015. "Sexuopharmaceuticals." In Patricia Whelehan and Anne Bolin (eds.), *The International Encyclopedia of Human Sexuality*. Bridgewater: Wiley, pp. 1115–1354.

Calasanti, Tony, and Neal King. 2005. "Firming the Floppy Penis: Age, Class, and Gender Relations in the Lives of Old Men." *Men and Masculinities* 8(1): 3–23.

De Berardis, Giorgia, Fabio Pellegrini, Monica Franciosi, Franco Pamparana, Patrizia

Morelli, Gianni Tognoni, and Antonio Nicolucci. 2009. "Management of Erectile Dysfunction in General Practice." *Journal of Sexual Medicine* 6(4): 1127–34.

Epstein, Steven, and Laura Mamo. 2017. "The Proliferation of Sexual Health: Diverse Social Problems and the Legitimation of Sexuality." *Social Science and Medicine* 188: 176–90.

Fairhurst, Eileen. 1998. "'Growing Old Gracefully' as Opposed to 'Mutton Dressed as Lamb': The Social Construction of Recognising Older Women." In Sarah Nettleton and Jonathan Watson (eds.), *The Body in Everyday Life*. London: Routledge, pp. 258–75.

Ferrero Camoletto, Raffaella. 2020. "Normal or Normative? Italian Medical Experts' Discourses on Sexual Ageing in the Viagra Era." In David Rowland and Emanuele Jannini (eds.), *Cultural Differences and the Practice of Sexual Medicine: A Guide for Health Practitioners*. Cham, Switzerland: Springer, pp. 221–33.

Ferrero Camoletto, Raffaella, and Chiara Bertone. 2012. "Italians (Should) Do It Better? Medicalisation and the Disempowering of Intimacy." *Modern Italy* 17(4): 433–48.

———. 2017. "Medicalized Virilism under Scrutiny: Expert Knowledge on Male Sexual Health in Italy." In Andrew King, Ana Cristina Santos, and Isabel Crowhurst (eds.), *Sexuality in Theory and Practice: Insights and Critical Debates from Europe and Beyond*. London: Routledge, pp. 196–209.

Ferrero Camoletto, Raffaella, Chiara Bertone, and Francesca Salis. 2015. "Medicalizing Male Underperformance: Expert Discourses on Male Sexual Health in Italy." *Salute e Società* 14(1): 183–205.

Giami, Alain. 2010. "La spécialisation informelle des médecins généralistes: l'abord de la sexualité." In Géraldine Bloy and François-Xavier Schweyer (eds.), *Singuliers généralistes: sociologie de la médecine générale*. Rennes: Presses de l'EHESP, pp. 147–67.

Giglio, Francesca. 2015. "Dalla medicina dei bisogni alla medicina dei desideri. Il caso dell'invecchiamento." *Anthropologica* (2015): 205–212. Retrieved 15 September 2019 from http://www.anthropologica.eu/dalla-medicina-dei-bisogni-alla-medicina-dei-desideri-il-caso-dellinvecchiamento/.

Gott, Merryn. 2005. *Sexuality, Sexual Health and Ageing*. Maidenhead, England: Open University Press.

Gott, Merryn, Elisabeth Galena, Sharron Hinchliff, and Helen Elford. 2004. "'Opening a Can of Worms': GP and Practice Nurse Barriers to Talking about Sexual Health in Primary Care." *Family Practice* 21(5): 528–36.

Gott, Merryn, and Sharron Hinchliff. 2003. "Barriers to Seeking Treatment for Sexual Problems in Primary Care: A Qualitative Study with Older People." *Family Practice* 20(6): 690–95.

Gott, Merryn, Sharron Hinchliff, and Elisabeth Galena. 2004. "General Practitioner Attitudes to Discussing Sexual Health Issues with Older People." *Social Science and Medicine* 58(11): 2093–2103.

Gross, Gregory, and Robert Blundo. 2005. "Viagara: Medical Technology Constructing Aging Masculinity." *Journal of Sociology and Social Welfare* 32: 85–97.

Gurevich, Maria, Usra Leedham, Amy Brown-Bowers, Nicole Cormier, and Zara Mercer. 2017. "Propping Up Pharma's (Natural) Neoliberal Phallic Man: Pharmaceutical Representations of the Ideal Sexuopharmaceutical User." *Culture, Health and Sexuality* 19(4): 422–37.

———. 2018. "Sexual Dysfunction or Sexual Discipline? Sexuopharmaceutical Use by Men as Prevention and Proficiency." *Feminism and Psychology* 28(3): 309–30.
Hinchliff, Sharron, Merryn Gott, and Elisabeth Galena. 2004. "'GPs' Perceptions of the Gender-Related Barriers to Discussing Sexual Health in Consultations: A Qualitative Study." *European Journal of General Practice* 10(2): 56–60.
Humphrey, Sarah, and Irwin Nazareth. 2001. "GPs' Views on Their Management of Sexual Dysfunction." *Family Practice* 18(5): 516–18.
Johnson, Ericka, Elba Sjögren, and Cecilia Åsberg. 2016. *Glocal Pharma: International Brands and the Imagination of Local Masculinity*. Routledge: London.
Jones, Ian Rees, and Paul F. Higgs. 2010. "The Natural, the Normal and the Normative: Contested Terrains in Ageing and Old Age." *Social Science and Medicine* 71: 1513–19.
Katz, Stephen. 2000. "Busy Bodies: Activity, Aging, and the Management of Everyday Life." *Journal of Aging Studies* 14(2): 135–52.
Katz, Stephen, and Tony Calasanti. 2015. "Critical Perspectives on Successful Aging: Does It 'Appeal More Than It Illuminates'?" *The Gerontologist* 55(1): 26–33.
Katz, Stephen, and Barbara L. Marshall. 2003. "New Sex for Old: Lifestyle, Consumerism, and the Ethics of Aging Well." *Journal of Aging Studies* 17(1): 3–16.
———. 2004. "Is the Functional "Normal"? Aging, Sexuality and the Bio-marking of Successful Living." *History of the Human Sciences* 17(1): 53–75.
Lamb, Sarah (ed.). 2017. *Successful Aging as a Contemporary Obsession: Global Perspectives*. Baltimore: Rutgers University Press.
Loe, Meika. 2001. "Fixing Broken Masculinity: Viagra as a Technology for the Production of Gender and Sexuality." *Sexuality and Culture* 5(3): 97–125.
———. 2004. *The Rise of Viagra: How the Little Blue Pill Changed Sex in America*. New York: New York University Press.
———. 2006. "The Viagra Blues: Embracing or Resisting the Viagra Body." In Dana Rosenfeld and Christopher A. Faircloth (eds.), *Medicalized Masculinities*. Philadelphia: Temple University Press, pp. 21–44.
Low, Wah-Yun, Chirk-Jehn Ng, Ngiap-Chuan Tan, Wan-Yuen Choo, and Hui-Meng Tan. 2004. "Management of Erectile Dysfunction: Barriers Faced by General Practitioners." *Age* 40: 40–55.
Mamo, Laura, and Jennifer R Fishman. 2001. "Potency in All the Right Places: Viagra as a Technology of the Gendered Body." *Body and Society* 7(4): 13–35.
Marshall, Barbara L. 2002. "'Hard Science': Gendered Constructions of Sexual Dysfunction in the 'Viagra Age.'" *Sexualities* 5(2): 131–58.
———. 2006. "The New Virility: Viagra, Male Aging and Sexual Function." *Sexualities* 9: 345–62.
———. 2007. "Climacteric Redux? (Re)medicalizing the Male Menopause." *Men and Masculinities* 9(4): 509–29.
———. 2008. "Older Men and Sexual Health: Post-Viagra Views of Changes in Function." *Generations* 32(1): 21–27.
———. 2009. "Rejuvenation's Return: Anti-aging and Re-masculinization in Biomedical Discourse on the 'Aging Male.'" *Medicine Studies* 1(3): 249–65.
———. 2010. "Science, Medicine and Virility Surveillance: 'Sexy Seniors' in the Pharmaceutical Imagination." *Sociology of Health and Illness* 32(2): 211–24.
———. 2012. "Medicalization and the Refashioning of Age-Related Limits on Sexuality." *Journal of Sex Research* 49(4): 337–43.

Marshall, Barbara L., and Stephen Katz. 2002. "Forever Functional: Sexual Fitness and the Ageing Male Body." *Body and Society* 8(4): 43–70.

———. 2012. "The Embodied Life Course: Post-ageism or the Renaturalization of Gender?" *Societies* 2: 222–34.

Martinson, Marty, and Claire Berridge. 2015. "Successful Aging and Its Discontents: A Systematic Review of the Social Gerontology Literature." *The Gerontologist* 55(1): 58–69.

Platano, Giacomo, Jurgen Margraf, Judith Alder, and Johannes Bitzer. 2008a. "Frequency and Focus of Sexual History Taking in Male Patients—A Pilot Study Conducted among Swiss General Practitioners and Urologists." *Journal of Sexual Medicine* 5(1): 47–59.

———. 2008b. "Psychosocial Factors and Therapeutic Approaches in the Context of Sexual History Taking in Men: A Study Conducted among Swiss General Practitioners and Urologists." *Journal of Sexual Medicine* 5(11): 2533–56.

Potts, Anne. 2005. "Cyborg Masculinity in the Viagra Era." *Sexualities, Evolution and Gender* 7(1): 3–16.

Potts, Anne, Victoria M. Grace, Nicola Gavey, and Tina Vares. 2004. "'Viagra Stories': Challenging 'Erectile Dysfunction.'" *Social Science and Medicine* 59(3): 489–99.

———. 2006. "'Sex for Life'? Men's Counter-Rhetoric on 'Erectile Dysfunction,' Male Sexuality and Aging." *Sociology of Health and Illness* 28(3): 306–29.

Ribeiro, Sofia, Violeta Alarcão, Augusto Almeida, Filipe Leão Miranda, Mário Dias Carreira, and Alberto Galvao-Teles. 2011. "General Practitioners' Knowledge, Perceptions and Barriers in the Management of Sexual Dysfunction." Retrieved 25 September 2019 from http://uepid.wdfiles.com/local–files/projectos/PosterIASRSexosl_finalissimo.pdf.

Ribeiro, Sofia, Violeta Alarcão, Rui Simões, Filipe Leão Miranda, Mário Carreira, and Alberto GalvãoTeles. 2014. "General Practitioners' Procedures for Sexual History Taking and Treating Sexual Dysfunction in Primary Care." *Journal of Sexual Medicine* 11(2): 386–93.

Rose, Nikolas. 2007. "Molecular Biopolitics, Somatic Ethics and the Spirit of Biocapital." *Social Theory and Health* 5(1): 3–29.

Rubinstein, Robert L., and Kate de Medeiros. 2014. "'Successful Aging,' Gerontological Theory and Neoliberalism: A Qualitative Critique." *The Gerontologist* 55(1): 34–42.

Sandberg, Linne. 2011. *Getting Intimate: A Feminist Analysis of Old Age, Masculinity and Sexuality*. Linköping: Linköping University Electronic Press.

———. 2013. "Just Feeling a Naked Body Close to You: Men, Sexuality and Intimacy in Later Life." *Sexualities* 16(3–4): 261–82.

Taylor, Abi, and Margot A. Gosney. 2011. "Sexuality in Older Age: Essential Considerations for Healthcare Professionals." *Age and Ageing* 40(5): 538–43.

Tiefer, Leonore. 1986. "In Pursuit of the Perfect Penis: The Medicalization of Male Sexuality." *American Behavioral Scientist* 29(5): 579–99.

———. 2006. "The Viagra Phenomenon." *Sexualities* 9(3): 273–94.

Twigg, Julia, and Martin, Wendy. 2015. "The Challenge of Cultural Gerontology." *The Gerontologist* 55(3): 353–59.

Walz, Thomas. 2002. "Crones, Dirty Old Men, Sexy Seniors: Representations of the Sexuality of Older Persons." *Journal of Aging and Identity* 7(2): 99–112.

Wentzell, Emily. 2013a. *Maturing Masculinities: Ageing, Chronic Illness and Viagra in Mexico*. Durham and London: Duke University Press.
——. 2013b. "Aging Respectably by Rejecting Medicalization: Mexican Men's Reasons for Not Using Erectile Dysfunction Drugs." *Medical Anthropology Quarterly* 27(1): 3–22.
Wentzell, Emily, and Jorge Salmerón. 2009. "You'll 'Get Viagraed': Mexican Men's Preference for Alternative Erectile Dysfunction Treatment." *Social Science and Medicine* 68(10): 1759–65.

CHAPTER 3

Repairing the Body and Improving the Nation
Corrective Plastic Surgeries for Protruding Ears in Brazil

MARCELLE SCHIMITT

The act of repairing is not always heroic or guided toward noble goals, as it can work toward the maintenance of antidemocratic and anti-humanistic projects (Jackson 2014). To repair is also to normalize, because it emphasizes a state we should follow (Ureta 2014). The goal to be reached, the "normal," represents both what is typical in terms of a pattern and what *should be*, presenting itself as one of the most potent ideological tools there is (Hacking 1990). Alternatively, as Foucault (1979a: 184) would say, it is "one of the greatest instruments of power at the end of the classical age." From this perspective, I present in this chapter a few reflections on otoplasties—ear surgeries—as reparative procedures that can be thought of not only as body enhancements but also as practices that materialize norms onto bodies, discourses, and policies, thus reproducing old apparatuses for human hierarchization that are tied to the improvement of the nation.

According to the Brazilian Ministry of Health (2019), "Differently than aesthetic plastic surgeries, reparative[1] plastic surgeries have the goal of correcting deformities ... reparative plastic surgeries aim to enhance or reinstate functions and also regenerate the [human] form as close to the normal as possible." This is a definition that constructs the act of repairing in relation to an ideal of normalcy and, one could say, of notions of what the body *should be like*. In such a context, reparative plastic surgery is also defined in contrast to aesthetic surgery—in other words, it is reparative because it is not aesthetic. However, the boundaries between aesthetic and reparative surgeries are not always clear, particularly in Brazil.

Gilman (1998) states that reparative or corrective plastic surgery was framed as being the extreme opposite of aesthetic surgery since it first appeared as a medical specialty. Even today, patients and doctors view the two kinds of plastic surgeries as the antitheses of one another, the first being a matter of health per se and the second as mere frivolity. Nonetheless, I propose that Brazil represents an exceptional case regarding the boundaries between the aesthetic and the reparative, mostly because the Public Health System (Sistema Único de Saúde [SUS]) offers both types of plastic surgery free of charge. I also argue that such boundaries have been shaped in multiple ways, particularly when we consider that the framing of a procedure as aesthetic or reparative depends on different contingencies. Whether the SUS offers the surgery—as the list of approved surgeries is constantly changing—and the patient's race, class, gender, and perceived psychological issues, such as self-esteem, well-being, body-image disorder, are all elements that come together to produce an aesthetic or reparative procedure. In other words, a network of actors constantly enacts the "aesthetic" and the "reparative," rendering different materialities onto themselves and onto the procedures they perform. These delimitations do not only emerge from social, historical, and political contingencies, but also make and enact realities. They emerge from difference and also produce it; they are the effect of specific, situated, and unpredictable interventions.[2]

The World Health Organization (1948) defines health as a "state of complete physical, mental, and social well-being and not merely the absence of disease or infirmity." Because it guides the perceptions of many plastic surgeons, this definition emerges as an axis through which one can follow different understandings concerning the limits between the reparative and the aesthetic. This notion informs a significant number of opinions from doctors to whom I spoke about the topic, encompassing several health concepts that otherwise seemed disassociated from one another: the organic/physical, the psychological/subjective, and the social. It is also possible to observe that ideals of self-esteem, quality of life, and well-being emerge as possibly integrative elements of these health domains. They thus become essential for a more situated understanding of the subject. I contend that, in the Brazilian context, the concept of health as something that is holistic and comprises the ideals of quality of life, self-esteem and well-being, normalcy, proportionality, and functionality ends up subsuming the body into notions of what it "should be," relating in a profound manner to a more general concept of bodily normativity.

Accordingly, I argue that the same surgical intervention can be enacted in multiple ways. In other words, variations of the same procedure enact different materialities and subjectivities. Hence, we can understand plastic surgery as a medical practice that surpasses a mere material modification of the body and affects the subjectivity of those who go through it. This conception allows us to comprehend such practices as enacting multiple material realities onto the body:[3] procedures that are both aesthetic and reparative, and forms of improvement that are simultaneously individual and collective. In this sense, we can think about plastic surgeries in terms of the materialization of ideological investments and not only as social constructions. Consequently, the limits regarding surgical interventions—understood here as discursive-material practices (as in Barad 2003)—are not settled. They can be undone by other interventions and social relations, and they can take on multiple forms according to the associations they establish.

These issues have substantial political and economic implications, and by addressing the unavoidable relationship between defining the "aesthetic" and the "reparative" to a wide range of contingencies I do not intend to overlook or underestimate the specific implications that neoliberal policies, for example, have in such circumstances. On that matter, Jarrín (2012) suggests that despite plastic surgeons' claims to benevolent and humanitarian ideals, "plastic governmentality" helps to create a neoliberal biopolitical regime in Brazil that turns public health into a profit-driven scheme. What I would like to convey throughout this chapter is that the logic that seems to operate in Brazil regarding plastic surgeries, whether they be aesthetic or reparative, "discursively" destabilizes the boundaries and distances between what is an aesthetic and a reparative surgery, while also shaping and materializing what is understood as bodily repair in Brazil.

Improving the Nation

In March 2019, Rio de Janeiro's mayor Marcelo Crivella announced the program Orelhinha Bonitinha (Beautiful little ears). According to the city's Health Observatory (2019), the initiative was a joint effort to perform several otoplasties—plastic surgeries that reshape, reposition, or change the proportion of ears[4] —in children aged seven years or older. The government offered surgeries in four different hospitals in the city that provide consultations via the Public Health System. To have access to the otoplasty, the child needed a referral from the National Regulation System (SISREG), and his/her parents or guardians had to register with the Family Clinic closest to their homes. Despite having children as its target, adults and adolescents could also register, considering that the program's goal was to address all patients waiting for the procedure within the Public Health System.

In an interview for Rio de Janeiro's city hall website, Crivella named *bullying* as the main reason for the program's creation. The mayor stated that otoplasties would "free" patients from the inconvenience or humiliation that could cause psychological scars during the "most beautiful part of childhood."

> The joint effort Orelhinha Bonitinha is an essential ally in the fight against bullying, since many children in schools suffer from it. We are going to perform surgery on thousands of children. However, it is all under strict controls, our plastic surgeons have mastered the technique, and everything is already set up. It is a surgery conducted under local anesthesia, just a small sedation, and the child goes home on the same day and has to wear a small hat [*touquinha*] for five days. But he/she will be free from bullying that could leave psychological scars during the most beautiful part of their childhood. I am sure that these surgeries will bring significant benefits to the city. (Marcelo Crivella, mayor of Rio de Janeiro)

Orelhinha Bonitinha is not, however, the first initiative of its kind in Brazil. Alvaro Jarrín (2015) briefly describes the case of a surgeon from the state of Ceará who, in 2007, started the philanthropic project Plastic Surgery in School. With private companies as its sponsors, the program's goal was to offer free otoplasty surgery for school-aged children. The initiative's founder claimed that children who needed surgical intervention and did not have it could suffer several developmental problems and not reach their full potential. The doctor also indicated the high incidence of "protruded" ears in Ceará State as an implication of a problem affecting people from the northeast of the country in particular.

According to Jarrín (2015), these children's representations were pathologized as a problem that caused not only personal stagnation but also that of a whole region—the northeast of the country. Here, one can readily notice something that was also evident in Crivella's discourse: the characterization of plastic surgery as beneficial for both individuals and populational improvement as well. Whether offered by the Public Health System or in partnership with private companies, the joint efforts gain a philanthropic aura when addressing an "abnormal" condition of not only a specific person but of a whole region and a very particular age group—school-aged children.

Also relevant for the construction of a humanitarian aura around plastic surgery and plastic surgeons was the work of Ivo Pitanguy (1926–2016), a Brazilian doctor known as "the king of plastic surgery," who developed a social project to provide free procedures to people from low-income households. He is also recognized as one of the reasons why, since the foundation of the Public Health System in 1988, public resources have been used to run medical residency programs in plastic surgery within public hospitals. The surgeon's former students are responsible for directing several of these programs, following Pitanguy's belief in plastic surgery as an essential humanitarian service that must be available to patients from different social classes and origins (Jarrín 2017).

Long before Ivo Pitanguy, the eugenicist and doctor Renato Kehl (1889–1974) already described plastic surgery as having a much more significant role than merely granting a better appearance to different body parts. Kehl graduated from Rio de Janeiro's School of Medicine in 1915 and founded several eugenic societies in Brazil. Among his many publications on the "improvement of the nation," beauty, and medicine, *A Cura da Fealdade* (The cure for ugliness) from 1923 stands out.[5] The work, published with the support of writer Monteiro Lobato, consisted of a beauty manual with the essential objective of disseminating eugenic and hygienic knowledge for the individual's well-being and, therefore, that of the species (Kehl 1923). Kehl believed that hygienic regimes, populational control, and plastic surgery were crucial elements to "cure the ugliness" of the Brazilian people. For the doctor, plastic surgeries to correct "malformations" concerned not only individuals but the whole nation. Thus, they should be broadly and continuously performed and not just in specific cases.

Considering this brief digression into Pitanguy and Kehl's ideas, I pose the following question: how do the ideas of these two doctors—notably the eugenic project of the latter—and the persistent defense of plastic surgeries as a path to achieve superior individual and populational aesthetics relate to "protruded ears" and the current otoplasties performed in children and adolescents? According to Castañeda (2003), Kehl (1923) described head and face asymmetries or deformations, and ear shape defects in particular, as indicatives of degeneration, mental or intellectual retardation, cretinism, and imbecility. Degeneration, from this perspective, would distance an individual from his or her originary qualities due to involuntary factors, particularly those of congenital or hereditary order. The surgeon already signaled ear size as evidence of dysgenics[6] in individuals and, consequently, in populations.

It is not only in Kehl's writings that one can find ear size as one of the body stigmas related to the ugly, the degenerate, the abnormal, and the malformed. Both Gould (1996), in *The Mismeasure of Men*, and Pedro Tórtima (2002), in *Crime e Castigo para além do Equador*, bring to the fore the correlations that Cesare Lombroso (1835–1909) developed between ears size and the "degenerated" or "criminal" character. In one of the passages of his book *Crime: Its Causes and Remedies*, from 1911, the association is very clear: "Upon examination I found that this man had outstanding ears, great maxillaries and cheek-bones, lemurine appendix, division of the frontal bone, premature wrinkles, sinister look, nose twisted to the right—in short, a physiognomy approaching the criminal type" (Lombroso 1911: 437).

By bringing a few statements from Lombroso, Kehl, Pitanguy, and Crivella for discussion along with projects like the Orelhinha Bonitinha and Plastic Surgery in School, I aim to reflect on the possible relations between plastic surgeries—particularly otoplasties performed in children— and a broader project to "improve the nation." In other words, these surgeries to repair "deformities" relate to eugenic notions dating from the beginning of the twentieth century and how they are currently inscribed in medical discourses. Throughout this chapter, I will present quotations from interviews I conducted with plastic surgeons who work for the Public Health System in order to develop an understanding of the matter. When analyzing these medical discourses[7] in parallel with the Orelhinha Bonitinha and Plastic Surgery in School programs, I compare the logic that they are "humanitarian"—such as the claim disseminated by Pitanguy—with a body enhancement logic that transcends the limits of the individual and is suggestive of a medical project that seeks the enhancement of the population, like the one Renato Kehl sought.

Repairing/Normalizing Protruded Ears

The Plastic Surgery League[8] from a university in the city of Porto Alegre[9] promoted an event where professors conducted several lectures for medical school students, one of them Davi, who is responsible for the medical residency program and taught a course on otoplasty. The doctor started his presentation by stressing the importance of understanding what a "normal" ear means in terms of position, form, and function. He also noted that every fold is essential aesthetically and functionally within one's ear, which makes it necessary for the surgeon to know each crease and its position meticulously. Davi asserted that since patients of otoplasty are commonly very young children who are still in school, professionals must be especially careful and particularly attentive to the ears' nerves because damaging them could cause chronic sensibility loss.

Davi explained that abnormalities in this body part could be of position, form, or size. Protruding ears, the most common of them, can be diagnosed in early childhood, and there is an agreement among doctors that treatment should start before preadolescence. Aside from this, congenital malformations such as microtia[10] and anotia[11] can also cause "deformity" and are harder to treat. In cases like this, surgeons usually use cartilage from another body part to reconstruct the ear or, as an alternative, use prosthetic ears that "stick" to the skin. Alternatively, the surgeon can use a device that aids him to fit the prosthesis within an aesthetically appropriate position. As Davi explained, with newborn babies, one can also choose to use ear molds starting in their first week of life until they are thirty days old. During this period, there is a significant level of hyaluronic acid[12] in the ear's cartilage, which makes the tissue more vulnerable to reshaping it. In the doctor's opinion, the technique of molding the newborn's ears—despite many perceiving it as an aggressive procedure—was highly recommended because it prevented, in most cases, future surgeries.

Davi's remarks on otoplasty lead us to comprehend the body as not bounded within itself, as the usage of prosthetics or molds illustrates. The ear the surgeon reconstructs/repairs through a process that is, in his own words, handcrafted allows us to think of the body beyond its organic materiality. Still, what stands out in his explanation is the nonfunctional character the auricular reconstruction suggests. As stated by the surgeon, ear repairing surgeries do not aid in recovering any hearing loss caused by microtia or anotia. Hence, despite not being aesthetic, the surgery does not help the ear to restore its primary function: hearing. Still, the classification of otoplasties as reparative procedures is prevalent, since the face has, according to several doctors, a primary "social function."

If, on one hand, the surgery's reparative character derives from the restoration of a given function—as a few surgeons mentioned—and, on the other, aesthetic surgeries would be those whose only goal is to enhance and harmonize features, where would otoplasties stand? Moreover, the fact that they are done very early in life, with its patients being mainly children, infers that otoplasties would not be so widely accepted as "merely" aesthetic procedures. With that in mind, I suggest we can reach an understanding of plastic surgeries as realities shaped by different relations and contingencies. In some cases, what conveys its repairing character is the reconstruction of a lost or absent function, and in others, it is the reinstatement of the desired form seeking a better harmony, balance, or normality of an organ or tissue. Consequently, these parameters alone cannot place otoplasties—or any other procedures—as aesthetic or reparative. In this context, the contingent character of the boundaries between what is reparative and what is aesthetic becomes profoundly evident.

In a talk with Aline, a medical resident in craniomaxillofacial surgery[13]—a specialty within plastic surgery—a few of these issues emerged:

> Otoplasty is a classic case of aesthetic surgery. It is performed on a six-, eight-year-old child who does not have any functional problem. The child has no hearing issue, but she has a little jug ear. Well, that is what ICD[14] is here for, right? The International Classification of Diseases. Many health insurances pay for the surgery. The parents let a six-year-old child go through general anesthesia, the risks of the procedure, the postoperative stress, missing school, all of that. So, the child loses in all aspects: the procedure's risks and the social losses of having the surgery. Well, why do some parents put their children through it? Is it simply

an aesthetic surgery? The child can hear, so she has a problem that is plainly not functional, at least in the auditory sense. But the face has a social function. So otoplasty is in a place somewhere in between the aesthetic and the reparative, right?

From Aline's statement, one can infer that the "social function" of the face is part of what shapes the reparative aspect of procedures. It is possible to observe how "functionality" upholds and at the same time shapes a significant number of procedures as reparative. In the surgeon's narrative, the "social" is a central element within the construction of the properties attributed to the face. In other words, if socialization is a constitutive part of human beings and a so-called abnormality deters us from having healthy social interactions, the reparative surgery is justified. Regarding the "social function of the face," it is interesting to observe what it might represent in such a context. We can notice how the idea of "function" expands, referring to something that goes beyond the individual or at least to something not confined to it. An organ or body part's functionality, which has been commonly perceived as relating to biological aspects, now encompasses an extremely relevant social component. This phenomenon is not new, so I will not elaborate on this aspect. However, it is pivotal to foreground how the "social"—just as the *psi* categories of self-esteem, quality of life, and well-being—is also engaged within the context of plastic surgery to provide a broader and more holistic justification for such procedures. The logic of promoting a normalized body in order to produce socialization within acceptable patterns closely resembles a few of Renato Kehl's and Ivo Pitanguy's principles on plastic surgery's significance to not only the individual but mainly to the social. In the context of otoplasties, as Aline mentioned, the ears' aesthetic properties have a "social function." Thus, such cosmetic procedures are perceived not as frivolous, but as necessary for achieving normalcy.

The "social stigma" associated with protuberant ears appeared as the main justification for otoplasties in children on two other occasions during my research. The first was in an interview with Paulo, plastic surgeon and chief of the plastic surgery department in a renowned hospital in Porto Alegre. The second was with Carina, a university professor and psychiatrist who researches, among other things, how surgeries impact patients' quality of life. In both cases, they mentioned bullying to explain why having an ear that diverges from the expected normality causes distress. The two passages below are clear in stating how it is another person's looks and comments that shape the discomfort:

> I performed surgery on a twelve-year-old girl who did ballet. Her father was my colleague and said, "I want my daughter to have a 'jug ear' surgery. She dances ballet and has to put her hair up for it." She had a concert and invited two friends and told them, "I will be on the third line on the right," and her friends replied,

"You don't have to tell us where you will be because we know. We just have to look for your ears." Her jug ears were a problem for her to do the one thing she likes most in life. No health insurance will pay for this kind of surgery, but we can do it through SUS [Public Health System]. Through SUS, we can operate on jug ears. (Paulo)

In the case of otoplasty, a person can go through years of therapy, but if he fixes his ears, he will no longer be bullied. [Plastic surgery] sometimes fixes things that years of therapy don't. And sometimes it can solve self-esteem issues. It can improve one's self-esteem. (Carina)

In his book *Making the Body Beautiful*, Sander L. Gilman[15] (2001) described how already, in 1910, William H. Luckett addressed the "hate relating to ears." In the American context of the time, there was an association between having big ears and being Irish or Jewish. Big ears were a repugnant sign of the difference they represented. In his article "A New Operation for Prominent Ears Based on the Anatomy of the Deformity," Luckett describes how one of his patients' classmates constantly harassed him for his ears, so much so that the doctor advised him to have surgery. In Luckett's understanding, the sufferings such interactions produced in both parents and children justified the surgical intervention: "The strife that a big-eared child sows among his classmates spreads so much unhappiness in the world that the surgeon's larger duty, as well as the needs of his patient, demands that he operate" (Gilman 2001: 127).

The similarities between Luckett's discourse in 1910 and Carina's and Paulo's in 2017 suggest the existence of continuities regarding justifications for otoplasties that endured for over a century. According to Gilman (1998), the idea that one could cure a "character" or psychological disease through bodily interventions was already present in the nineteenth century. The author suggests that "curing the physically anomalous is curing the psychologically unhappy—this view provides the key to any understanding of the power of all surgery to alter the psyche. The 'beautiful' becomes the 'happy'" (Gilman 1998: 7). Doctors, patients, and several authors who have studied the matter present justifications that resemble Gilman's logic. I subscribe to this as well, to a certain extent.

Nonetheless, I would like to highlight the associations between the idea of "individual repair" and ideas that are inscribed within a broader scope of body "normalization," as one can note in Crivella's, Pitanguy's, and Kehl's discourses. Healing or repairing bodies through otoplasties is also deeply connected to the aesthetic and moral improvement of the nation. Thus, to repair is also to normalize; and to normalize goes beyond regulating bodies, because it produces the "normal" for the entire nation. In this sense, while they repair, otoplasties also reproduce the stigma they aim to mend.

Repairing the Children for the Future of the Nation

In order to think about otoplasties—particularly those performed on children—in relation to a more extensive project of repairing, improving, and normalizing populations, I return to Renato Kehl. The eugenicist saw medicine as a possibility to manage the social and to enhance it. It was not by chance that one of his publications from 1926, called "Health bible," presents medicine as the "science of the social." In this perspective, children were beings whose physical and moral plasticity enabled more straightforward medical and state interventions. Thus, it was imperative to teach them good manners and how to preserve their bodies from a young age. Based on these premises, Kehl, a member of the National Department of Public Health (Departamento Nacional de Saúde Pública—DNSP), developed scientific books and school textbooks on hygiene. In 1923 he signed a contract with publisher Livraria Francisco Alves to publish a hygiene manual titled "Fairy Hygia." It was the first of its kind to address mothers and teachers on how to teach hygiene to children. As pointed by Espírito Santo and colleagues (2006), by the end of the nineteenth century into the beginning of the twentieth century, medical activities prioritized family-oriented actions. In this context, doctors saw children as "health soldiers" and as the way to get through to other family members: "[Children were] the seed to achieve the desired image of the adequate adult in the near future for the Brazilian society" (Espírito Santo, Jacó-Vilela and Ferreri 2006: 23).

Whether through hygienic manuals or actual surgical interventions, children still occupy a position in which they are seen as more malleable today. According to Foucault (1979a), particularly in the seventeenth century, the focus of concern expanded, going beyond natality matters to address how to manage children's lives properly. If health is an essential goal for family units in this context, children's health becomes even more crucial. Family, in this sense, becomes a unique instrument for the government of populations, and the control and vigilance over children's bodies are put in place (Foucault 1979b).

The urgency to intervene as soon as possible is also present in plastic surgeries that correct protruded ears. As Davi's course showed, children can start using molds to correct ear deformities in their first days of life, indicating that the younger the body, the more "malleable" it is. There seems to be a will for crafting normalcy: it is necessary to sculpt what nature failed to materialize and thus protect the children from future suffering. The urgency to normalize children is also related, in a sense, to the imperative of giving back their childhood and to restoring a worry-free state of well-being so commonly idealized for this stage of life.

The urgency to surgically intervene can undoubtedly be justified as improving the lives of those who suffer from the condition, but it can also be inscribed within the realm of a broader regulation of bodies. The assumption that infant bodies are more malleable, plastic, and accessible is not new, as one can see in Renato Kehl's assumptions and those of many before him. The belief that treating the individual is equivalent to caring for the nation is just as old. Otoplasties performed in children, and particularly those done by the Public Health System (SUS) or philanthropic projects, are a path through which we can trace a few understandings on the broader subject of repairing as a strategy for normalizing bodies and producing the norm.

It is important to stress that I do not intend to affirm that the aforementioned body enhancements/bodily repairs directly materialize eugenic conceptions from the nineteenth and twentieth centuries in contemporary Brazil. Neither do I affirm that otoplasties cannot have positive effects on children's lives. Nonetheless, the reflections offered here lead us to the following questions: Why are "jug ear" surgeries the ones offered free of charge? Why for this specific age group? How does the ear size become something that causes strangeness, discomfort, and suffering? I certainly contend that from these questions one can better understand the extent of such procedures in the Brazilian context.

Brazil is currently the second-largest consumer of plastic surgeries in the world. According to the International Society of Aesthetic Plastic Surgery (2017), in 2017[16] alone more than 1.4 million aesthetic procedures were performed in the country. Considering that the number of reparative surgeries performed by the Public Health Service (SUS) is not available for that year, the estimate is that the total number of plastic surgeries is higher than even in the United States, the top country for the number of yearly plastic surgeries. In 2016 the Brazilian Plastic Surgery Society (Sociedade Brasileira de Cirurgia Plástica 2017) conducted the national census on plastic surgery. Its results showed that in that year, SUS performed 16.3 percent of plastic surgeries (free of charge), health insurance companies covered the costs of 19.8 percent, and private consultants performed 53.3 percent of them. Of all the procedures, 55,953 were otoplasties. According to the census, 3 percent of all plastic surgeries in Brazil were performed in children from zero to twelve years old, an increase of 44 percent when compared to 2014.

The number of plastic surgeries performed in Brazil can be understood through different logics and has been commonly analyzed from the perspective of cultural aspects related to the "cult of the body," "concerns about being in shape," and the constant search of individual enhancement. Throughout this chapter, I chose to disclose a less discussed facet of this phenomenon: reparative procedures performed mainly in school-age children. By bringing together eugenic conceptions of plastic surgeries from the nineteenth and twentieth centuries, I intended to elaborate not only on broader ideas on "repairing," but also on the boundaries between "reparative" and "aesthetic" surgeries.

By presenting this discussion, I do not question the children's or their parents' suffering. Nor do I question the good intentions of plastic surgeons who aim to ease the possible social discomforts "protruded ears" may cause. My goal was rather to look at, analyze, and better understand the entanglements between our conception of body normality and a more comprehensive project of a nation's improvement, as well as the ways through which these entanglements express and produce effects, particularly in otoplasties performed in children.

Marcelle Schimitt is an anthropologist and PhD candidate in social anthropology at the Federal University of Rio Grande do Sul. She is a member of the research group Living Sciences: Knowledge Production and Heterogeneous Articulations. Her research focuses on the blurred boundaries between aesthetic and reconstructive plastic surgeries in Brazil. She is currently researching about public policies for people with cleft lip and palate from a critical view of surgical procedures to repair facial abnormalities.

Notes

1. In Portuguese, the term *cirurgia plástica reparadora* refers to reconstructive plastic surgery. I opted to do a literal translation in order to convey the argument of this paper. Hence, throughout this chapter, I will use the term "reparative plastic surgery" to refer to what is commonly known as reconstructive plastic surgery.
2. Such propositions are based on the perspectives of many authors, such as Barad (2003); Haraway (1992, 2004); Law (2004); Mol and Law (2002); Mol (2002); M'charek (2010).
3. When addressing the "body multiple," I refer to the perspective of Annemarie Mol (2002).
4. Designation of otoplasty from the Brazilian Plastic Surgery Society's (SBCP) website. Also, according to SBCP, "if salient or deformed ears bother you or your child, you may want to consider plastic surgery. Ear surgery—also known as otoplasty—may improve the ears' shape, position, or proportion."
5. Besides "The cure for ugliness," Renato Kehl also published other books on eugenics: "Health bible" (*A bíblia da saúde*; 1926), "Eugenics and social medicine" (*Eugenia e medicina social*; 1920), "Shall we improve and prolong life: The eugenic valorizing of men" (*Melhoremos e prolonguemos a vida: a valorização eugênica do homem*; 1923).

6. Term frequently used by Renato Kehl to designate those who do not fit into eugenic physical, moral, and intellectual patterns.
7. I interviewed several professionals who work with plastic surgery in four different hospitals in the city of Porto Alegre that work through the Public Health Service (SUS). A few passages from these interviews are used in this chapter. The interviewed were medical students, residents, and plastic surgeons and chiefs of the plastic surgery department of the hospitals. During the research, I also participated in and observed events organized by the Plastic Surgery Leagues of two universities in the city. Professionals and students' names were modified and the names of universities and hospitals omitted in order to prevent them from being recognized.
8. The Academic Leagues are groups organized mostly by students to address subjects of a specific subject within medical specialties. They are also founded on the academic triad of teaching, research, and extension programs.
9. Porto Alegre has a population of approximately 1.5 million people and is the capital of Rio Grande do Sul State, Brazil's southernmost state.
10. Microtia is a congenital deformation in the auricular cavity that prevents it from developing.
11. Anotia is the congenital absence of one or two ears.
12. Substance found on skin, joints, and cartilage.
13. Craniomaxillofacial is the medical specialty that treats paranasal alterations on the face, jaw, maxilla, and the inside of the mouth.
14. The ICD, *International Statistical Classification of Diseases and Related Health Problems*, presents codes referring to the classification of disease and abnormal health aspects. The World Health Organization (WHO) publishes the list, which is in its tenth edition. The current edition has classification Q17.5—also known as "protuberant ears"—as the deformity Aline cited.
15. Historian from the United States who studies, among other things, the history of medicine. He presented the notion of "passing," which is now widely used in debates on plastic surgery.
16. This is the last published study that presents data concerning repairing surgeries performed in Brazil.

References

Barad, Karen. 2003. "Posthumanist Performativity: Toward an Understanding of How Matter Comes to Matter." *Signs: Journal of Women in Culture and Society* 28(3): 801–31.

Brazilian Ministry of Health. 2019. *Cirurgia plástica reparadora*. Retrieved 3 August 2019 from http://www.saude.gov.br/atencao-especializada-ehospitalar/especialidades/cirurgia-plastica-reparadora.

Castañeda, Luzia Aurelia. 2003. "Eugenia e casamento." *História, Ciência e Saúde—Manguinhos* 10(3): 901–30.

Espírito Santo, Adriana Amaral do, Ana Maria Jacó-Vilela, and Marcelo de Almeida Ferreri. 2006. "The Image of Children in the Theses of the Medical College of Rio de Janeiro (1832–1930)." *Psicologia em Estudo* 11(1): 19-28.

Foucault, Michel. 1979a. *Discipline and Punish: The Birth of the Prison.* Harmondsworth: Penguin Books.
———. 1979b. *Microfísica do Poder.* Rio de Janeiro: Edições Graal.
Gilman, Sander L. 1998. *Creating Beauty to Cure the Soul: Race and Psychology in the Shaping of Aesthetic Surgery.* Durham, NC: Duke University Press.
———. 2001. *Making the Body Beautiful: A Cultural History of Aesthetic Surgery.* Princeton, NJ: Princeton University Press.
Gould, Stephen Jay. 1996. *The Mismeasure of Man.* New York: W. W. Norton.
Hacking, Ian. 1990. *The Taming of Chance.* New York: Cambridge University Press.
Haraway, Donna Jeanne. 1992. "The Promises of Monsters: A Regenerative Politics for Inappropriate/d others." In Lawrence Grossberg, Cary Nelson and Paula A. Treichler (eds.), *Cultural Studies.* New York: Routledge, pp. 295–337.
———. 2004. *The Haraway Reader.* New York: Routledge.
Health Observatory. 2019. *Prefeitura do Rio oferece cirurgia para correção de "orelha de abano."* Rio de Janeiro. Retrieved 31 July 2019 from http://observatoriodasauderj.com.br/prefeitura-do-rio-oferece-cirurgia-para-correcao-de-orelha-de-abano/.
International Society of Aesthetic Plastic Surgery. 2017. *ISAPS International Survey on Aesthetic/Cosmetic Procedures Performed in 2017.* Retrieved 25 October 2020 from https://www.isaps.org/wp-content/uploads/2018/10/ISAPS_2017_International_Study_Cosmetic_Procedures.pdf.
Jackson, Steven J. 2014. "Rethinking Repair. In Tarleton Gillespie, Pablo J. Boczkowski, and Kirsten A. Foot (eds.), *Media Technologies: Essays on Communication, Materiality, and Society.* Cambridge, MA: MIT Press, pp. 221–39.
Jarrín, Alvaro. 2012. "The Rise of the Cosmetic Nation: Plastic Governmentality and Hybrid Medical Practices in Brazil." *Medical Anthropology* 31(3): 213–28.
———. 2015. "Towards a Biopolitics of Beauty: Eugenics, Aesthetic Hierarchies and Plastic Surgery in Brazil." *Journal of Latin American Cultural Studies* 24(4): 535–52.
———. 2017. *The Biopolitics of Beauty: Cosmetic Citizenship and Affective Capital in Brazil.* Oakland: University of California Press.
Kehl, Renato. 1923. *A Cura da Fealdade: Eugenia e Medicina Social.* São Paulo: Monteiro Lobato & Co-Editores.
———. 1936. *A Fada Hygia: Primeiro Livro de Hygiene.* Rio de Janeiro: Livraria Francisco Alves.
Law, John. 2004. *After Method: Mess in Social Science Research.* New York: Routledge.
Lombroso, Cesare. 1911. *Crime: Its Causes and Remedies.* Boston: Little, Brown.
M'charek, Amade. 2010. "Fragile Differences, Relational Effects: Stories about the Materiality of Race and Sex." *European Journal of Women's Studies* 17(4): 307–22.
Mol, Annemarie. 2002. *The Body Multiple: Ontology in Medical Practice.* Durham, NC: Duke University Press.
Mol, Annemarie, and John Law. 2002. "Complexities: An Introduction." In John Law and Annemarie Mol (eds.), *Complexities: Social Studies of Knowledge Practices.* Durham, NC: Duke University Press, pp. 1–22.
Pitanguy, Ivo. 1998. "Especial: Ivo Helcio Jardim de Campos Pitanguy." Special issue, *Médicos.*
Sociedade Brasileira de Cirurgia Plástica. 2017. *Censo 2016: Situação da Cirurgia Plástica no Brasil—Análise Comparativa das Pesquisas 2014 e 2016.* São Paulo. Retrie-

ved 25 October 2020 from http://www2.cirurgiaplastica.org.br/wp-content/uploads/2017/12/CENSO-2017.pdf.

Tórtima, Pedro. 2002. *Crime e Castigo para além do Equador*. Belo Horizonte: Inédita.

Ureta, Sebastián. 2014. "Normalizing Transantiago: On the Challenges (and Limits) of Repairing Infrastructures." *Social Studies of Science* 44(3): 368–92.

World Health Organization. 1948. "Constitution of the World Health Organization." Geneva. Retrieved 25 October 2020 from https://www.who.int/about/who-we-are/constitution.

CHAPTER 4

The Itinerant Beauty Brigade
Repairing Social Fractures through the Apapacho Estético

EVA CARPIGO

The Mexican "Itinerant Beauty Brigade"[1] (Brigadas de Belleza Itinerantes) is a group of volunteers that offers aesthetic treatments for free to vulnerable, isolated, or marginalized populations in Mexico City. I met and followed this group during 2016–17, using an ethnographic field methodology, which included filming their events and recording intimate interview sessions.

My contribution brings a counterexample that diverges from previous analyses of beauty practices, particularly in a humanitarian context. The existing scholarship found that dynamics of domination and imperialism or logics of inherent racism and eugenics were centrally constitutive of aesthetic services in humanitarian contexts. Alvaro Jarrín (2015) argues that Brazilian plastic surgery expresses a eugenic cultural project to whiten the ethnic origins of black Brazilians. Foucault's theoretical paradigm of biopolitics is often solicited to critique aesthetic practices, which are accused of forcing a process of normalization or "standardization" of body appearance. In this perspective, Mimi Thu Nguyen (2011) analyzes the initiative Beauty Without Borders as an expression of liberal imperialism of the United States in Afghanistan.

With my contribution, I didn't choose to analyze the Beauty Brigade within the paradigm of biopolitics, nor did I choose to see the Beauty Brigade as an experience that "hides"—or reveals—a structural/cultural dominating force that shapes subjects' decisions, practices, and bodies. Instead, I was curious to understand why people engage in this experience and what benefits they get from it. Thereby, the main questions explored in this chapter are "Which are the anthropological factors that can explain the success of the Beauty Brigade?" and "How do its participants feel about partaking in it?"

In order to answer these questions, I'll first present the social context in which the Beauty Brigade emerged. This perspective will help me argue why the Beauty Brigade is an initiative that restructures social bonds. As observed before by Peter Kropotkin (2013) and Pablo Servigne and Gauthier Chapelle (2017), cooperation between the members of a group (and/or of several groups) is an efficient social strategy that takes place in hostile environments. In this perspective, the Beauty Brigade can be read as an experience of humanitarianism that responds to the paradigm of mutual aid and social resistance.[2] Secondly, I'll expound on the characteristics of the Beauty Brigade. Finally, I'll show how the Beauty Brigade's activities can repair affective consequences of social isolation, exclusion, and invisibility of vulnerable groups, while they allow participants to relieve emotional distress and symbolically evacuate it.

Mexico City: A Fragmented Social Context

Mexico is a North American country that has been plagued by social crises and a spike in violence for more than twenty years.[3] Mexican society is overall deeply divided, as there is "a very strong social hierarchy, wherein a few big families are pitted against the middle classes and the huge mass of the poor" (Musset 2017: 96). Mexican society is deeply fractured into social classes and experiences an increasing level of daily violence (and consequently feelings of insecurity, mistrust, and isolation of citizens).

Mexico City, also called by its inhabitants "the monstrous city" (*la ciudad monstruo*), is located seventy-five hundred feet above sea level and surrounded by active volcanoes. It is the third most populated city on the American continent (after New York and São Paulo), with twenty-one million inhabitants in its urban area. While living in Mexico City, I observed and listened to reports of multiple forms of everyday violence: kidnappings for extortion, muggings (*asaltos*), sexual assaults, and robberies. In Mexico City, one does not feel safe and must be constantly on alert.

The city's growth has been unchecked, as a result of pervasive corruption in the real estate and construction sectors and due to the expansion of the suburban barrios (reminiscent of the Brazilian favelas). People move to the city from the surrounding areas or more remote regions to look for work and a better life (Musset 2017: 86). Agier describes the context in this manner: "A whole world of poorly housed individuals, runaways, unemployed, or at best workers engaged in a precarious process of upward social mobility, makes up an urban mass that is seemingly inert, invisible, and hopeless" (Agier 1999: 8).

It would be naive to claim that Mexicans have become "used" to these conditions of violence and social precarity. Amid this insecurity, individuals still feel tension, anxiety, and fear for themselves as well as for their loved ones. Criminality may strike members of all classes, but those without the means to increase their safety (by living in protected residences or traveling in secured vehicles) are particularly at risk. Insecurity comes in waves and affects certain areas depending on the situation of drug trafficking and of the political and criminal influence networks at a given time. If the police in a neighborhood is corrupted, it will grant more leeway to criminals, who will take advantage of the situation to expand their territory and ramp up trafficking.

In addition to this social insecurity, environmental variables also impact the quality of life of Mexico City's residents: earthquakes, floods, water shortages, and power cuts regularly disrupt everyday life. The city was built on an ancient lake, and many buildings are at risk of collapsing during an earthquake, which has led to tragedies, most recently in September of 2017.[4] Since then, every time the seismic alert (*alerta sismica*) is heard in the city, indicating that an earthquake is happening, it spreads panic and apprehension among Mexico City's inhabitants. In this context, citizens experience the public space, and the urban context, under the paradigms of anxiety, mistrust, and fear.

On the other hand, as in any other city, Mexico's city inhabitants suffer from the disaggregating force of the "individualistic demon."[5] This paradigm is represented by many sociologists as the main culprit for social fragmentation, also called the "liquification" of societies (Bauman 2004, 2006a, 2006b, 2007). Criminality, natural disasters, social precarity, and (urban) individualism can be read as threats, or disaggregation factors, experienced daily by Mexicans. An anthropology of threat[6] should analyze the circumstances in which members of a group feel insecurity and fear, as well as the representations of what threaten subjects or a group's integrity, but also the strategies used by the group to protect its members and pacify these feelings.[7]

It can seem paradoxical, but at the heart of extremely individualistic and fragmented systems, bottom-up initiatives of mutual aid arise. People organize into collectives to reinforce social bonds and (re)establish social networks. The communitarian brigades are an example of resistance to these threatening forces of social disaggregation. There is a lengthy history, of at least fifteen or twenty years, whereby Latin America people organize in *brigadas*. Since around 2013, in Mexican zones affected by drug trafficking, popular armed groups arose who call themselves "self-defense brigades."[8]

But there are also nonviolent groups called "solidarity brigades," which can be defined as experiences of internal humanitarianism.[9] These projects aim to ameliorate the exclusion of some groups (especially economically vulnerable populations) from a wide range of services, from medical or juridical services to aesthetic care. Most of the brigades are composed of voluntary groups of citizens.

The Itinerant Beauty Brigade: A Space to Recover

The Itinerant Beauty Brigade is a group of volunteers who offer free aesthetic care to vulnerable populations in Mexico City.[10] It started in 2014 as a vision of the charismatic hairstylist Diego Sexto, after he met some unemployed women who couldn't afford a haircut.[11] Since then, the Beauty Brigade grew and became structured as a concept.[12] Around 250 volunteers have participated at least one Beauty Brigade, 15 of whom form a main core who are present one Sunday per month (see Figure 4.1). Volunteers are mostly beauty professionals (makeup artists, hairdressers, barbers, beauticians), experienced or in training. They are men and women (cisgender and transgender) from Mexico City's lower middle classes. Some of them identify with the LGBTQ community. They have gradually come to identify with the role of *brigadista* or *brigadier*, a distinctive identity that is printed on their aprons and is even tattooed on their bodies.

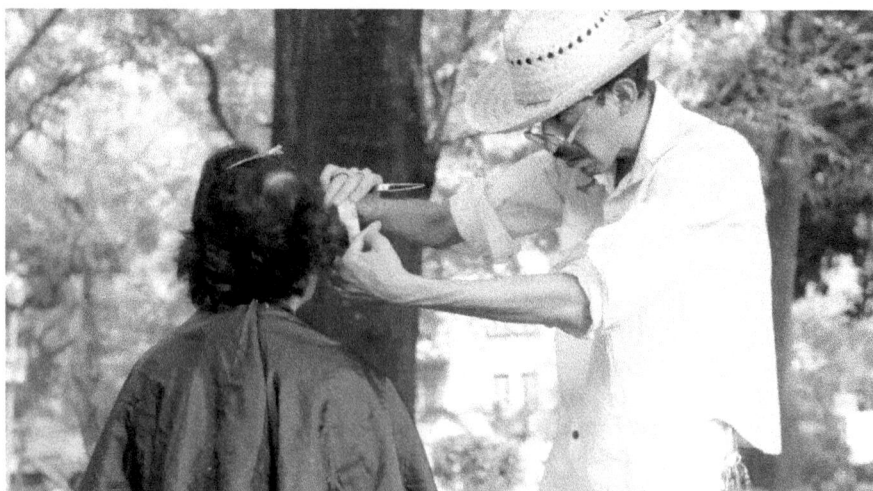

Figure 4.1. Diego Sexto, the founder of the Itinerant Beauty Brigade, is an itinerant hairdresser. He works in a park in Mexico City. Mexico, 2017. Photo by the author.

The Beauty Brigade operates in the urban area of Mexico DF, which makes it a somewhat local initiative,[13] but targets a wide spectrum of populations: people with chronic conditions (scleroderma, lupus, fibromyalgia, AIDS, cancer), disabled people, victims of violence, elderly sex workers, women who have experienced abortion, teenage mothers and their children, prisoners, homeless persons, maids, taxi drivers, artists, journalists, and victims of acid attacks.[14] The range of aesthetic treatments proposed by the Beauty Brigade are hair cleaning and scalp massages, hair dying, haircuts, skin care and facial massages, eyebrow care, makeup, manicure, and image counseling.[15] Volunteers don't accept funding from government or political parties;[16] however, they receive donations in the form of beauty products (hair dyes and other hair care products) from several private companies.

After this brief description of the Beauty Brigade, it is useful to understand the context in which this initiative arose. The Beauty Brigade was born in an urban context, which is not neutral, but has specific sensorial and social connotations. Especially in a big metropolis as Mexico City, inhabitants experience a sensory proximity that can be highly stressful. As described by Georg Simmel, modern "neurasthenic individuals" (urban inhabitants) are visually, auditorily, and olfactorily overstimulated (2013).[17] Citizens (try to) avoid tactile contact with other citizens to preserve themselves and to reduce stimulations such as friction. In urban contexts, "the senses of the citizen are mobilized to create distance and avoid touching each other in one way or another," as noticed by Philippe Simay (Simmel 2013 : 34). In this scenario, beauty practices are often proposed and demanded as services that "pacify the senses" and "relax" stressed subjects. Aesthetic treatments offer citizens the opportunity to "escape" symbolically and sensorially the ordinary urban intermingling. In this perspective, beauty institutes are intimate and circumscribed spaces to recover from the aggressivity of the "outside" world.[18] As Morgan Cochennec noticed:

> A [beauty] institute finds itself out of the social world: a space of intimacy, it implements an inward-looking dynamic and it concentrates all the activities on the person. ... The constitution of a space apart from the social world is symbolically important. The space of the aesthetic is always presented by its official spokespersons as a place "out of the world" and "out of the time." The [beauty] institute is ordinarily presented as a safe haven and a place of sensuousness, in which outside tensions and social logics don't exist: its borders protect the clients from the violence of the outside. (Cochennec 2004)

Conceived as an urban oasis, the beauty institute is welcoming, intimate, and warm. It offers a moment to abstract from productive/professional activities and familiar responsibilities, while one is able to regenerate and relax. In this space one can enjoy a special moment, usually represented as a self-oriented "gift." The Beauty Brigade has the same welcoming characteristics of the beauty institute described by Cochennec. It is a safe place, pleasant and benevolent. Nevertheless, its workspace is nomadic. Volunteers intervene wherever they are solicited: in public spaces (such as in prisons, libraries, museums) or in private spaces (such as nursing homes or hairdressing studios lent by volunteers). Even if this nomadic workspace implies a logistical challenge, the Beauty Brigade adapts to the situation. The venues are refitted for their arrival. Whenever possible, music is played, and flowers and balloons are used for decoration, to build a colored and pleasant ambiance (see Figure 4.2).

Beauty Brigade events often take place in big rooms. Consequently, recipients don't benefit from an objective intimacy with the beauty operator.[19] Nevertheless, this is alleviated by the division of the big space into many little areas, within which each team is able to provide specific services (e.g., makeup, hair coloring, facial masks). This helps to re-create areas of intimacy within which recipients feel a special attention toward themselves.[20]

It is important to say that the Beauty Brigade is not only a space where recipients can relax, like in traditional beauty institutes. The Beauty Brigade is also a space of recreation. Whenever possible, volunteers sing some popular Mexican songs to recipients, they dance together, and they share a

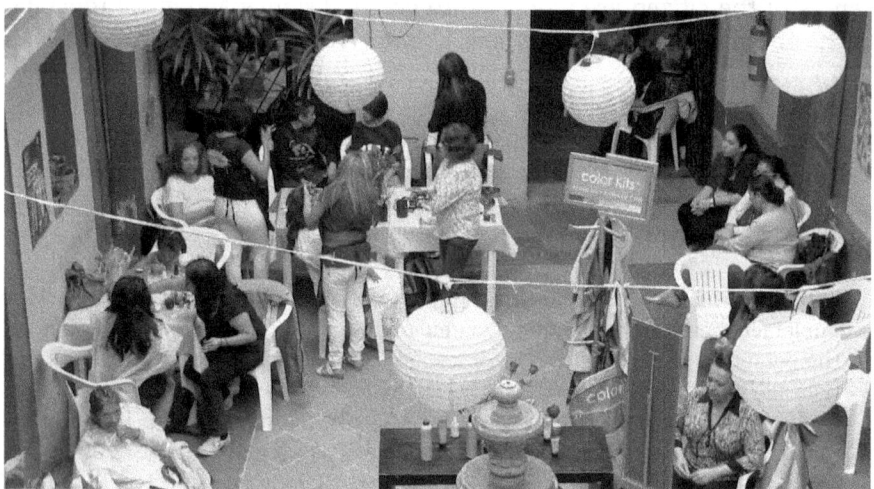

Figure 4.2. Itinerant Beauty Brigade at Casa Xochiquetzal, a refuge for elderly sex workers. Venues are refitted, and little areas (for makeup, nails, face masks, haircuts, image consulting) are created in the courtyard. Mexico City, 2016. Photo by the author.

meal. These elements indicate that their intention is to re-create an ambiance similar to a family party. A familiar dimension is accentuated by organizing the events on Sunday, the day that is traditionally spent with family. This manner of enjoying collective reunions and sharing excitement during the activities reflects a Mexican form to reinforce intimate relationships. In this context, through the collective and festive dimension a subject can psychologically regenerate.

The Familia Brigadista

> The brigade is a group that does not just bring a service to individuals; it creates a community and provides a mutual aid.
> —Terkita, makeup artist and volunteer

"Where and when do the social relationships that occur during the act of repairing something manifest themselves?" (Martinez and Laviolette 2019). Within the Beauty Brigade there are three main socializing dynamics that reinforce social bonds: between volunteers, between recipients, and between recipients and volunteers.

Volunteers often define the Beauty Brigade as a family: *la familia brigadista*. This strong identification of volunteers with the brigade is a positive unexpected result of different factors. In part this is a consequence of the good leadership of Diego Sexto. He plays an important role in managing the group, thanks to his charisma, but also due to his ability to create occasions that deepen intimacy—for example, eating together or having a night drinking pulque.[21] During these convivial moments, volunteers have the opportunity to get to know each other better and share about their experiences in the brigade. Another factor is the emotional nature of the experiences shared in the Beauty Brigade, which creates deep ties between participants.

To plan the logistics of a Beauty Brigade, as well as for internal mutual aid purposes, volunteers communicate through social media, especially Facebook and WhatsApp.[22] Within the paradigm of collaborative learning they share techniques and expertise. The most experienced hairstylists interact with apprentices, and they work together with the same objective. To recognize and to thank the most deserving *brigadista*, volunteers do pools to offer the "scissors of equality," a pair of professional scissors, or other professional-grade items. This symbolic recognition, which is delivered in a public ceremony during the Beauty Brigade, constitutes a reinforcement and an encouragement in order to stay committed and identify with the group. The *familia brigadista* also includes members of their "original" families (children, parents, friends, or *comadres*) who help the volunteers with logistics (preparation of the events or distributing tacos).[23] The experience as a volunteer strengthens their personal and professional networks and in some cases unites the two spheres.

The Beauty Brigade is also an opportunity for recipients to share a recreative moment. In this space-time of beauty care, they can "leave behind" or "forget" for a moment the heavy concerns of daily life, to share pleasure and complicity in coquetries (see Figure 4.3). During the event they laugh, share "small talk" with each other, exchange advice and opinions, and, of course, compliment each other about the aesthetic change that they go through. Recipients share the same "restoring" process, as well as emotions linked to this moment. For them, the Beauty Brigade constitutes a fortunate occasion to socialize with people who experience the same causes of vulnerability and valorize themselves mutually.

> When I look around me right now, I say to myself: how many sisters I have! All of us [women with scleroderma] look like each other. The shape of the mouth or the nose, we look like each other. We are like sisters. . . . We are as a family. Here [in the brigade] you look at the girl at your side and you say to her, "Oh! You are becoming very beautiful! What they have done to you! That is the nicest part. Here you can trust people; they don't criticize you [for your appearance]. (A woman with scleroderma, speaking to a volunteer in a Beauty Brigade's event)

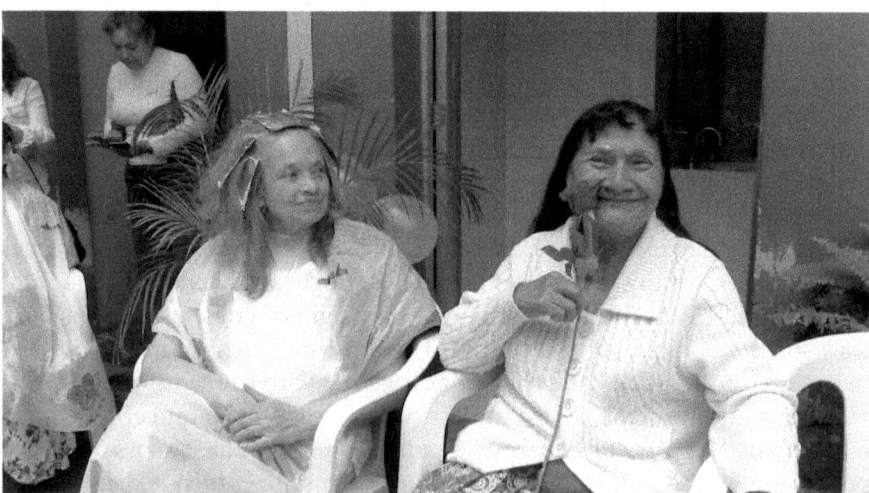

Figure 4.3. Women from Casa Xochiquetzal, elderly sex workers, participants at a Beauty Brigade. Mexico City, 2016. Photo by the author.

Thanks to the Beauty Brigade, recipients can find a renewed complicity. These kinds of activities reinforce their identification as a group. In these occasions, they valorize each other through compliments, as a sort of mutual encouragement.

We also see that with the passage of the time, a special relationship can emerge between volunteers and recipients. The Beauty Brigade's meeting produces quite strong affective bonds, especially if the brigade comes regularly to visit one group or association. The second time that volunteers went to Casa Xochiquetzal,[24] a refuge for elderly sex workers, women were expecting them with a lot of excitement. When the brigade finished and the *brigadistas* promised to come back again after a few months, this announcement filled the residents with joy and happiness:

> I want to thank them [the Beauty Brigade] for their attention to come and groom us. . . .[25] Today is the second time that they come! The last time I liked very much the way they "made me up" and the way they cut my hair. I want to thank them for their attention, because we are old and often our families abandon us! Our own families. But then, there are some people [such as volunteers] that come to visit us, they help us, they cut our hair, they groom us. There are also other people who came and gave us school classes. All these details are very appreciated! For me they are very important. I am grateful for this. Thank you, for taking pictures of us [she smiles]. (Maria, a resident of Casa Xochiquetzal, a refuge for elderly sex workers, in Mexico City)

The visit of the *brigadistas*, especially for people who don't have family anymore (as most of the elderly women of Casa Xochiquetzal), is affectively very important to recipients. With their mere presence, volunteers show to recipients that somebody still cares about them. Furthermore, volunteers assume the responsibility to visit vulnerable groups regularly to reinforce relationships and bring them affection, hope, and warmth.

Empathy in Sharing Vulnerability

In contrast to many initiatives in humanitarian fields, within the Beauty Brigade the separation between givers and recipients is not well defined. As Diego Sexto has said to me many times, "You can't call recipients *beneficiados* [beneficiaries]. Everybody (recipients and volunteers) benefits from the experience in Beauty Brigade." On many occasions, Lula—the psychologist and animator of the Beauty Brigade—repeated this concept. Everybody benefits from the empathetic exchange with "the Other."[26] Since these moments are always charged with emotion for all parties involved, all participants experience deep memories and feel closer to one another. This meeting is meant to be transformative for both parties.

In Casa Xochiquetzal, Lula asked both recipients and volunteers to gather and then to move positions within the room only when they feel called by her affirmations. Lula exclaimed, "Move if you suffered by shortage! Move if you suffered by dishonesty! Move if you suffered by failure! Move if you suffered by loneliness! Move if you suffered by violence!" Almost all the participants moved around the room. She concluded, "We can realize that we all have emotions, and we all have suffered by some negative emotion [or precarious situation]." That discourse allows all participants to enter into an empathetic relationship with all the other participants.

Another factor that probably increases the empathy between participants is sharing a similar sociographic background. Both volunteers and recipients come mostly from the lower-middle classes of Mexico City. They are exposed to some similar factors of risk and of vulnerability, like muggings, street violence, and unemployment. Some volunteers have been exposed to situations of economic precarity or of discrimination, or they have disabilities. For example, Diego Sexto had experienced poliomyelitis when he was a child, and Micky has a disabled hand. This produces a "mirror effect" between volunteers and recipients, favoring the identification between the two parts.

The empathetic contact with receivers can awake a volunteer's social consciousness. Nevertheless, an excess of empathy is counterproductive and can be emotionally unaffordable. As Griselda testified:

> This one time, when we went to the [prison] "reclusorio Oriente," I must confess that I felt very bad. Because in the end I was crying with these girls! And that is not good, because we are supposed to sustain them! And then, you melt with their histories. When I saw their child, ahhh! I started to cry. As a mother myself, I said "My child! How they can live here [in prison]?" Then Lula told me to stay strong! Because we came to sustain these girls and not to cry. There I understood that we should be prepared to face these situations and prevent ourselves from having this [emotional] impact. In another brigade I met an elderly woman and she told me her life. In some way that story made me remember the relationship with my parents, right? How poor they are, they stay all alone ... and I ended crying with her.

Lula, the psychologist of the Beauty Brigade, organizes moments of talk (mixed or non-mixed), in which volunteers can reflect on their emotions and, as a consequence, open their eyes to their own vulnerability. Sometimes they also organize sessions of self-care, as tai-chi sessions and sweat lodges (*temazcal*) (see Figure 4.4).[27]

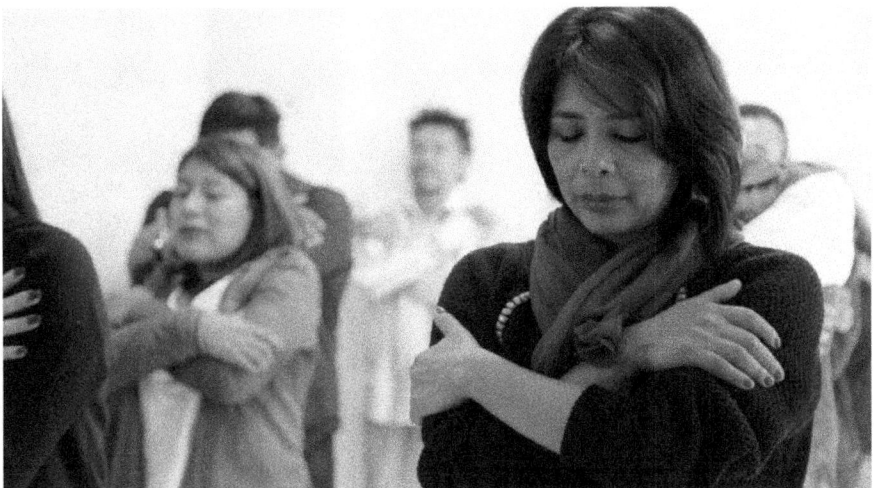

Figure 4.4. A session of self-care for Itinerant Beauty Brigade's volunteers. Mexico City, 2016. Photo by the author.

Overcoming Inhibitions

Sometimes achieving empathy with recipients is not an easy process. A heavy silence can prevail between volunteer and recipients instead of a dialogue. While they are getting their hair cut, recipients may exhibit signs of distress: they may lower their eyes, they may look deeply sad, and they may fail to respond to the hairdresser's questions or jokes. These behaviors may indicate that they cannot "let go," and they stay reserved. Some people are not used to this kind of intimacy, which is inherent to aesthetic procedures. In some cases, they haven't seen themselves in a mirror or haven't been to a hairdresser in decades. Others are wary of contact due to their illness, which may affect their skin, giving them hypersensitivity.

Volunteers may feel reluctant with people with disabilities and rare diseases. They may be scared of contagion of some illness. They may feel powerless when dealing with hard life stories of people they meet. They may also become resigned to the fact that they will not be able to properly communicate with recipients. But instead of forcing the recipient to talk or to smile, they should learn patience and be respectful toward the histories of suffering "written in the recipient's body."

Lula (psychologist) and Berenice (pedagogue) build a narrative that ritualizes the interactions between participants (see Figure 4.5). Their aim is to create a benevolent space in which emotions can be expressed and judg-

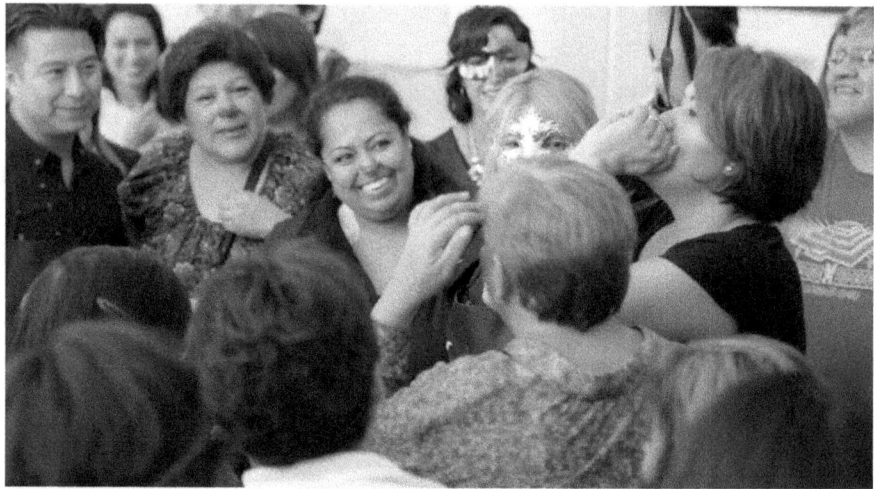

Figure 4.5. Lula and Berenice animate the encounter between volunteers of the Beauty Brigade and people with scleroderma. Mexico City, 2017. Photo by the author.

ments be inhibited. They coordinate some animations in which participants "break the ice" and "open their heart" to the other.

Cathartic Exchanges

When recipients walk into the Beauty Brigade's space, they usually light up. Their expression changes to one of moderate excitement, and a smile appears on their face with the prospect of a change in their look. Actually, changing their appearance has a symbolic correspondence with changing their own self-image. While receiving personal attention for a whole day, they can see their beauty come out, as if it was their hidden strength and their hidden potential. As a positive consequence of the process, they feel valued and socially included again.

> It's interesting and important to recognize how brigadistas, who have no knowledge of the disease, commit to making us feel better. Maybe they don't realize that beyond the beauty care services they offer, they make us feel included. (Sandy, a young woman with scleroderma)

The meeting between the *brigadista* and the recipient retains an ordinary beauty operator-client relationship. Recipients are asked what they would like to have in terms of hair coloring, haircut, or manicure style, while *brigadistas* can make some suggestions. Likewise, laughter and jokes help the protagonists break the ice and foster intimacy. During the beautification process, they engage in conversation and start to speak about their personal lives. Volunteers usually ask recipients to tell them their story. For example, a *brigadista* approached a woman with scleroderma and said, "Please, tell me your story. I will do a manicure, and I will be your psychologist [little laugh]."

Volunteers can also share their story and experience with recipients. There is a particular cathartic function in these interactions, as people express their emotions while talking, laughing, or crying. This cathartic function of the dialogue between volunteers and recipients can have some therapeutic psychological repercussions.

Apapacho Estético: An Affective Paradigm in Beauty Care

> You know, if you have a friend
> In whom you have confidence
> And if you wish to get good results
> Your soul must blend in with his
> And you must exchange presents
> And visit him often
> —Hávamál, old Norse poem cited in Marcel Mauss's essay, *The Gift*

When I assisted with the Beauty Brigade's services, I tried to understand and illustrate the sensations experienced by recipients. I focused on the expressivity of their face and body while receiving a shampoo, a facial, or makeup: closed eyes, relaxed foreheads, little smiles on their lips, completely relaxed cheeks or hands.[28] Those images describe a complete, personal, introverted pleasure, and even if it lasts only a few seconds, recipients seem deeply involved and willing to "go within." Volunteers create the conditions to "let go" and "just feel." In these moments recipients forget the "alert" mode, experienced in daily life, to completely surrender themselves to the care (see Figure 4.6).

I realized that in the interactions between volunteers and recipients, something larger than the mechanical act of beautification happened. The answer came when participants mentioned the concept of *apapacho*. This word comes from the native Nahuatl language and refers literally to a caress.[29] In daily life Mexicans use the world *apapacho* especially when a sad person needs to be reassured and cuddled. They would say that the person needs an *apapacho*. Sometimes Mexican define the *apapacho* as a "hug with the soul." In fact, *apapacho* is mostly tactile. It implies a hug or some other

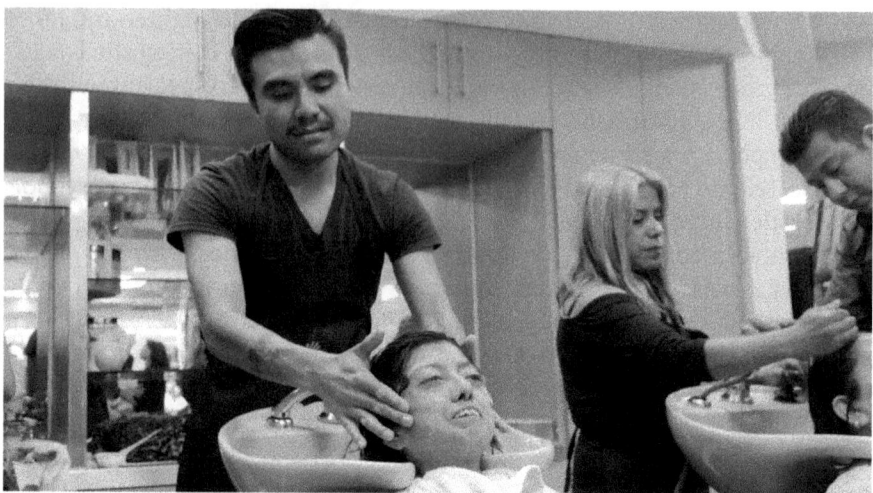

Figure 4.6. Volunteers of the Itinerant Beauty Brigade are doing a scalp massage for women with scleroderma. Mexico City, 2017. Photo by the author.

physical contact. In the semantic of *apapacho* is the notion to surround someone with one's presence and warmth.

But *apapacho* can be understood also as a deep and empathic heart movement toward the other. To give an *apapacho*, one is meant to feel empathy with another's distress. *Apapacho* has the power of "lowering masks" and deeply connecting people. *Apapacho* is a form of free care, because anyone can offer, through a hug, proximity and reassurance. Its consequences are that of transforming internal feelings of fear and suffering into self-confidence and trust in oneself and in others.

This word is used by the Beauty Brigade as *apapacho estético*. The *apapacho estético* can be translated as the act to reassure and "heal" trough aesthetic treatments. In *apapacho estético*, the senses are "awakened" through pleasant activities such as makeup, facials, or hair cleaning with scalp massage. This sensory dimension allows volunteers to build an intimate bond with people in distress. This aesthetic "caress" is meant to reassure and to make recipients feel safe. The beautification of a recipient's body is not intended by *brigadistas* as a mere physical work on appearance, but it's represented as a movement toward the recipients with the objective to reassure them and bring them some warm presence.

The *apapacho estético* is a sensory encounter that can relieve sadness and despair, repair the sensation of distress, and reinforce self-confidence through the act of beautification. The *apapacho estético* is also a particular way to approach recipients. Volunteers don't address uniquely and primarily the person's body, but the embodied subject as a whole. Their aim is to emotionally reassure recipients through a sensitive approach and encourage a cathartic and healing process implicit in the act to transform one's appearance.

> It seems like we give them a very positive, sort of nostalgic, energy. At the end of the day, they're very happy that we came to "hug" them [apapacharlos] and spend time with them.[30] (Fanny, volunteer hairstylist)

> I put my arms around people, and while I'm doing it, I can feel that I'm giving them a good kind of energy. If the person was laughing right before that, from one second to the next she might burst into tears. There's a connection between us. The person feels "hugged" [apapachada] and protected! (Terkita, volunteer makeup artist)

As was expressed by Terkita, the *apapacho estético* also has the effect of "lowering masks." It helps to let sadness and suffering emerge and, at the same time, evacuate. Often, these heavy feelings are repressed or disguised "behind a smile." The *apapacho* has the power to let people express their feelings, while they are listened to by a benevolent person who can reassure them.

Following Luz Gabriela Arango, aesthetic work on the body can be understood as a form of care, because "it cares for one's appearance, for one's self-presentation and it stresses important stakes about dignity and the place of people in society" (2013: 181). In fact, through the beautification recipients are seeking a symbolic recognition of their dignity and their value as human beings. They want to be aesthetically appreciated "as anyone else," no matter their illness, disability, social condition, or profession. Sandy, a young woman with scleroderma, remarked, "It's their way of coming closer to us that comforts us. They give us a lot of love and we feel equal to them." The following dialogue reveals a similar recognition of the recipients' dignity:

> Woman with scleroderma: I have alopecia, so I always wear a hat or a wig on my head. When I go to the beauty institute, I usually go with a hair stylist that I know. But other people who are waiting, they look at me, they observe me. When I go on public transportation, people look at me as if I was a strange bug [*bicho raro*]. But now [in the Beauty Brigade] I feel good eyes on me, I can show myself! I can let the stylist do a dying and everything.
>
> Ulyses [*brigadista*]: We are here for a reason. Here we are all comfortable, no?
>
> Woman with scleroderma: Yes, it's what I say: we are in a family. . . . Here we are in confidence, no one is judging us.

The *apapacho estético* allows recipients to reinforce their self-confidence but also the confidence in society at large. In other words, the *apapacho* is an affective and sensitive tool used by *brigadistas* to rebuild individual trust in society.

We can analyze the *apapacho* into the paradigm of the gift, theorized by Marcel Mauss (2010). What counter-gifts are given by the recipients of the *apapacho*? A first gesture of reciprocity consists in accepting this proximity, this exchange of conversation and physical contact with the volunteers. When this happens, the volunteer may then experience the satisfaction of having partaken in a cathartic, healing act.

Sometimes the rituals are structured to offer the recipients the possibility of being reciprocal. At Casa Xochiquetzal, right before the brigade, Lula puts a little bit of hand cream in the hands of recipients. This cream is presented as a "gift" which recipients should give to volunteers through a little hand massage. This first tactile contact helps them to "break the ice," and it constitutes an anticipated reciprocity. Follow this logic, volunteers' services are already intended as a counter-gift (see Figure 4.7).

When participants arrive at the end of the beautification process, they take the "after" pictures all together, and luckily recipients are often happy with the results.[31] This picture testifies to something more than merely individual physical change; it testifies to a collective process of reunification (see Figure 4.8).

The enthusiasm of being part of this whole human experience of the Beauty Brigade, can lead some volunteers to develop a social sensibility in their own professional day-to-day practice. This is the case of Terkita,

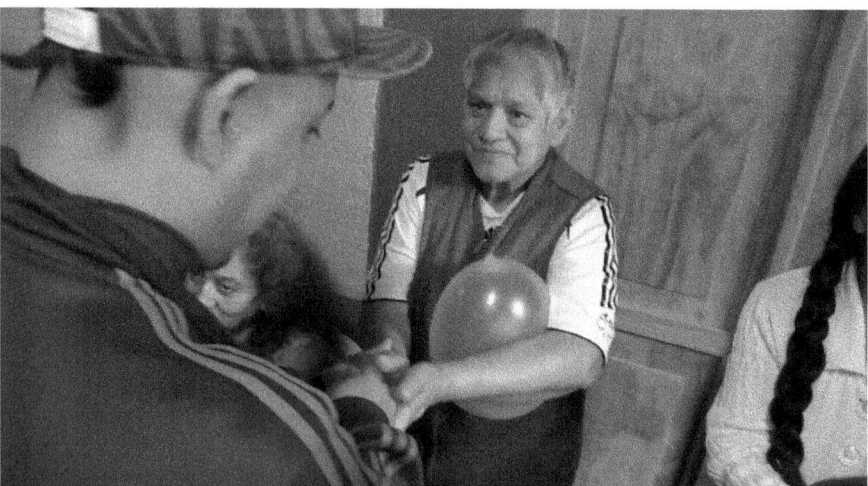

Figure 4.7. Albert, hairstylist volunteer of the Itinerant Beauty Brigade, is receiving the symbolic "gift" from a Casa Xochiquetzal resident: hand massage and benediction. Mexico City, 2016. Photo by the author.

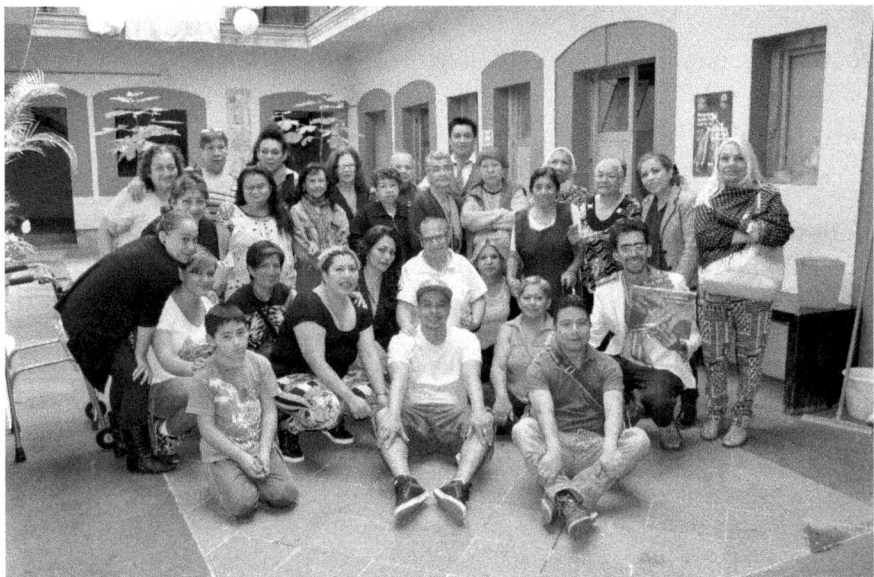

Figure 4.8. Closing picture of a Beauty Brigade in Casa Xochiquetzal (house for elderly sex workers in Mexico City). Mexico City, 2016. Photo by Francisco Cano Z.

a volunteer who decided to open her own "inclusive beauty institute" the IBYCIM (Instituto de Belleza y Cultura Incluyente México).[32] This institute offers disabled people (e.g., those with Down syndrome, blind people, deaf people) the opportunity to learn beauty skills, in order to be autonomous and make up themselves or to become a professional.

Conclusion

The fragmentation of Mexican urban society, and the consequent exclusion of some particular groups, is one social problem affecting especially the lower-middle classes in Mexico City. As citizens from the lower-middle classes, both volunteers and recipients of the Beauty Brigade experience daily insecurity and physical and psychological vulnerability. In this scenario, like other brigades all over Latin America, the Beauty Brigade arises as a self-managed bottom-up initiative of mutual aid. Its main values are that of solidarity, inclusion, benevolence, and horizontality. The Beauty Brigade creates a safe space in which participants can socialize, which contrasts with the urban "outside" world, where insecurity, aggressiveness, discrimination, and indifference are mostly dominant.

The Beauty Brigade has many virtuous repercussions for all its participants. Its horizontal predisposition allows people to "open" themselves to others and develop mutual empathy. The sociological proximity between volunteers and recipients of the Beauty Brigade reinforces mutual recognition and mutual understanding. As underlined by Arango, the relationship between the beauty operator and clients is reinforced by the proximity of social status. Between two subjects belonging to "popular classes, [where] the proximity of status and of conditions of life is bigger, the emotional work can entertain an atmosphere of confidence in which the hairstylist can play the role of the confidant who listens and shares opinions about the problems of daily life of her/his client" (2013: 183).

Furthermore, the Beauty Brigade "enables the recreation of social relationships" (Martinez and Laviolette, 2019) because it favors multiple forms of socialization. The Beauty Brigade's volunteers learn progressively the value of fraternity.[33] That is possible because within the Beauty Brigade, they find a noncompetitive atmosphere in which they can collaborate and share professional competences. Social networks are platforms used by volunteers to communicate and support each other in day-to-day life.[34] Those positive implications allow them to stay committed to the group and identify as a family: *la familia brigadista*.

Recipients benefit from this experience in multiple ways too. First, they can benefit from an aesthetic service for free. Second, thanks to the Beauty Brigade, they can escape from their daily routine and experience a moment of relaxation, but also of recreation and festivity. Third, they socialize with other participants, enlarging their affective network. Eventually, they are progressively included in the *familia brigadista*, as a heterogeneous group that valorizes everyone's differences and particularisms. Fourth, through the *apapacho estético* they can feel dignified as any other member of society and trust again in others. Fifth, they can express their distress and benefit from a cathartic-healing effect (speaking, laughing, crying). In this sense, the beautification process is meant to repair, rebuild, and reinforce self-esteem and social bonds.

Within the Beauty Brigade, aesthetic treatments are a privileged way to express the will to be "integrated in" and "recognized by" society. Especially for particularly marginalized people, aestheticization is a struggle for visibility.

For the cultural anthropologist Francesco Remotti (2003, 2006, 2013), aesthetic procedures have an *anthropopoïetic* role: they shape "humanness." That is to say, beautification can be read as a cultural tool used to resolve the feeling of "incompleteness" (for Remotti, inherent in human condition) or to alleviate the feeling of invisibility that concerns particularly marginalized groups (Carpigo 2016). The process of beautification can be lived as the first step to (re)integrate into society or (re)socialize into a particular group. Through beautification, people erase the "signs of exclusions" inscribed on their body, as observed by Sander Gilman with cosmetic surgery for the early twentieth-century US immigrants (2000). The desire to improve their appearance expresses the desire of social recognition.

In the Itinerant Beauty Brigade, the paradigm of the *apapacho estético* should be read as an affective movement through the others, in order to fend off and soothe their suffering. This affective strategy of care can short-circuit the "individualistic demon" and the isolation threats so pervasive in urban social structure. The *apapacho estético* renews the sense of hope,[35] because it awakes the desire to stay committed with and to others.

The participation in Itinerant Beauty Brigade is a technical, emotional, and moral challenge for all its participants. Volunteers experience it as an opportunity to grow as a professional and also as a human being, improving values of tolerance, solidarity, sharing, and humility.

In a social scenario impregnated with violence and injustices, mistrust and terror, the Beauty Brigade engages in a pacific performance of resistance and inclusion. Nevertheless, to fully enjoy the experience, all participants (volunteers and recipients) should overcome their fears and inhibitions. Volunteers should overcome disgust, avoiding paternalism and navigating other forms of prejudice pertaining to the groups they come to meet.[36] Recipients' main challenge is to trust volunteers, even if they are apprentices, disabled people (e.g., blind people), or people with any other specificity (e.g., transgender). The Itinerant Beauty Brigade creates a safe and supportive ambiance, in which participants can overcome inhibitions or fears and embrace affectively the alterity.

Acknowledgments

Thank you very much to all members of the Beauty Brigades and the photographers Mercy Alejandra Portillo Alcocer and Francisco Cano Z. I thank all the partners who funded this research (and the documentary *Belleza Humanitaria*): Embassy of France in Mexico, CEMCA, UAM-Xochimilco, Martha Uc, Ciencine Productions, and La Maroma Productions. Thanks also to Jean-Yves Bart, Katia-Myriam Borth, Rhiannon Kevis, and Christophe Humbert for the reading and the correction of this text.

Eva Carpigo is a PhD candidate in anthropology at the University of Strasbourg (France) and Universidad Autonoma Metropolitana (Mexico DF). Her PhD research is about cosmetic surgeons in France and Mexico. She co-organized a seminar on aesthetic practices called "Body and Beauty" (Corps et beauté) in 2018–19: https://corpsbeaute.hypotheses.org.

Notes

1. I will call it Beauty Brigade, for convenience. See their website, http://brigadasdebellezaitinerante.org; their Facebook page, https://www.facebook.com/brigadasdebellezaitinerante/; and their Twitter account, https://twitter.com/brigadasbelleza, last accessed on 24 June 2019.
2. The work of James C. Scott (1992) analyzes the "secret discourse" of dominated people as a performative way to express political positions of resistance in relation to their social order. In the case of Beauty Brigade, the social resistance is expressed through the body. The investment on the body's appearance, to "stay beautiful," is intended as a way to incorporate visibility and so affirm the right to be present—and visible—in society. The beautification corresponds to the desire of marginalized people, to affirm their right to be visible, recognized, and dignified in society.
3. Over two hundred thousand individuals have died since 2006 of drug trafficking-related causes. The number of missing people (*desaparecidos*) and mass graves linked to the cartel wars, with the complicity of corrupt politicians and police forces, keeps rising. According to the 2019 Global Peace Index (https://urlz.fr/ekVV), Mexico is one of the lowest countries on the peace index in the world (place: 140/163). According to the 2020 Mexican Peace Index (https://urlz.fr/ekVR), "Homicides have multiplied drastically in the last five years. Since 2015 homicides have risen 86 percent, and in the last year [2019], more than thirty-five thousand people have been murdered. This is the highest level of violence ever registered. The conflicts inside the criminal organizations and between them have increased, spreading high levels of violence. Homicide is the main cause of death in people ages fifteen to forty-four years, and the fourth for children under fourteen years ... Lack of security is the largest worry for Mexicans, before unemployment, inflation, corruption, and impunity." Some professions have been increasingly at risk, such as journalists and politicians, who are constantly threatened and killed for their social engagements.
4. An earthquake struck Mexico on 19 September 2017 with a magnitude of 7.1, causing 369 deaths. Source: https://www.bbc.com/mundo/noticias-america-latina-45544734, last accessed 6 August 2019.
5. A metaphorical expression I choose to indicate individualism.
6. An anthropology of threat was preconized in a symposium by Francis Affergan (Anthropologie de la menace), https://urlz.fr/elwU. In Mexican popular representations of urban geography, danger increases when traversing particular urban areas (as lonely places or neighborhood of "traffics" (as, for example, Tepito in Mexico City). Danger increases also everywhere after the sunset. During the night the world transforms; people should remain in their houses while spirits (as the Llorona legend tells) and criminals are walking down the streets. An anthropology of the night is explored by Jacques Galinier and Aurore Monod Becquelin in *Las cosas de la noche. Una mirada diferente* (2016).

7. There are lots of body techniques and logistic strategies used by Mexico City's inhabitants to avoid physical danger of being attacked. First of all, they choose accurately the way in which they transport. Often Mexicans use "magic" protections from potential threats (e.g., amulets worn as jewelry, saints' iconic representations, reiki symbols).
8. The "self-defense brigades" (Brigadas de Autodefensa) were created by citizens to defend themselves from drug traffickers and/or corrupt national army soldiers. This is shown by the documentary "La vida de autodefensas 'documental,'" YouTube video, https://www.youtube.com/watch?v=ihb6d1gftqk, retrieved 17 August 2019.
9. Observing internet sources, for about fifteen years there are traces of the existence of pacific "solidary brigades" (e.g., medical, legal, ecological). Even if pacific in nature, the military etymology of "brigade" suggests a close-knit group organized to resist. They share a mission, which consists usually in supporting isolated populations in remote areas where the state doesn't arrive/intervene. Their members are generally young volunteers guided by experts.
10. Care is intended as "a species activity that includes everything that we do to maintain, continue, and repair our 'world' so that we can live in it as well as possible. That world includes our bodies, ourselves, and our environment, all of which we seek to interweave in a complex, life-sustaining web" (Fisher & Tronto 1991: 40).
11. Diego Sexto is himself an itinerant hairdresser (*peluquero itinerante*), which means he follows/perpetuates an old Mexican tradition of street hairdresser working in markets (*tianguis*) and parks.
12. The Itinerant Beauty Brigade volunteering differs from humanitarian development projects such as those observed by Laëtitia Atlani-Duault (2005), shepherded by large GOs and NGOs. A Beauty Brigade is not a formalized group, and there is no membership fee or member status.
13. Volunteers come from various areas of Mexico City but also from the surrounding area of the state of Mexico. Some travel for over two and a half hours to lend a hand.
14. That list is not exhaustive; the Beauty Brigade is constantly searching for new partners to offer their services.
15. Image counseling coaches on which colors should be adapted to wear, in accordance with skin and eye color, to improve one's attractiveness.
16. The Mexican government is considered to be corrupted, populist, and clientelist.
17. It is always topical, even if Simmel lived in Berlin at the beginning of the twentieth century.
18. That was also noticed by Loïc Wacquant for sports halls. Situated in a violent quarter, Chicago's boxing club constitutes "an island of security, of order and organization, where social interactions forbidden on the 'outside' become possible again. The sports hall offers a protected place of sociability, relatively closed, where anybody can find a break from the pressure of the streets and of the ghetto, a world where exterior events have little hold and penetrate difficultly" (Wacquant 1989: 41).
19. The category of "beauty operator" was formulated repeatedly in the research seminar "Corps et beauté" 2018–19 (https://corpsbeaute.hypotheses.org). It refers indicatively to any professional or nonprofessional recognized as reference

or as an expert (by the group of reference) in modifying body appearance and aestheticizing the body.
20. In Mexico, beauty institutes (especially if cheap) can be very tiny and unisex. All kinds of people are gathered in a little space, while services are visible to everybody (pedicure, manicure, haircut, shave, makeup). In spite of this aspect, a sort of privacy was respected anyway, thanks to the discretion of aestheticians and clients, who try to not observe intrusively each other.
21. Pulque is a traditional Mexican drink, made from fermented agave.
22. Networks of solidarity mobilize when members struggle for health or economic reasons or have been victims of a robbery, flood, or earthquake.
23. For example, hairstylist Micky comes to brigades with his son, who helps him with the logistics of the "color area" (dying area). Makeup artist Terkita comes with her mother, who helps distribute tacos to all volunteers. Hairstylist apprentice Ulyses invited his *comadre*, who helps the volunteers in the shampoo area and with logistic tasks.
24. Aztec Xochiquetzal goddess was presented as the "patron saint," protector of beauty, flowers, love, and both sex workers and beauty professionals.
25. The term used was *arreglarnos*, which literally means "repair," "arrange," "fix" us.
26. I use the expression "the Other" because, in this context, two groups recognize each other as "different" (at least professionally).
27. *Temazcal* is a traditional Mexican sweat lodge. Mexicans do it to "purify" the body from negative energies while it connects to the earth. Usually, this experience is done in a group.
28. As pointed out by Chiara Pussetti (2011), in ethnography it can be difficult to illustrate an emotion or a feeling, experienced by interlocutors, because "the emotional experience has an apparent immediacy and concreteness, yet a way of receding into a conceptual and investigative haze" (Pussetti 2005: 6, quoting Knapp 1958: 55).
29. From the Uto-Aztecan family, Nahuatl is the most widely spoken native language in Mexico. According the online dictionary of the Academia Mexicana de la lengua, *Diccionario breve de mexicanismos de Guido Gomez de Silva*, apapacho comes from the *nahua* verb *papatzoa*, from *patzoa, pachoa*. It means "caress" (https://bit.ly/34j3Kol, retrieved 23 September 2019).
30. In these quotations, I choose to translate *apapachar* with the verb "to hug."
31. I documented some who were unhappy with the result, which happened with an apprentice. When recipients are unsatisfied, some experienced volunteers can retouch the results.
32. IBYCIM (Instituto de Belleza y Cultura Incluyente México), https://www.facebook.com/IbycimMexico.
33. These exceptions, linked to personal "egos" and envy, mostly present in novices who are socialized in the spirit of competition, which prevails outside the brigade.
34. If some volunteer needs urgent help (because his or her salon was robbed or flooded), they organize internal fundraisings and send money or materials.
35. The association of aesthetic practices and hope was developed by Coleman and Moreno Figueroa (2010).

36. Disgust can appear at the sight of the skin lesions of patients with visible illnesses, and paternalism when facing with people with disability.

References

Agier, Michel. 1999. *L'invention de la ville. Banlieues, township, invasions et favelas*. Paris: Éditions des archives contemporaines.
Arango, Luz Gabriela. 2013. "Soin de l'apparence. Travail émotionnel et service au client." *Association Multitudes* 1(52): 180–85.
Atlani-Duault, Laëtitia. 2005. *Au bonheur des autres. Anthropologie de l'aide humanitaire*. Paris: Société d'ethnologie.
Bauman, Zygmunt. 2004. *L'Amour liquide, De la fragilité des liens entre les hommes*. Arles: Éditions du Rouergue.
———. 2006a. *La Vie liquide*. Arles: Le Rouergue/Chambon.
———. 2006b. *Vies perdues: La modernité et ses exclus*. Paris: Payot.
———. 2007. *Le présent liquide*. Paris: Seuil.
Carpigo, Eva. 2016. "Beauty at the Service of Humanity: A Review of the Therapeutic Value of Aesthetic Treatments." In *Beauty: Exploring Critical Perspectives*. Oxford: Interdisciplinary Press. Published online in July 2019 by Brill.
Cochennec, Morgan. 2004. "Le soin des apparences. L'univers professionnel de l'esthétique-cosmétique." *Actes de la recherche en sciences sociales* 4(154): 80–91.
Coleman, Rebecca, and Mónica Moreno Figueroa. 2010. "Past and Future Perfect? Beauty Affect and Hope." *Journal for Cultural Research* 14(4): 357–73.
Fisher, Berenice, and Joan Tronto. 1991. "Toward a Feminist Theory of Care." In E. Abel and M. Nelson (eds.), *Circles of Care: Work and Identity in Women's Lives*. Albany: State University of New York Press, pp. 36–54.
Galinier, Jacques, and Aurore Monod Becquelin. 2016. *Las cosas de la noche. Una mirada diferente*. Mexico: CEMCA.
Gilman, Sander. 2000. *Making the Body Beautiful: A Cultural History of Aesthetic Surgery*. Princeton, NJ: Princeton University Press.
Kropotkine, Pierre (Kropotkin, Peter). 2013. *L'entraide*. Paris: Éditions Topos/H. Trinquier.
Jarrín, Alvaro. 2015. "Towards a Biopolitics of Beauty: Eugenics, Aesthetic Hierarchies and Plastic Surgery in Brazil." *Journal of Latin American Cultural Studies* 24(4): 535–52.
Knapp, Peter H. 1958. "Conscious and Unconscious Affects." *Psychiatric Research Reports* 8: 55–74.
Martinez, Francisco, and Patrick Laviolette. 2019. *Repair, Brokenness, Breakthrough: Ethnographic Responses*. New York: Berghahn Books.
Mauss, Marcel. 2010. *Sociologie et anthropologie*. Paris: Presses Universitaires de France.
Musset, Alain. 2017. *Le Mexique. Que-sais-je?* Paris: Presses Universitaires de France.
Pussetti, Chiara. 2011. "Emozioni." In Cecilia Pennacini (ed.), *La ricerca sul campo. Antropologia, oggetti e metodi*. Roma: Carocci Editori, pp. 257–86.
Remotti, Francesco. 2003. "Interventions esthétiques sur le corps." In Francis Affergan et al. (eds.), *Figures de l'humain. Les représentations de l'anthropologie*. Paris: Éditions de l'EHESS, pp. 279–306.

———. 2006. *Prima lezione di antropologia*. Bari: Edizioni Laterza.
———. 2013. *Fare umanitá. I drammi dell'antropo-poiesi*. Bari: Edizioni Laterza.
Scott, James C. 1992. *Domination and Resistance: Hidden Transcripts*. New Haven, CT: Yale University Press.
Servigne, Pablo, and Gauthier Chapelle. 2017. *L'entraide. L'autre loi de la Jungle*. Paris: Éditions LLL, Les liens qui libèrent.
Simmel, Georg. 2013. *Les grandes villes et la vie de l'esprit*. Prefaced by Philippe Simay. Paris: Petite Bibliothèque Payot.
Thi Nguyen, Mimi. 2011. "The Biopower of Beauty: Humanitarian Imperialisms and Global Feminisms in an Age of Terror." *Journal of Women in Culture and Society* 36(2): 359–83.
Wacquant, Loïc J. D. 1989. "Corps et âme." *Actes de la recherche en sciences sociales*. 80(2): 33–67.

PART II
RESHAPING

CHAPTER 5

Shaping the European Body
The Cosmetic Construction of Whiteness

CHIARA PUSSETTI

Inspired by the anthropology of the body, critical medical anthropology, and gender and colonial/postcolonial studies, in this chapter I analyze the relationship between normative notions of beauty in Portugal, new paradigms of body (re)shaping, and aspirations of social integration among immigrant populations in the Greater Lisbon area. Based on my recent fieldwork conducted with immigrants and Afro-European women in Portugal aged between thirty and fifty, I investigate local beauty standards, aspirations, and cosmetic practices designed to shape an "ideal European body," as a specific form of bio-investment aimed at producing socially valued bodies in order to climb the social ladder or to boost chances of success.

Secondly, considering beauty as a project steadily "under construction" and focusing on what people say a perfect or "flawless" beauty should look like, I specifically explore the aesthetic labor enacted by these women as a way of adaptation to local and global circuits of representation. As beauty is about creating difference through artifice and shaping valuable bodies in a classed, aged, sexualized, gendered, and racialized way, I display that also bodies that are generally perceived as "white" are racialized, even if this racialization is not openly admitted nor interpreted politically.

The final purpose of this chapter is to highlight how beauty and cosmetic procedures are not only deeply "gendered" and "classed," but also "racialized" and "racializing," reproducing and reinforcing both symbolic boundaries and social inequalities.

The Beauty and the Blush

> "Mirror, mirror on the wall, who's the fairest of them all?"
> — The Brothers Grimm, *Snow-White*

Marcia Ann Gillespie, who in her essay "Mirror Mirror" analyzes the Euro-American narrative that constructs the "white" ideal of beauty as hegemonic, states that "our" (Eurocentric) magic mirror continues to proclaim that Snow White is indeed the fairest in all the land. Madonna—Gillespie continues—the "Queen of Pop," an intelligent and ambitious woman, soon understood that in order to reign she had to "reach for the bleach and peroxide" and discolor her hair (2003: 202). Many celebrities followed her example. In the realms of the famous, "the hair, eyes and skin color tend to progressively and lighten and the blonde is still the apogee" (2003: 202).

The results of the 477 qualitative online survey returns taken in Portugal in the context of the EXCEL project don't seem to contradict Gillespie's conclusions.[1] In responding to the challenge of stating a personal ideal of feminine beauty, the results of this first national survey evince a collective image of a thin, light-skinned, ethereal, elegant, beautiful, and not overly sensual woman. Highlights include Kristen Jaymes Stewart (who happened to play Snow White in the 2012 film *Snow White and the Huntsman*), Cate Blanchett (who shall be remembered as the glowing Galadriel, the "lady of light" in Tolkien's saga, with her long platinum hair), Charlize Theron (who in the latest Dior's campaign of the J'adore Absolu fragrance emerges naked, like a modern-day Cleopatra, from a pool of liquid gold, in a scenery reminiscent of Jean-Auguste-Dominique Ingres's *Turkish Bath*), and Emma Watson (who played Belle in the 2017 film *Beauty and the Beast* and appeared in ads for Lancôme's skin-lightening product Blanc Expert).

Among the survey participants, women were more likely to choose iconic references such as the ethereal Tilda Swinton (the candid Snow Queen in *The Chronicles of Narnia*), Julianne Moore, or southern Brazilian supermodel Gisele Bündchen (descendant of German immigrants), considered "the most beautiful girl in the world" in *Rolling Stone* magazine's 14 September 2000 issue. Aesthetically beautiful does not correspond, however, to sexually attractive or erotically desirable. These elegant women are something to be admired, not someone to have sex with; they are untouchable, something only to be gazed upon, classy but not sexual.

When, by contrast, we ask which women better represent icons of sensuality, the profile changes considerably. Here the highlights are Jennifer Lopez, Beyoncé, Rihanna, Grace Jones, Penélope Cruz, Shakira, and Kim Kardashian. What separates the first group of "beautiful and classy" from the second group of "sexy" women is not simply a clear "global colorline"

(Lake and Reynolds 2008). All women in the second group—even brunettes who in Portugal are considered "white"—are classified as sexy, erotic, "exotic," and "ethnic" beauties, beyond the traditional white/black binary. They are "white but not quite" (Santana Pinho 2009) and thus unable to gain legitimate entrance into the category of "elegant and classy" women. They represent, however, "whiteness of different colors" (Jacobson 1998), emphasizing the extreme fluidity and instability of whiteness as a category that expands and contracts depending on nationality, class, gender, age, and sexual orientation.

When directly questioned in interviews about "ethnic" beauties, the choices fall almost exclusively on heavily whitewashed women, with clear contact lenses, extensions, and blond hair. In the few answers that mention less "vanilla" women such as Grace Jones, Naomi Campbell, Lupita Nyongo, or the American Somali fashion model Iman, their beauty is immediately exoticized: they are described as "panthers" or "gazelles." And these voluptuous "wild" animals from the jungle, "butterflies," "exotic birds," "giraffes," and "tigresses," associated with nature and earth, become African queens that will never be the kind of queen that rules over Snow White's kingdom.[2]

"White" women are the beautiful ones, and the other women are the desired ones. Establishing alternative forms of femininity (Morris 2016) implies that "there is a standard model of beauty form which anything else is a deviation" (Deliovsky 2008: 55). As Sally Markowitz claims, "The femininity of non-white women, far from being heightened, is likely to be denied. . . . It is not difficult, after all, to find a pronounced racial component to the idea of femininity itself: to be truly feminine is, in many ways, to be white" (2001: 390).

"Mirror, mirror on the wall who's the fairest of them all? . . . Most of the time, when the question is raised from a black girl"—Gillespie claims (2003: 202)—"the answer is: isn't you." "Ethnic" girls are not "the classic beauty"; Snow White continues to reign, and other women can be only the sexy witches. According to my interviewees, the true queens that shall occupy the throne with Snow White are the golden goddesses; they "glow," their skin is "bright" and "radiant," they are "sunny" and have a special aura.

According to Richard Dyer, who in his book *White* examines the reproduction and preservation of whiteness in visual culture from the fifteenth to the end of the twentieth century, "To glow still remains a key quality in idealized representations of white women" (1997: 32). The iconographic construction of whiteness in the eighteenth century[3] reproduces the complexion of the "blushing Roses" European woman, often juxtaposed with her "exotic" black servant, positioned at her feet, so as to give value to a superior and desirable whiteness (Rosenthal 2004). The "erotic-exotic" servant or colonized woman (as I highlighted in other articles: Pussetti 2015a,

2015b, 2019; Pussetti and Barros 2012a, 2012b) is portrayed as sensuously passive and mysterious, submitted prone to the white and masculine domination.[4] Many authors have highlighted how the representations of African and Asian women in eighteenth- and nineteenth-century Orientalist art evoked the sensuality, docile submission, exoticness, and allure of difference of the "others" by race and culture. The attractive and lascivious image of the colonized woman highlights at the same time the virtue, chastity, honor, purity, and elegance of the European lady, honest bride and angel of the house (see, e.g., Said 1979; Dobson 1991; Barkan 1992; Lewis 1996; Manderson and Jolly 1997; Yegenoglou 1998).

The female beauty ideal as light-permeated, virtuous, pure, and "whitified" (Ware 1992 Poitevin 2011), which my research highlights, becomes a contemporary apex in an aesthetic hierarchy that crosses a good part of European history and is dependent on, and fed by, the presence of "other bodies" and contact with them. Building on the long-standing colonial ideologies that value European culture, aesthetics, and their moral underpinnings, these "shades of difference" (Glenn 2009) classify bodies, not only creating a pigmentocracy between civilized Europe and the colonies' territories, but also hierarchizing the population within Europe.[5]

Though historical indications of colorism existed before the onset of colonialism and preferences for fair skin as a social marker of aristocratic heritage, high class, social status, or caste predate colonialism and the introduction of Western notions of beauty (Cogenau 2015), images derived from colonial legacies have had (and continue to have) a profound impact on the (re)production of what is considered a normal/desired/legitimate "European body." We are obviously not talking about a real body, but rather representations and fantasies of "Europeanness," the construction of a fictional identity or European style, constantly reproduced in order to consolidate borders and exclude otherness. This image, however, produces real effects on people's lives, and it literally shapes the body both of immigrants, of "Europeans of color"—who represent other color-coded symbolic economies—and also of "white" Europeans (in particular of non-privileged social classes).

Though the presence of racialized canons is clear in the interviews, underpinning the entire discourse, "race" and "racialization" are never openly discussed. A major challenge that emerges in fieldwork, when dealing with whiteness as a racialized construct, is that white beauty as a constructed norm insistently refuses to be analyzed. When directly questioned, the response of my (white) interviewees is always—naively, or assuming a clear defensive attitude—that "race" has nothing to do with their answers. "White" femininity appears as a depoliticized, "unraced" norm, against which all difference is measured.

If "race" and "racism" are never openly addressed, the theme of a "European body" emerged spontaneously as a central topic in almost all my interviews.[6] Speaking of Portugal as a "white" nation—despite decades of immigration, despite the complexity of colonial and post-colonial relations, and despite of the presence of Afro-Portuguese citizens—the interviewees drew a line that neatly defines what is the European ideal of beauty. To answer the question "What is considered beauty in Portugal today?" one of the interviewees, a well-established professional makeup artist, says:

> In the old days you had that pattern of beauty, the elegant European woman.... But today that is changing. We have so many influences.... It is almost an aggression. And that way we lose the European style that distinguished us.... Brazilian, African, and Russian women arrived. And now we have lost the notion of what being beautiful, elegant, sophisticated is; we have lost our European references, we have lost our culture. We have long gone over the limit; bad taste is now entrenched in Portugal.

In the words of a beauty consultancy and makeup school manager:

> You have that syndrome on the internet, on YouTube. It is almost an aggression: television, music, a continuous disturbance, it actually disrupts.... People even feel bad for not being able to become what the internet shows ... and so they think they have to change, change their look ... they lose their references, our European references.

The insistence on the idea of eroticized beauty patterns penetrating the confines of the European body due to the migration flows of people, images, music, icons, as well as access to social networks, Instagram and YouTube, coupled with the growing importance of influencers, is a constant in the interviews.

The contrast manifested in this interview between, on the one hand, the paradigm of "good taste, elegance, and sobriety" in defining the Portuguese ideal of beauty in Portugal and, on the other hand, the influences that "come from abroad" (such as migrants, or through the internet or TV) is a theme that insistently reappears in every interview. Like a virus, penetrating and invading the permeable "European body," these models have contaminated the taste of Portuguese people, infecting them with flashiness. A young fashion stylist comments:

> It's an exaggerated visual: a lot of curves, lips and chest, wide hips, enormous nails, fake eyelashes, hair extensions, super tanned. And the people who adopt these references are suburban people. You see those women with nails up to here ... you see that more in the periphery. They work in Lisbon, they are Portuguese, but they live in the periphery, with the Brazilians, the Africans ... it's

actually the neighbours that bring that, and over there the people come together, grow similar. In the elites you don't see that. Even if they like it, they'd never admit it to their friends.

In the words of a famous image consultant:

> There is a new wave of beauty: Kardashians, Anitta, something we didn't have ten years ago. Sure, it also depends on the context.... That is what they want in the suburbs. The upper classes in Portugal continue to enjoy a woman with an elegant figure, simple, natural, a luminous skin free of blemishes, with a fresh peach healthy blush... you know, the ideal European urban woman.

Here, another important distinction comes into play: class distinction. The upper-class woman has all the characteristics of elegance and of the European style. In lower classes, the reference models come "from outside." Your style is a class indicator; all my interviewees emphasize a clear distinction between the darker, poorer population and the paler, wealthier class.

The words of another interviewee reinforce the idea of an idealized European beauty:

> The higher classes in Angola and Brazil want to appear European, with super perfect white skin, without even a tiny blemish. In the old days, white women were ashamed to be white; today they are proud, because a tan is no longer in fashion. Being very tanned these days doesn't work... cosmopolitan women, those who know the world, who are informed, know perfectly well what damage the sun causes, the risks of melanoma, of photo-aging. Cultured women more and more want to have a very healthy skin. We let the Brazilians sunbathe... in Europe there is a different consciousness about health that has permeated society. Whiter people look healthier. It means they care about themselves.

Most of my interviewees point out that such aesthetic evaluations cannot be divorced from the racial hierarchies produced by centuries of European and, in this specific case, Portuguese colonial expansion and from the intersections of this past and racist attitudes in the present (Gorjão Henriques 2018). The beauty standards of my interviewees converge with genderism, classism, and racism in ways that select certain bodies as "sloppy," "ordinary," "working-class," "marginal," "suburban," as well as giving them a misleading positive value (the exoticized, eroticized, and hypersexualized body). Examining how appearance is conceptualized in intersection with social class, nationality, profession, and whiteness, the interviewees suggest that the reasons behind the decision to adopt or undertake particular forms of "exotic-looking"[7] cosmetic interventions are linked to the acquisition of an "erotic capital"—beauty, sex appeal, charm, dress sense, liveliness, and fitness—to get ahead in life.

But how is this so highly desired European body imagined? What are its shape, its color, its defining characteristics? In the words of an Argentinian makeup artist, who at the moment trains makeup artists for a famous cosmetic brand:

> I came to Portugal with an image in my head of European beauty, fashion, the elegance ... wanting to be like that. I think it's also that idea ... then, when you're here, you see that it's not quite like that. It's only a fantasy. It's natural in a human being, [it] happens to everyone. Even here in Portugal ... Portuguese women are not like French women—which Portuguese people consider more [truly] European than themselves. They are not so ... elegant. Search in Instagram: in the lower classes you find a false beauty, which is what I call Kardashianization. In the upper classes, it is exactly the opposite: Portuguese women attempt to be thin, classy, like French women.
>
> We think, for instance, that [a woman who] takes care of herself does so with more style: only red lipstick ... some eyeliner, a more classic, more fifties look, the hair up. We who came from abroad try to learn from and adapt to the European style: for instance to do what in the profession we call *classy or sleek makeup*, which is a super-minimalist kind of makeup that makes the skin appear glowing and radiant, but it's as if the person had no makeup at all.
>
> European women represent the very classical beauty: slim figure, tall, blond hair, and blue eyes. It is an ideal! Many Portuguese girls color their hair blond. And it's not just hair coloring ... they also put in blue or green lenses, and they use a foundation that is one or two shades lighter too. A perfect fair complexion is a classic sign of beauty and good health.
>
> When you imagine the "ideal beauty," you are visualizing the typical tall, slender, white, and blond archetype: high cheekbones, lips full, but not *too* full, a narrow nose, large eyes, and in general fair skin. Brazilian and African women have an exaggerated visual. Russian women are closer to the typical blond beauty model. But they too are very loose, very forward, in sexuality, in beauty. ... It's not that it's right or wrong ... but, please, not in a real lady!
>
> Oh, sorry! It's not about you, of course: it's obvious you're classy and totally European!

The interactions between researcher and research participants cannot produce neutral data. The color of my skin, eyes, and hair and my facial features are immediately associated in Portugal with the phenotype of Eastern Europe. This connection placed me in the stereotypical category of a "Russian woman." While it is an aesthetically appreciated phenotype, Eastern women are often associated with sex work and considered—at least in the popular imagination—as having a corrupting influence on Western morals. My appearance pushed me into a kind of phantasmal sphere of second-class citizenship.

If Europeanness has always been a (racialized) construction—even for women who perceive and define themselves as white—apparently my body doesn't fully perform this ideal. If aesthetic economies classify bodies, differentiating who counts as beautiful and valuable, then beauty labor serves the purpose of creating difference through artifice. Consequently, the bodies perceived as "not quite European" can be seen as performatively "making up Europeanness" through stylization, cosmetic alteration, and fashion practices. Europeanness is thus not something that simply is, but it is rather something to be done. Through what Elias, Gill, and Scharff define as "aesthetic entrepreneurship" (2017: 5), anyone can create a body that is read as European and, hence, endowed with capital. The "Europeanization," necessary to an easier integration, can be performatively enacted by cultivating a personal style, through a motivated process of self-making or of aesthetic self-shaping. This appearance investment (Gough, Seymour-Smith, and Matthews 2016) is not limited to the physical body but also involves ways of dressing, personality, diction, relationships, and lifestyle (Elias et al. 2017: 37).

Following the argument of Anika Keinz and Paweł Lewicki in the thematic issue *Who Embodies Europe?* (2019), in the last three years I have explored the desires and strategies deployed by non-white Portuguese and immigrant women to conform to the European body, in order to acquire a specific "aesthetic capital" (Hunter 2011)—embedded in promises of cosmopolitanism, success, and wealth (Mahé and Gounongbe 2004).

The literature dedicated to the growth of investment in biological capital highlights the recent rise and flourishing of a lucrative aesthetic and plastic surgery "ethnic" market in Europe, destined to transform bodies of "inadequate" color or appearance according to ideals of beauty, modernity, and success.[8] According to Perry (2006), Glenn (2008), and Hunter (2005, 2011), the growth of this specific cosmetic market around the globe can be attributed to the constant mass-marketing of contemporary images of "white beauty and lifestyle," which builds on the long-standing colonial ideologies that emphasize the superiority of European culture.

The media have recently drawn attention to skin-whitening practices following the death of some refugees in the reception center of Bussolengo (Verona, Italy), after excessively consuming skin-whitening products in 2016.[9] As the investigations began, the Italian police seized several products containing toxic chemical agents such as mercury chloride and hydroquinone, sold at very affordable prices to immigrants and refugees and marketed as providing clearer, more European skin. It was the opening of a Pandora's box. The practice of skin bleaching for cosmetic purposes in immigrant communities (Mahé 2014) became a matter of public interest. Many blog articles began to appear, and on 28 May 2019 *La Stampa* (Italy's most popular and recognized daily newspaper) dedicated its central pages to bleaching creams, described as the "European obsession of immigrant Nigerian women" ("L'ossessione europea delle donne nigeriane").[10]

As summarized in the article by Pryanka Kalra (2017), for "the ugly immigrant" (Heinö 2014: 148) never considered "beautiful enough" and always in need of "European citizenship," the "yearning for lightness" (Glenn 2008) depends on a desire for social integration.[11] To be beautiful involves, however, labor, costs, pain, and heightened risks.[12] The wish to attenuate the racial markers that separate them from societal standards of "beauty" or "visual neutrality" can be interpreted as tied to the determination to fit into the European standards of the socially valued body.

What are people's motives, desires, and aspirations around shaping an ideal European body? What is the pattern of beauty that's actually desired? What kind of aesthetic labor is in action? Are Europeanness and whiteness commodities that can be possessed, bought, and performed? What are people willing to do in order to get the right shades of whiteness and Europeanness? Is Europeanness a superficial form of styling, or a "style of skin"?

The Beauty and the Bleach

In this section I present ethnographic data about the emergence, in the Greater Lisbon area, of a new market in cosmetic products and treatments aimed at altering physical features that are considered socially undesirable or else devalued according to Euro-centered beauty standards. The aesthetic medicine professionals whom I interviewed defined as "ethnic aesthetic" any intervention geared toward altering "ethnic traits or racial markers" that are considered inharmonious or inadequate according to contemporary beauty patterns. The most sought-after ethnic interventions, the interviewed surgeons say, are eye or nose reshaping or skin whitening. In particular, they mention blepharoplasty or surgery to correct the Asian eyelid (double eyelid), which can sometimes be performed in conjunction with epicanthoplasty (the removal of the inner corner fold in the eye). They also mention rhinoplasty, both in black and Asian individuals, for thinning the nose, making it more salient, defining the tip, and reducing the nasal wings. To quote a health professional in one of the best-known private clinics in the city, this kind of surgery serves to

> create a more open, vivacious, attractive look, which looks less tired and allows for easier application of makeup. Ethnic rhinoplasty improves the wide and flat look of the nose, reducing the disharmony of an excessively wide nose, thus creating a more elegant and delicate look.

With regards to skin, she mentions:

> [There are] hyperpigmentation problems, typical in black skin, which tends to cause spots and irregularities, with excessive darkening. However, the customers that ask for a reduction in discoloration spots or dark skin spots (dermatosis papulosa nigra), in general also want to be given a "whitening." The neck in particular... it looks somewhat dirty, don't you think? With fractioned laser, with a peeling with depigmentation agents, we achieve a better skin.

In the discourse of the physicians interviewed, the use of expressions such as "excessive or exaggerated racial features," in contrast to "classical European beauty," is frequent. The medical discourse and the language of aesthetics both naturalize and re-biologize the idea of "race," dislocating its implications from the historical, political, and social processes that gave birth to it.[13]

A critical reading of colonial medicine's notions of bodily health and European moral superiority is fundamental to understand how certain ideologies are (re)produced today by the contemporary practices—scientific, economic, and cultural—of the aesthetic industry. The main purpose of this chapter, however, is not to reconstruct a genealogy of ethnic aes-

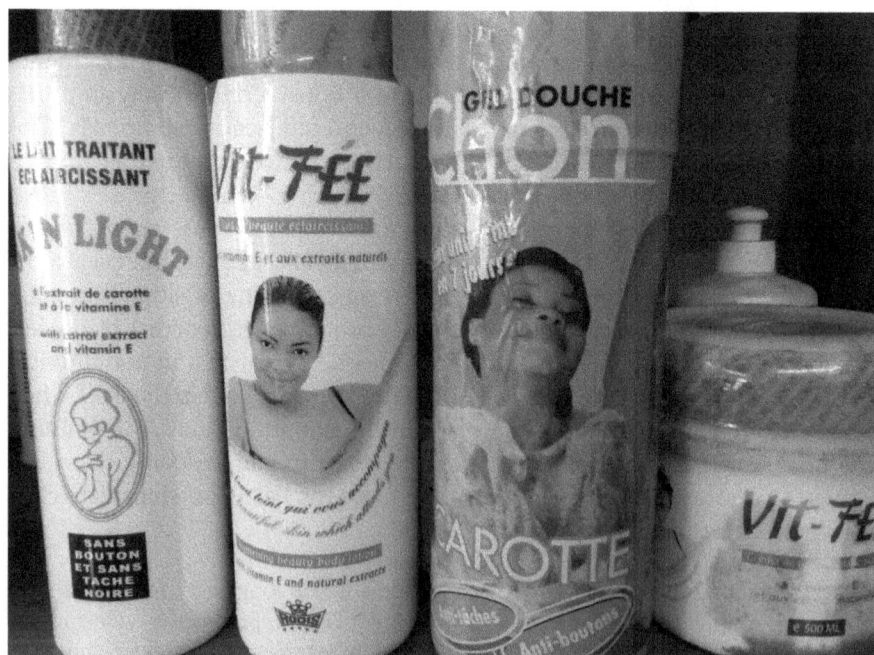

Figure 5.1. Skin-lightening products available at a beauty store in Rua dos Anjos, Lisbon. Photo by the author.

thetic medicine, but rather to highlight the contemporary manifestations of that colonial heritage in interventions that aim to alter "ethnic" characteristics—such as skin bleaching; hair straightening, uncurling, and coloring; and Westernization of the eyes, nose, lips, and facial contours, among others.

In this first phase of this ethnographic study, interviews were conducted primarily with immigrant women and Portuguese women who descend from citizens of every continent.[14] By discussing with them the reasons behind their decision to undertake cosmetic interventions, I have tried to observe their everyday negotiation of gender, ethnic appearance, and social class. I started investigating the interplay between these three variables to better understand the relation between desire and consumption practices, as well as aspirations of inclusion and social mobility, something that Alvaro Jarrín defines as "aesthetic economies" (2015: 535).

If, in fact, the purpose of aesthetic intervention is to correct physical defects and to improve appearance—and therefore self-esteem and quality of life—then the first question we must ask is what we actually consider a defect. The aesthetic industry proposes a set of hegemonic patterns of beauty, avowedly defined as "Caucasian," thereby codifying any exceptions to the norm as imperfections that can be corrected, literally, through specific products or the surgeon's scalpel.

The convergence of new cosmetic biotechnologies and old colonial ideologies has spawned a substantial market for products and procedures, in which consumers can buy "racial capital" in beauty salons and in "ethnic" products stores, as well as in private aesthetics clinics, according to their means.

The female respondents in this project do not seem to consciously express a direct relationship between their aesthetic practices and the desire to alter "ethnic traits." Even when directly confronted with questions about hegemonic patterns of "white" beauty, even those that presented conspicuous body modifications,[15] respondents mention that their ideal of beauty isn't "white," but rather is represented by black celebrities such as Beyoncé, Rihanna, Nicky Minaj, Iman, Trina McGee, Lil Kik, or Keri Hilson.[16]

The youngest Afro-descendants whom I interviewed (from eighteen to twenty-five years of age) mention aesthetic alterations (such as skin bleaching, hair straightening or extensions, fake eyelashes or nails, or wearing a wig) as "style" or "fashion" choices—something that has to do with being considered cool, glamorous, sexy. Despite European social survey data and academic studies indicating that there is a large percentage of the Portuguese who believe in the biological existence of races and who have clearly racist attitudes (Vala, Brito, and Lopes 2005; Rosário et al. 2017; Ramos, Pereira, and Vala 2019), the question of racial discrimination never clearly surfaces in the discourse of my young interviewees. In the words of Sara, a young Afro-European who works as a blogger and fashion influencer:

> It is solely a question of image, how to paint your hair or choosing a certain hairstyle. Or how to tan, how to do makeup. It's not about race, it's about beauty. Chiara, do you paint your hair blond because you are ashamed of your natural color? No! It's because you like it, and it suits you. It's to distinguish yourself from others. To stand out. In the same way as when you wear certain clothes, accessories that draw attention more, to create a style that marks you out. Lately I have whitened my skin, cut and discolored my hair. Next time I'll do lots of braids, the thin ones, down to my ass. Or else I'll grow out my hair, make a fabulous Afro, like a lioness, which is very "fashionable." I never go out without doing makeup and thoroughly thinking through what I'm going to wear. They are aesthetic choices, it's nothing that has to do with race or with problems because I'm black. Mine is an African beauty. To whiten your skin is just like putting on makeup. That way, I can have more followers. All women, black and white, can relate and follow me as an example of style.

She clearly does not want to be "like" a white woman, nor chemically remove the colonial imprinting that continues to mark her black skin through discriminatory stereotypes and racist ideologies still present in Portuguese society. What she wants is to be charming, pretty, elegant, stylish—to feel free to use and manipulate various cultural styles according to context and timing. Today a more European style, tomorrow "some other style," while at the same time defending an ideal of "authentic African beauty" (Ahmed 1998). The practices that Sara engages in—oscillating between affirming identity politics and subjectivation defined by consumer culture—are "self-fashioning practices." Sara mixes and combines *cultural styles* as creative and strategic "intentional communication" (Hebdige 1979). In the words of Ferguson:

> Cultural style is first of all a performative competence.... Thus it is not simply a matter of choosing a style to fit the occasion, for the availability of such choices depends on internalized capabilities of performative competence and ease that must be achieved, not simply adopted. Cultural style thus implies a capability to deploy signs in a way that positions the actor in relation to social categories. (1999: 96)

Both the supposed "European body" and the "African body" depend on a mise-en-scène, which comprises the habits as well as the adequate material and symbolic props that accompany them. In the words of Luana, a young Angolan-born woman who was clearly amused in the face of my provocation:

Not everything is to be seen in black and white [*laughing*]. I don't want to be white at all, God forbid! I just want to be glamorous, like Beyoncé, Mariah Carey, Alicia Keys, Halle Berry, or Rihanna! Beautiful women, powerful and black! Did they whiten their skin? Did Rihanna's eyes change color? Is the hair real? Who cares? They bought the hair and now it's their hair. They are empowered women, who have the money, the time, and who can afford the luxury of changing their eye color if they feel like it! They are women who can do anything: what nature didn't give them, they can buy. To have style is not a question of "races." In the same way that some prefer a rap style, or hip-hop, or funky.

My fieldwork highlights the complexity of the relationship—never made explicit directly and often even denied—between these "cultural styles" and the idea of acquiring "aesthetic capital" as a "passport to privilege" (Dyer 1997: 44), as the hope of integration, and as the promise of cosmopolitanism, modernity, and success.

If younger women discuss "style" at length, more mature women (often first-generation migrants), who possibly carry with them stronger experiences of discrimination and social exclusion, explain that acquiring "white social capital" facilitates integration in their host country, thus in-

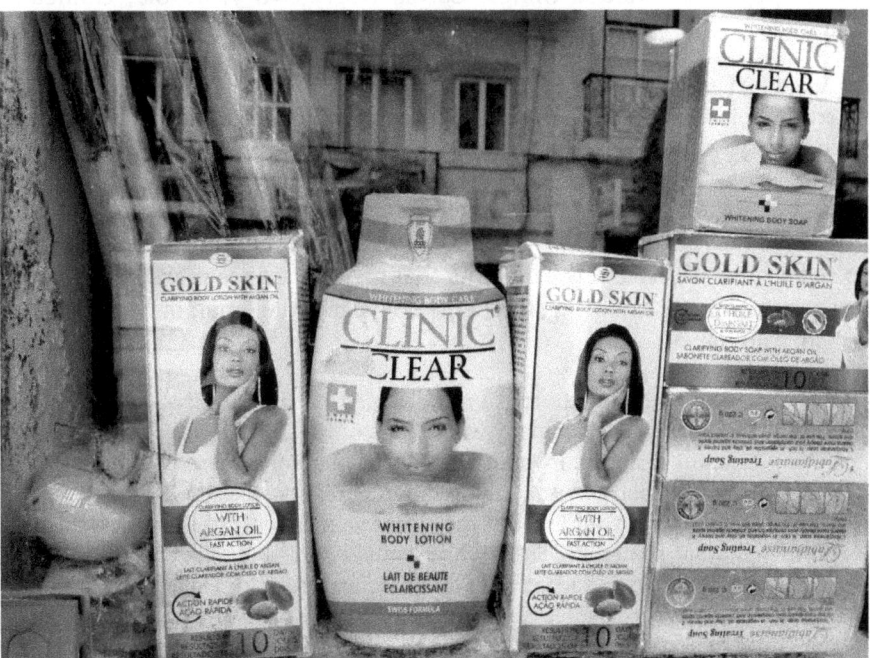

Figure 5.2. Products available at an African beauty salon in the Almirante Reis Avenue, Lisbon. Photo by the author.

creasing their chances of professional upward mobility and better marriage perspectives.

Some of the interviewees mentioned that certain anatomical characteristics, such as skin and especially hair (Banks 2000), are historically imprinted in a negative way by colonial rhetoric, arguing, however, that the desire to alter such characteristics does not mean to erase one's identity. Rather, such alterations are meant solely to increase their chances of success in professional and relationship contexts. As mentioned by Manu, a 32-year-old Angolan makeup artist:

> When there is a cosmetic alteration, whether it's skin bleaching, painting and straightening the hair, having extensions done, not getting fat, not having wrinkles, having painted nails, wearing certain clothes, speaking competently and elegantly, and so on, it's always to better fit into social expectations, regardless of our national or social origins.

The beauty, health, and fitness industries all produce hierarchies connected to gender, class and race, thereby selecting certain bodies as models of "health" and "good looks," while relegating others to the box of old, sloppy, undervalued things. Carola (forty-two years old, Guinean), remarked:

> Adapting here wasn't easy at first. Sometimes you have the feeling of being different, of not belonging here, of not being like the others. And so you try to change in order to achieve a greater well-being.

By employing the expression "well-being," Carola extends the traditional notion of health to include satisfaction with one's own life when it comes to self-expectations and the benefits that an appearance more befitting the host environment can bring. Rachel, a 26-year-old woman of Mozambican origin, told me:

> Beauty is half your wealth. Had I not changed my appearance a little, I would not have worked at the company where I am now [Rachel is a representative for Avon]. And, for instance, I would not now have a Portuguese boyfriend [laughing]. Portuguese men like something different, exotic, like the long thin braids [cornrows] down to your ass. But they want women with style, with sophistication. They want something like a white woman dipped in milk chocolate [laughing]! The ones that don't adapt will make hamburgers at McDonald's, in the back, in the kitchen, where people can't see them. Even in being proud of your origins, nobody wants to have the look of a servant.

Despite stating that she is proud to be black and that she agrees with me in thinking the aesthetic industry promotes a "white" ideal, to the point of not having adequate products for other possible skin tones,[17] at the same Rachel conforms to a "Western" gaze that values a Europeanized "exotic beauty." Her hair is chemically straightened, her skin bleached with high-quality products, and she wears a foundation that's considerably lighter than her natural skin tone:

> Where there is supply, there is demand. Others might even tell you that they don't use these products, or that the people using them are a friend of a friend, or a distant cousin [*laughing*]. But all stores carry them—and mind you, they have them in large amounts—so this means someone buys them. Others will tell you that they only use it here and there for a few darker blemishes. Believe me, this is addictive. You start with one blemish, and all of a sudden it's the whole face, the neck . . . and those who can, they keep going.

Alexa (Cape Verdean, twenty-eight years old) said:

> When I was a child, besides my mother, who always used these creams—all other models of beauty to which I aspired, which I saw on TV or in the movies, were not like me. They toned their skin, surely, like my mother did. Just like the women in the movies that boys loved: J. Lo, Alicia Keys, Whitney Houston. They have fine lines, delicate nose, clear skin. . . . They are lighter and more white-like than me.

Many of the interviewees say that they were introduced to this practice by their own mothers, by close family members, or by people in their closest group of friends. They grew up seeing the women in the household taking care of their bodies—the same products, the same smells, and the same gestures.

Alexa's words are corroborated by another black woman, Portuguese, separated from her husband, who works in a design store and the hipster center of town:

> I started it to remove some blemishes and some acne scars. I started taking better care of my skin. Then another blemish, a few darker spots in the forehead . . . and then you start to get lighter, and in Facebook photos you don't need to touch up so much, you start enjoying being like that . . . but it's not a question of wanting to change to become white, that's absurd! Why do you use red lipstick, for instance? Do you have an issue with the color of your mouth? It's a choice, it's freedom and beauty. Many people buy it, you find it in any store in the city center, at Martim Moniz, Almirante Reis . . . or in the outskirts . . . have you ever been to the Babylon shopping mall?

Even if these practices are not conspicuous, even if there is a degree of compunction or hesitancy in admitting to the use of these cosmetics, skin-bleaching products are extremely common, economical, and easily available at various hotspots in the city center: in grocery stores, in shopping malls, in beauty salons and African, Chinese, and Indian hair salons of Martim Moniz and Almirante Reis Avenue. Among these, the most common are Fair & White, Caro White, Black/White Bleaching Cream, Supreme White Intense, Beneks' Fashion Fair, Crusader Medicated Soap or the best-selling Whitenicious (produced and promoted by Cameroonian-born model and entrepreneur Dencia, famous by the publicity slogan "White means pure"), and Fair & Lovely (produced by Hindustan Unilever and originally present in the Indian, Bangladeshi, Malaysian, Indonesian, Singaporean, Brunei, Thai, Sri Lankan, and Pakistani markets since 1975).

In none of these stores can you find any type of warning or awareness-raising notices about the collateral effects and potential health risks associated with the continuous use of substances such as hydroquinone, corticosteroids, mercury, kojic acid, monobenzone, niacinamide, and other melanin suppressors. Without any kind of pharmacological oversight from Infarmed,[18] without any oversight in terms of the health safety of individual components, and without authorization according to the European Cosmetics Regulation, several products that are illegal (in Portugal, law no. 1223/2009) due to high concentrations of hydroquinone (a substance forbidden in Europe since 2001), corticosteroids, and mercury[19] (mostly originating from India, China, or West Africa) can be easily purchased in ethnic stores. The hustle and bustle of Martim Moniz is the ideal setting for a parallel market in illegally imported substances.

Ana, a woman from Praia (Santiago island, Cape Verde) who works in a Lisbon shopping mall, says:

> In Indian stores there are good products, better than in the African salons. Indians have good pharmacists and they know how to advise you on what to use to remove pigmentation quickly. I use the cream two, three times a day on my face. It bleaches well, but it can cause skin irritation and scaling, and it makes the skin really sensitive to the sun, so you have to use a very strong sunblock. . . . After a few months it's better to stop, give it some time. But not too long, otherwise the skin will become darker again.

Susana, another woman born in Mindelo (São Vicente island, Cape Verde), intervenes:

> I, on the contrary, have never thought about bleaching my skin. I am lucky, and my skin is already quite clear. When my daughter was born she was so beautiful, super-clear skin; she looks like a little angel. As for the hair . . . the hair has always been a problem, in fact. My mother, who is one of those much whiter Cape Verdeans with very pretty curly hair, like Brazilians have, spent her days trying to tame, straighten, braid my hair. Even now, she insists I should do something. If

Shaping the European Body 109

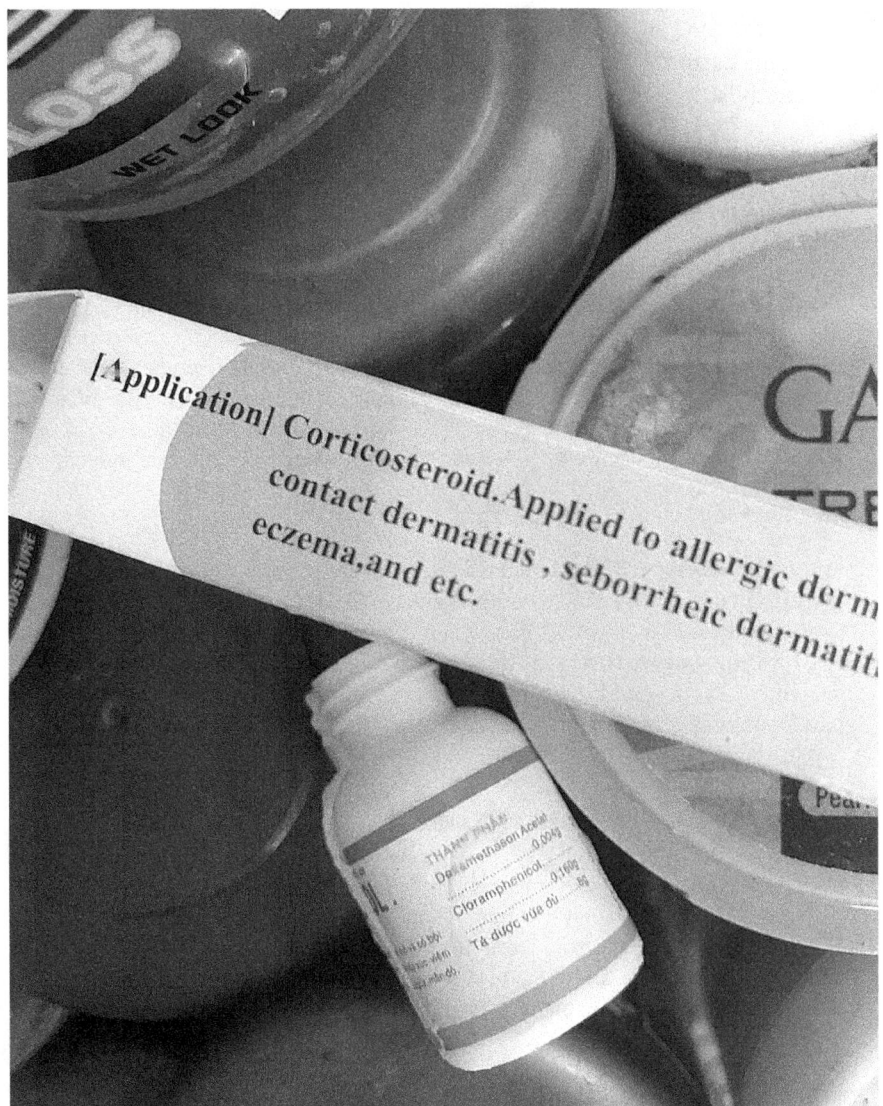

Figure 5.3. Skin-lightening product with corticosteroids in a small Pakistani market in Avenida Almirante Reis, Lisbon. Photo by the author.

I am careless for a moment, she immediately tells me: Oh child! It's not like you! You look like one of the girls that never left the village.

We mustn't forget that in the body of any black woman, any choice of style, fashion, aesthetic treatment, or even relationship ends up being politicized and the target of evaluations or judgment, even within the Afro-descendent community itself. Jessica, a young Portuguese born in Guinea and an activist in a black feminist group, explains:

> I tried using these creams once, a cream that a friend bought in Dakar. She said it was only to improve the look of acne scars, which were bothering me. But my face started changing color. I thought: Holy smokes! I'm becoming white! God forbid! [*Laughs.*] I stopped immediately and I started trying to convince my friend to stop using that crap. Especially if she wants to join this movement ... she would be the target of attacks, she would be shamed ... one must love to learn one's own negritude. Because people already criticize you if you straighten your hair, if you date a white guy, if you frequent circles of white friends ... it triggers the impression that you're reproducing familiar "whitening" dynamics. Which is undoubtedly an important historical question. But when you can't even choose how you do your hair or who you date, then it's a lot of surveillance indeed!

Vanda, a young Afro-European, said:

> In school, I always felt that white colleagues were prettier. We all want to be appreciated, right? You know what they always liked about me in school? My ass! [*She says this with a laugh, but also with a degree of bitterness.*] I wasn't the pretty girl. I was the one with the sexy, tight ass that boys commented on out loud, saying what they imagined they'd do to me ... I was mortified with shame ... they said I was as sexy as an animal ... they called me the "sexy beast."

The Beauty and the Beasts

> "All animals are equal, but some animals are more equal than others."
> ... No question, now, what had happened to the faces of the pigs.
> The creatures outside looked from pigs to men,
> and from men to pigs, and from pigs to men again.
> But already it was impossible to say which was which.
> —George Orwell, *Animal Farm*

Feminist and disability studies have thoroughly analyzed the political and normative dimensions of beauty hegemonic standards in body modification practices, shifting the focus from the individual to the social dynamics in which they are enmeshed (see, e.g., Bordo 1993; Davis 1995; Weitz 2003; Toffoletti 2007; Heyes and Jones 2009; Eilers, Grüber, and Rehmann-Sutter 2014). They have argued that beauty practices are an exercise in patriarchal power that disciplines, normalizes, and medicalizes the female body.

Several authors question the impact of European or Western beauty standards on nonwhite bodies in different countries in Africa, Asia, or South America. However, the way "race" shapes the bodies of women who perceived themselves as "white" has not been a major focus of anthropological research. The pressure to adopt styles and attitudes consistent with an imposed "pure white" feminine aesthetic affects all the women—especially those who by origin, social class, neighborhood of residence, or profession are considered as "not European enough."

Lightening and depigmenting skin products are sold in every perfumery, drugstore, and pharmacy in several European countries (especially the United Kingdom, due to the high South Asian population, and Germany and France, due to massive population from North Africa and from Africa south of Sahara) and in southern European countries like Portugal, Italy, Greece, and Spain, considered more tenuously European than others and known by the discriminant acronym "PIGS." Stereotypically perceived by the northern European gaze as "swarthy bronze looking," tanned and with "olive skin"—a mixture of "Arabs," "Middle Eastern," or "North Africans"—the PIGS[20] are somewhat exotic and outside of the European standard. PIGS are stereotyped as lazy and untrustworthy people who waste money on "wine and women"—as stated two years ago Jeroen Dijsselbloem, the chairman of Eurogroup, in a German newspaper. Echoing long-standing colonial ideologies, PIGS are characterized as lazy, unprofessional, corrupt, too emotional, "hot" and sensual Latin lovers, temperamental, and more open and warm than the rest of Europe. In short, they are a kind of second-class European citizens that are not able to keep up with their more sophisticated northern neighbors (Satzewich 2000; Mamadouh 2017; Sierp and Karner 2017).

This image—which continues to shape modern European everyday realities—is based on a silent but powerful discourse on European cultural hierarchies that conflates essentialized national representations with lifestyles, class, sexuality, beauty ideals, and skin color. Europeanness is a construction, a work in progress that "inheres in subjectivity, as well as in bodies, social relationships and social activities. . . . It is simultaneously structural and personal" (Knowles 2008: 168–69). How, for what reasons, and through which stylization practices someone might be fully integrated in the category "European"—and what are the consequences of being included or not in that category—is a complex historical narrative, intimately connected to the social construction of whiteness.[21] Alastair Bonnett provides a critical history of the conflation of European and white identities, highlighting that the excessive idealization of this identification is related to the gradual marginalization of less-white people through ethnic and class hierarchies: "The history of the Europeanization of whiteness is narrative of the ability to marginalize and forget other forms of white identity and to create, assert and disseminate a particular vision of human difference" (Bonnett 1998: 1029).

This conflation of whiteness and Europeanness continues to signal social and cultural capital to this day. A flawless white skin remains a key benchmark for standards of physical beauty, social integration, and class worth. Quoting Laura, forty-two years old, a dermatologist:

> You know, there is this idea that the Portuguese are the darkest-skinned people in Europe. While that could be true, most of that idea comes from the fact that when most tourists go to Portugal is precisely when the Portuguese are most tan. Until recently Portuguese people were considered as *pigs: ugly, dirty, and bad.* Today we are finally investing in ourselves ... we care about the health of our skin, we remove sun spots, age spots, freckles, and skin hyperpigmentation using several cosmetic products and technologies such as peeling or laser. Today we can buy the best products on the market and we can get a healthier, bright, radiant and perfect skin.

In Lisbon's pharmacies, supermarkets, and perfume stores, products for skin depigmentation are positioned in the most visible displays, at consumer eye level. In a single week of research in pharmacies, perfume stores, and supermarkets in the center of Lisbon, I assembled an incredible list of famous skin-bleaching products whose name is associated with "pure," "white," or "clean" beauty (table 5.1).

Table 5.1. List of products found in the main perfumeries of the city center of Lisbon.

White Perfect (l'Oréal)	White Active (l'Oréal)
White Lucent (Shiseido)	Blanc Expert (Lancôme)
Whitening (Dove)	Even Better White (Clinique)
Derma White Brightening (Clinique)	Anew Clinical Luminosity Pro Brightening (Avon)
Le Blanc Serum Blanchissant (Chanel)	White Essentiel (Chanel)
Whitening Model Effect (Chanel)	White Caviar Illuminating and Whitening Lotion (La Prairie)
Intensive Whitening (La Prairie)	Illuminating Pearl Infusion (La Prairie)
Pigment White Brightening (Filorga)	White Objective (Bioderma)
Pigment Control (Talika)	Nuxe Intensive Whitening (Nuxe)
Whitening Light (Garnier)	White Complete (Garnier)
Blanc de Perle (Guerlain)	Perfect White Excellence (Guerlain)
Brightening Orchidée Impériale White (Guerlain)	Even Brighter (Eucerin)

Shaping the European Body   113

Fluide Éclaircissant (Vichy)	Intensive Whitening (La Prairie)
Illuminating Pearl Infusion (La Prairie)	Pigment White Brightening (Filorga)
White Objective (Bioderma)	Pigment Control (Talika)
Nuxe Intensive Whitening (Nuxe)	Whitening Light (Garnier)
White Complete (Garnier)	Blanc de Perle (Guerlain)
Perfect White Excellence (Guerlain)	Brightening Orchidée Impériale White (Guerlain)
Even Brighter (Eucerin)	Fluide Éclaircissant (Vichy)
Crescent White (Estee Lauder)	Supreme Light + (Estee Lauder)
White Prestige (Dior)	DiorSnow White Reveal (Dior)
Ideal White (Vichy)	Ideal White (Carita)
Blanc Divin (Givenchy)	Fine Fireness (Neutrogena)
Depiderm White (Uriage)	White Light (Diego dalla Palma)
Advanced White Radiance (Lancer)	Snow White Cream (Secret Key)
Pure White (Rahul Phate)	Sérum White Diamant (Eisenberg Paris)
Whitening Corrector Intense (Eisenberg Paris)	Whitening Treatment (GlamGlow)
Pure Cleansing Lotion Clarifiant (Juvena of Switzerland)	Illuminating Porcelain Flower (Perfect Focus, Douglas)
Light as Air Mask (Aqua Focus, Douglas)	Miracle Glow (Instant)
Blanc de Creme (Erborian Korean Skin Therapy)	Porcelain Skin (Tri-Luma)
Enhanced Brightening Pearl Skin (Foreo)	Special White (Collistar)
Deep Clean Brightening (Neutrogena)	Clean Whitening (Sensi)
White Glow (Lotus)	White Radiance (Olay)
Skin Revival Superheroes White (Oskia)	Magic White Ice (Arcona)
Refined White (Molton Brown)	Diamond White (Natura Bissé)
White Marble (Erno Laszlo)	White Brilliance Porcelain (Murad)
Essential White (Yon-Ka Paris)	Purely White Skin (Jurlique)
Wedding Dress White Cream (It's Skin)	Positively Radiant (Aveeno)
Lightening White (Swiss Perfection)	B.RIGHT! Whitening Skincare Set (Benefit)
Perfecting White (Boscia)	Lightening Pigment Gel (NeoStrata)
Lumilogie (Lierac)	Pigment Zero (MartiDerm)
Pigment Expert (ISDINceutis)	Melaperfect (Darphin)
Blanc Pureté Sublime (Galénic)	Beauty without spots (Sesderma)

A quick look at the names of the products listed suffices to notice the association of the idea of whiteness with extremely positive elements. White skin is "beautiful," "perfect," "classy," "better," "excellent," "prestigious," "ideal," "pure," "clean," "healthy," "divine," "magical," a true "miracle." The elements associated with white skin are quite precious and/or pure, such as "snow," "diamonds," "pearls," or "porcelain." If we attempt to enlarge our search, to include not only products that explicitly employ the words "white" or "whitening," but also those that employ definitions such as "brightening," "glowing," "fairness," "lightening," or "illuminating," the list grows significantly longer, but the underlying message is always that of whitening as a strategy of skin *improvement.*

Mass media is incredibly pervasive in our society; constant and readily available, it permeates our everyday lives. The global beauty industry, the same as the fashion and music industries, presents (in magazine covers, advertisements, music videos, Instagram, and so on) a whitewashed ideal of beauty. The most famous cosmetic product brands—which can normally be found in perfume stores, pharmacies, and supermarkets—carry messages in their names as well as in their publicity slogans that reinforce existing stereotypes. The message conveyed is that of whitening as a strategy for aesthetic as well as moral optimization. An analysis of the moral economies (Fassin 2009) associated with such hegemonic aesthetic norms can in fact reveal how positive moral characteristics and positive values are associated with light-skinned individuals (Dion et al. 1972; Eagly et al. 1991). Social studies show that individuals corresponding to dominant aesthetic patterns are also considered more intelligent (Kanazawa and Kovar 2004), healthier (Jones et al. 2001), more competent and more efficient in a professional setting (Ruetzler et al. 2012), more captivating and engaging in social settings (Hope and Mindell 1994), but also that they are considered purer, more sincere, and more honest—in short, better people.[22]

This idealized representation of beauty first of all promotes a standard body type with high regulatory capacity and, therefore, instrumental in practices of exclusion and discrimination of "other bodies" that do not conform to the ideal. The diversity of "other bodies"—not white, not blond, not skinny, not tall, without fine features, not normative—becomes a "defect" that needs to be corrected. Secondly, evoking the virtue, chastity, honor, purity, and elegance of the European lady, it classifies bodies, not only creating a color line between civilized Europe and the "Rest," but also hierarchizing the population within Europe.

In this sense beauty is a (racialized) construction for all women, including Portuguese women who perceive and define themselves as white who continue to use products that are at once "racially labeled," "racialized" (based on colonial ideas of racial hierarchies), and "racializing" (reproducing these race-based hierarchies and the embodied effects of structural racism). All my interviewees, in one way or another, are compelled to adopt a "whitified" style coherent with an imposed middle-class, cisgender feminine aesthetic, through a specific "appearance investment" called by Elizabeth Wissinger the "European glamour labor" (2015: 3). Understanding the biopolitical, affective, and visceral dimensions of beauty imposes a critical rethinking of the historical, social, and economic relations involved, of the transnational flows of values, images, and desires, and of the different shades, lexicons, and narratives on the basis of which people incorporate discriminatory and racializing patterns. It is necessary and urgent today to reconsider women's aesthetic choices through the lens of style, aesthetics, and agency, their narratives and intimate moments regarding modifications and experiences of their bodies. Understanding how women actively negotiate their beauty expectations and desires involving nationality, race, gender, class, political orientation, and more is a first step toward an aesthetic decolonization of bodies, images, and desires.

Acknowledgments

The research presented in this chapter is part of and supported by the project EXCEL: The Pursuit of Excellence; Biotechnologies, Enhancement and Body Capital in Portugal (PTDC/SOC-ANT/30572/2017), financed by the Portuguese Foundation for Science and Technology and led by Chiara Pussetti (website: www.excelproject.eu).

Chiara Pussetti is currently auxiliary researcher at Institute of Social Sciences of the University of Lisbon. Over the last eighteen years, she has lectured at graduate and postgraduate levels in Italy, Portugal, and Brazil and has researched and published extensively on the subjects of migration, health care, gender, body and emotions, social inequality, suffering, and well-being in urban contexts. She is also principal investigator of the project EXCEL: The Pursuit of Excellence; Biotechnologies, Enhancement and Body Capital in Portugal (PTDC/SOC-ANT/30572/2017).

Notes

1. While conducting questionnaires and qualitative surveys on a national scale has proved to be important for revealing beauty trends and ideals in Portugal, ethnography provided the central tool of research, employing participant observation, informal and semi-structured interviews, and life histories. In the first phase of fieldwork, I have undertaken participant observation in private clinics, beauty salons, and cosmetic product stores, and I have conducted indepth interviews with 12 men (7 health professionals and 5 fashion and beauty

professionals) and 42 women (6 health professionals, 14 beauty professionals, and 22 patients/consumers). I have also gathered 12 life stories connected to "ethnic" aesthetic practices, according to a person-centered ethnography method. All interviews were conducted under the guidelines, codes of conduct, and ethical procedures commensurate with anthropological and ethnographic research standards. Participation in this study is always entirely voluntary, and all participants are informed about the contents and objectives of the research, as well as the intended outputs.
2. The theme of the exotic and erotic body of the "Black Venus"—that is at once scandalously attractive, monstrous, threatening, available, voracious, icon of sexuality, and a metaphor for the colonial penetration of virgin, wild lands—is one of the most common topics in all colonial literature.
3. These images are entrenched within colonial narratives, both in their representations sculpted from "snow-white ivory" (white material from the tusks and teeth of animals, gained by controlling foreign lands) and in the portraits of semitranslucent and delicate porcelain). Porcelain—also called "white gold"—was extremely valued for its delicacy and for its exotic origins. Marco Polo first brought it to Europe, from China, in the fourteenth century (Gleeson 1999).
4. Delacroix's famous painting *Women of Algiers in Their Apartment* represents a milestone for Orientalism in the arts and for the construction of the eroticized, voyeuristic male gaze and the projection of the "Western" fears, fantasies, and desires.
5. A critical understanding of the tropical climate etiology and colonial medical construction of the "Caucasian corporeal health and moral superiority" is a key to analyzing the exclusive cultural and economic privileges the European body accrues (Frankenberg 1993; Dávila 2003; Carbonell Laforteza 2015). At the same time, to address colonial literature on ethnic features and dark skin tone and texture as signs of savagery, inferiority, uncontrolled and libertarian hypersexuality, dysgenic malformations, racial degeneration, lack of corporeal hygiene, faulty morphological structure, and degenerative idleness is fundamental to understanding the disadvantaged social position of several immigrants and ethnic minorities today.
6. Namely, professional makeup artists, image consultants, fashion producers, modeling agency managers, models, managers at cosmetics companies, hairstylists, aestheticians, and managers at spas and cosmetic medicine centers.
7. Such as, for instance, BBL (Brazilian butt lift) surgery, "Latina" melanin tanning injections, or breast implants (Arrizón 1999; Edmonds 2010; Lloréns 2013).
8. The American Society of Plastic Surgeons defines as "ethnic medicine and cosmetic surgery" the practice of altering the physical traits of Africans, Asians, Latin, and Middle Eastern people. The use of the term "ethnic" in a medical context to describe any aesthetic procedure targeting "nonwhite" people raises interesting questions from an anthropological perspective (Boodman 2007; Heyes 2009; Wen 2013).
9. The percentage of people who have suffered the collateral effects of voluntary depigmentation is dramatically high (Vassallo 2009). The negative effects of mercury on human beings are well documented and include not only damage to the skin, but damage to the central nervous system and retarded neurological development in children (Fattori 2007).

10. Simoncelli Lorenzo, "Fra creme sbiancanti e mix letali di pillole, l'ossessione europea delle donne nigeriane, *La Stampa*, 28 May 2019.
11. In other works I have addressed the contemporary consequences in the health and aesthetic industry of colonial medical literature on ethnic features and dark skin tones as signs of savagery, inferiority, tropical pathology, pigmentation disorder, faulty morphological structure, environmental pollution, and racial degeneration (Pussetti 2015a, 2015b, 2019).
12. The use of skin-bleaching products has reached pandemic proportions, becoming one of the most severe dermatological public health problems around the world. This ranges from creams to lotions, pills, injections, intravenous drips, suppository, soaps, baking soda, bleach or even lye, as well as chemical agents like mercurous chloride and hydroquinone, often applied also to children (Souza 2008).
13. For reflections on the reintroduction of race as a biological entity in aesthetic clinical practice and in the cosmetic industry, see Whitmarsh and Jones 2010; Morning 2011; Roberts 2011; Bliss 2012; Pollock 2012; Inda 2014; Duster 2015.
14. At this stage of fieldwork, I've focused primarily on women for two reasons: on the one hand, because of the greater ease in creating trust and empathy and, on the other hand, because they are the biggest consumers of aesthetic products and procedures.
15. Such as skin bleaching, hair extensions and straightening, and surgical correction of facial lines. However, only two individuals, among all the interviewees, underwent rhinoplasty for reducing the nasal wings, as well as nasal tip projection and refinement, and they reported only functional motivations such as improvement in breathing and reducing allergic sinusitis.
16. In the first interviews conducted among women of Indian or Chinese origin, they mention as their ideal models of beauty some Bollywood actresses (among the most mentioned are Kajol, Priyanka Chopra, Shilpa Shetty, Rekha, and Bipasha Basu) and Chinese models and actresses (Yang Mi, Fan Bingbing, Godrey Gao, Zhang Ziyi, Fan Bingbing, Lin Xinru). Of that list, all have had aesthetic procedures such as chemical skin bleaching and Westernizing blepharoplasty.
17. The first person to launch a makeup line with forty tones of foundation was Rihanna, who owns the company Fenty Beauty.
18. The National Authority of Medicines and Health Products (Infarmed) is tasked with the regulation and oversight of medication and health products in Portugal (including medical devices, as well as cosmetic and bodily hygiene products), according to the highest standards in public health safety, thereby ensuring the quality, efficacy, and safety of such products, and guaranteeing that citizens and health professionals can access them.
19. See "Illegal Skin Lighteners," Southwark Council website, retrieved 26 April 2019 from https://www.southwark.gov.uk/business/trading-standards-and-food-safety/illegal-skin-lighteners; Westerhof and Kooyers 2005.
20. "PIGS" is a derisive acronym currently used in economics and finance. The PIGS acronym originally refers, often derogatorily, to the economies of the southern European countries of Portugal, Italy, Greece, and Spain.
21. For a brief review of recent works on the social construction of "whiteness" in literary, historical, and ethnographic research, see, e.g., Roediger 1991; Ware 1992; Frankenberg 1993; Jacobson 1998; Rosenthal 2004; Poitevin 2011; Fox,

Moroşanu, and Szilassy 2015; Garner 2016; Bambra 2017; and Lewicki 2019.
22. Garnham (2013: 44) explains how, in contemporary society, the body "becomes the surface of inscription for the choices one makes and can be read in terms of its virtue. Looking 'good' or an attractive appearance thus signifies the ethical subject." The connection between morality and beauty is forged from the earliest age: in children's stories, the ugly is always the bad, and the bad—even if apparently beautiful—ultimately reveals that, beyond an illusion, they actually look terrible (Baker-Sperry and Grauerholz 2003; Baumann 2008; Bazzini et al. 2010; Lorenzo, Biesanz, and Human 2010).

References

Ahmed, Sara. 1998. *Differences that Matter: Feminist Theory and Postmodernism*. Cambridge: Cambridge University Press.
Arrizón, Alicia. 1999. *Latina Performance: Traversing the Stage*. Bloomington: Indiana University Press.
Baker-Sperry, Lori, and Liz Grauerholz. 2003. "The Pervasiveness and Persistence of the Feminine Beauty Ideal in Children's Fairy Tales." *Gender & Society* 17(5): 711–26.
Bambra, Gurminder K. 2017. "Brexit, Trump, and 'Methodological Whiteness': On the Misrecognition of Race and Class." *British Journal of Sociology* 68(S1): 214–32.
Banks, Ingrid. 2000. *Hair Matters: Beauty, Power, and Black Women's Consciousness*. New York: New York University Press.
Barkan, Elazar. 1992. "Rethinking Orientalism: Representations of 'Primitives' in Western Culture at the Turn of the Century." *History of European Ideas* 15(4–6): 759–66.
Baumann, Shyon. 2008. "The Moral Underpinnings of Beauty: A Meaning-Based Explanation for Light and Dark Complexions in Advertising." *Poetics* 36(1): 2–23.
Bazzini, Doris, Lisa Curtin, Serena Joslin, Shilpa Regan, and Denise Martz. 2010. "Do Animated Disney Characters Portray and Promote the Beauty-Goodness Stereotype?" *Journal of Applied Social Psychology* 40(10): 2687–709.
Bliss, Catherine. 2012. *Race Decoded: The Genomic Fight for Social Justice*. Stanford, CA: Stanford University Press.
Bonnett, Alaister. 1998. "Who Was White? The Disappearance of Non-European White Identities and the Formation of European Racial Whiteness." *Ethnic and Racial Studies* 21(6): 1029–55.
Boodman, Sandra. 2007. "Cosmetic Surgery Goes Ethnic." *Washington Post*, 29 May 2007. Retrieved 3 December 2016 from http://www.washingtonpost.com/wp-dyn/content/article/2007/05/25/AR2007052502387.html.
Bordo, Susan. 1993. *Unbearable Weight: Feminism, Western Culture, and the Body*. Berkeley: University of California Press.
Carbonell Laforteza, Elaine Marie. 2015. *The Somatechnics of Whiteness and Race: Colonialism and Mestiza Privilege*. Surrey, Burlington: Ashgate.
Cogenau, Oana. 2015. "Travelling Ideologies: A Story of Whiteness." *Linguaculture* 2: 15–32.

Dávila, Jerry 2003. *Diploma of Whiteness. Race and Social Policy in Brazil, 1917–1945.* Durham and London: Duke University Press.
Davis, Kathy. 1995. *Reshaping the Female Body: The Dilemma of Cosmetic Surgery.* New York: Routledge.
Del Giudice, Pascal, and Pinier Yves. 2002. "The Widespread Use of Skin Lightening Creams in Senegal: A Persistent Public Problem in West Africa." *International Journal of Dermatology* 41(2): 69–72.
Deliovsky, Kathy. 2008. "Normative White Femininity: Race, Gender and the Politics of Beauty. *Atlantis* 33(1): 49–59.
Diaz, Félix. 2018. *Body Image as an Everyday Problematic: Looking Good.* New York: Routledge.
Dion, Karen, Ellen Berscheid, and Elaine Walster. 1972. "What Is Beautiful Is Good." *Journal of Personality and Social Psychology* 24: 285–90.
Dobson, Joanne. 1991. "Portraits of the Lady: Imagining Women in Nineteenth-Century." *American Literary History* 3(2): 396–404.
Duster, Troy. 2015. "A Post-Genomic Surprise: The Molecular Reinscription of Race in Science, Law and Medicine." *British Journal of Sociology* 66(1): 1–27.
Dyer, Richard. 1997. *White.* London: Routledge.
Eagly, Alice H., Richard D. Ashmore, Mona G. Makhijani, and Laura C Longo. 1991. "What Is Beautiful Is Good, but . . . : A Meta-analytic Review of Research on the Physical Attractiveness Stereotype." *Psychological Bulletin* 110: 109–28.
Edmonds, Alexander 2010. *Pretty Modern: Beauty, Sex, and Plastic Surgery in Brazil.* Durham, NC: Duke University Press.
Eilers, Miriam, Katrin Grüber, and Christopher Rehmann-Sutter. 2014. *The Human Enhancement Debate and Disability: New Bodies for a Better Life.* Manchester: Palgrave Macmillan.
Elias, Ana Sofia, Rosalind Gill, and Christina Scharff (eds.). 2017. *Aesthetic Labour: Rethinking Beauty Politics in Neoliberalism.* Manchester: Palgrave Macmillan.
Fassin, Didier. 2009. "Les Économies Morales Revisitées." *Annales. Histoire, Sciences Sociales* 64(6): 1237–66.
Fattori, Vittorio. 2007. "Evaluation of Toxicity on the Developing Nervous System Induced by Some Environmental Contaminants: Methyl Mercuryn and Polychlorinated Biphenyls (PCBs)." PhD dissertation. Università di Bari.
Ferguson, James. 1999. *Expectations of Modernity: Myths and Meanings of Urban Life on the Zambian Copperbelt.* Berkeley: University of California Press.
Forth, Christopher E. 2012. "Feature: Race, Bodies and Beauty: Fat, Desire and Disgust in the Colonial Imagination." *History Workshop Journal* 73: 211–39.
Fox, Jon E., Laura Moroşanu, and Eszter Szilassy. 2015. "Denying Discrimination: Status, 'Race,' and the Whitening of Britain's New Europeans." *Journal of Ethnic and Migration Studies* 41(5): 729–48.
Frankenberg, Ruth. 1993. *Race Matters: The Social Construction of Whiteness.* Minneapolis: University of Minnesota Press.
Garner, Steve. 2016. *A Moral Economy of Whiteness.* London: Routledge.
Garnham, Bridget. 2013. "Designing Older rather than Denying Ageing: Problematizing Anti-ageing Discourse in Relation to Cosmetic Surgery Undertaken by Older People." *Journal of Aging Studies* 27(1): 38–46.
Gillespie, Marcia Ann. 2003. "Mirror Mirror." In Rose Weitz (ed.), *The Politics of Women's Bodies.* New York: Oxford University Press, pp. 201–95.

Gleeson, Janet. 1999. *The Arcanum: Extraordinary True Story of the Invention of European Porcelain.* New York: Transworld.
Glenn, Evelynn Nakano. 2008. "Yearning for Lightness: Transnational Circuits in the Marketing and Consumption of Skin Lighteners." *Gender & Society* 22(3): 281–302.
———. 2009. *Shades of Difference: Why Skin Color Matters.* Stanford, CA: Stanford University Press.
Gorjão Henriques, Joana. 2018. *Racismo no País dos Brancos Costumes.* Lisboa: Tinta da China.
Gough, Brendan, Sarah Seymour-Smith, and Christopher R. Matthews. 2016. "Body Dissatisfaction, Appearance Investment, and Wellbeing: How Older Obese Men Orient to 'Aesthetic Health.'" *Psychology of Men & Masculinity* 17(1): 84–91.
Hebdige, Dick. 1979. *Subculture: The Meanings of Style.* London: Routledge.
Heinö, Andreas Johansson. 2014. "Sex and Sin in a Multicultural Sweden." In M. Demker, Y. Leffler, and O. Sigurdson (eds.), *Culture, Health, and Religion at the Millennium Sweden Unparadised.* New York: Palgrave Macmillan, pp. 133–54.
Heyes, Cressida. 2009. "All Cosmetic Surgery Is 'Ethnic': Asian Eyelids, Feminist Indignation, and the Politics of Whiteness.' In Cressida J. Heyes and Meredith R. Jones (eds.), *Cosmetic Surgery: A Feminist Primer.* Burlington: Ashgate, pp. 191–205.
Heyes, Cressida J., and Meredith R. Jones (eds.). 2009. *Cosmetic Surgery: A Feminist Primer.* Burlington: Ashgate.
Hope, Debra A., and Jodi A. Mindell. 1994. "Global Social Skill Ratings: Measures of Social Behavior or Physical Attractiveness?" *Behaviour Research and Therapy* 32(4): 463–69.
Hunter, Margaret. 2005. *Race, Gender, and the Politics of Skin Tone.* New York: Routledge.
———. 2011 "Buying Racial Capital: Skin-Bleaching and Cosmetic Surgery in a Globalized World." *Journal of Pan African Studies* 4(4): 142–64.
Inda, Jonathan Xavier. 2014. *Racial Prescriptions Pharmaceuticals, Difference, and the Politics of Life.* Burlington: Ashgate.
Jacobson, Matthew Frye. 1998. *Whiteness of a Different Color: European Immigrants and the Alchemy of Race.* Cambridge, MA: Harvard University Press.
Jarrín, Alvaro. 2015. "Towards a Biopolitics of Beauty: Eugenics, Aesthetic Hierarchies and Plastic Surgery in Brazil." *Journal of Latin American Cultural Studies* 24(4): 535–52.
Jones, Benedict, Anthony C. Little, Ian S. Penton-Voak, Bernard P. Tiddeman, D. Michael Burt, and David I. Perrett. 2001. "Facial Symmetry and Judgements of Apparent Health: Support for a 'Good Genes' Explanation of the Attractiveness-Symmetry Relationship." *Evolution and Human Behavior* 22(6): 417–29.
Kalra, Pryanka. 2017. "'The Ugly Refugee'—Brown Skin and White Beauty Standards." *Friktion*, 9 September. Retrieved 5 May 2018 from https://friktionmagasin.dk/the-ugly-refugee-brown-skin-and-white-beauty-standards-38d0246ec2bd.
Kanazawa, Satoshi, and Jody L. Kovar. 2004. "Why Beautiful People Are More Intelligent." *Intelligence* 32: 227–43.
Keinz, Anika, and Pawel Lewicki. 2019. "Who Embodies Europe? Explorations into the Construction of European Bodies." *Anthropological Journal of European Cultures* 28(1): 7–24.

Knowles, Caroline. 2008. "The Landscape of Post-Imperial Whiteness in Rural Britain. *Ethnic and Racial Studies* 31(1): 167–84.
Lake, Marilyn, and Reynolds, Henry. 2008. *Drawing the Global Colour Line: White Men's Countries and the Question of Racial Equality*. Melbourne: Melbourne University Publishing.
Lewis, Reina. 1996. *Gendering Orientalism: Race, Femininity and Representation*. London: New York: Routledge.
Lloréns, Hilda. 2013. "Latina Bodies in the Era of Elective Aesthetic Surgery." *Latino Studies* 11(4): 547–69.
Lorenzo, Genevieve L., Jeremy C. Biesanz, and Lauren J. Human. 2010. "What Is Beautiful Is Good and More Accurately Understood: Physical Attractiveness and Accuracy in First Impressions of Personality." *Psychological Science* 21(12): 1777–82.
Mahé, Antoine, and Ari Gounongbe. 2004. "The Cosmetic Use of Bleaching Products in Dakar, Senegal: Socio-economic Factors and Claimed Motivations." *Sciences Sociales et Santé* 22(2): 5–33.
Mahé, Antoine. 2014. "The Practice of Skin-Bleaching for a Cosmetic Purpose in Immigrant Communities." *Journal of Travel Medicine* 21(4): 282–7.
Mamadouh, Virginie 2017. "National and Supranational Stereotypes in Geopolitical Representations of the European Union." *L'Espace Politique* 32(2): 7–32.
Manderson, Lenore, and Margaret Jolly (eds.). 1997. *Sites of Desire/Economies of Pleasure: Sexualities in Asia and the Pacific*. Chicago: University of Chicago Press.
Markowitz, Sally. 2001. "Pelvic Politics: Sexual Dimorphism and Racial Difference." *Signs* 26(2): 389–414.
Morning, Ann. 2011. *The Nature of Race: How Scientists Think and Teach about Human Difference*. Berkeley: University of California Press.
Morris, Michael 2016. "Standard White: Dismantling White Normativity." *California Law Review* 104(4, article 3): 948–78.
Perry, Imani. 2006. "Buying White Beauty." *Cardozo Journal of Law and Gender* 12: 579–607.
Poitevin, Kimberly. 2011. "Inventing Whiteness: Cosmetics, Race, and Women in Early Modern England." *Journal for Early Modern Cultural Studies* 11(1): 59–89.
Pollock, Anne. 2012. *Medicating Race: Heart Disease and Durable Preoccupations with Difference*. Durham, NC: Duke University Press.
Pussetti, Chiara. 2015a. "Corpos indóceis. Sexualidade, planeamento familiar e etnopolíticas da cidadania em imigrantes africanos." In Joana Bahia and Miriam Santos (eds.), *Corpos em Trânsito: Socialização, Imigração e Disposições Corporais*. Porto Alegre, Brasil: Suliani Letra & Vida Editora, pp. 105–27.
———. 2015b. "The Fallopian Dilemma: African Bodies, Citizenship and Family Planning." *Journal of Racial and Ethnic Health Disparities* 2(1): 21–33.
———. 2019. "From Ebony to Ivory 'Cosmetic' Investments in the Body." *Anthropological Journal of European Cultures* 28(1): 64–72.
Pussetti, Chiara, and Victor Barros. 2012a. "Outros corpos: imigração, saúde e etnopolíticas de cidadania." *Forum Sociológico* 22: 38–70.
———. 2012b. "The Care of the Immigrant Self." *International Journal of Migration, Health and Social Care* 8(1): 42–51.
Ramos, Alice, Cícero Pereira, and Jorge Vala. 2019. "The Impact of Biological and Cultural Racisms on Attitudes towards Immigration Public Policies?" *Journal*

of Ethnic and Migration Studies 46(3): 574–92. https://doi.org/10.1080/13691 83X.2018.1550153.
Roberts, Dorothy. 2011. *Fatal Invention: How Science, Politics, and Big Business Re-create Race in the Twenty-First Century*. New York: New Press.
Roediger, David R. 1991. *The Wages of Whiteness: Race and the Making of the American Working Class*. London: Verso.
Rosário, Edite, Tiago Santos, and Sílvia Lima, 2017. *Discursos do racismo em Portugal: essencialismo e inferiorização nas trocas coloquiais sobre categorias minoritárias*. Lisboa: Estudos OI n.44.
Rosenthal, Angela. 2004. "Visceral Culture: Blushing and the Legibility of Whiteness in Eighteenth Century British Portraiture." *Art History* 27(4): 563–92.
Ruetzler, Tanya, Jim Taylor, Dennis Reynolds, William Baker, and Claire Killen. 2012. "What Is Professional Attire Today? A Conjoint Analysis of Personal Presentation Attributes." *International Journal of Hospitality Management* 31(3): 937–43.
Said, Edward. 1979. *Orientalism*. New York: Vintage Books.
Santana Pinho, Patricia. 2009. "White but Not Quite: Tones and Overtones of Whiteness in Brazil." *Small Axe* 13(2): 39–56.
Satzewich, Victor. 2000. "Whiteness Limited: Racialization and the Social Construction of 'Peripheral Europeans.'" *Histoire sociale / Social History* 33(66): 271–89.
Sierp, Aline, and Christian Karner. 2017. "National Stereotypes in the Context of the European Crisis." *National Identities* 19(1): 1–9.
Souza, Melanie Miyanji. 2008. "The Concept of Skin Bleaching in Africa and Its Devastating Health Implications." *Clinical Dermatology* 26: 27–29.
Toffoletti, Kim. 2007. *Cyborgs and Barbie Dolls Feminism, Popular Culture and the Posthuman Body*. London: I. B.Tauris.
Vala, Jorge, Rodrigo Brito, and Diniz Lopes. 2005. *Expressões dos Racismos em Portugal*. Lisboa: Imprensa de Ciências Sociais.
Vassallo, Giovanni. 2009. "The Use of Skin Whitening Products among African People: Research in Italy and the Congo." *JENdA: A Journal of Culture and African Women Studies* 14: 145–52.
Ware, Vron. 1992. *Beyond the Pale: White Women, Racism and History*. New York: Verso.
Weitz, Rose. 2003. *The Politics of Women's Bodies*. New York: Oxford University Press.
Wen, Hua. 2013. *Buying Beauty: Cosmetic Surgery in China*. Hong Kong: Hong Kong University Press.
Westerhof, Wiete, and T. J. Kooyers. 2005. "Hydroquinone and Its Analogues in Dermatology: A Potential Health Risk." *Journal of Cosmetic Dermatology* 4: 55–59.
Whitmarsh, Ian, and David S. Jones (eds.). 2010. *What's the Use of Race? Modern Governance and the Biology of Difference*. Cambridge, MA: MIT Press.
Wissinger, Elizabeth A. 2015. *This Year's Model: Fashion, Media, and the Making of Glamour*. New York: New York University Press.
Yegenoglou, Meyda. 1998. *Colonial Fantasies: Towards a Feminist Reading of Orientalism*. Cambridge: Cambridge University Press.

CHAPTER 6

Reshaping Masculinities and the Beauty Industry in Colombia

ALEJANDRO ARANGO-LONDOÑO

By the end of the interview, Jorge, a 34-year-old divorced man, told me that he would not mind getting that liposuction if he had the money. If so, he could attract more beautiful women. This was actually not an uncommon response during my interviews with different men who were somehow involved in the beauty market. In this chapter, I consider the ways in which male bodies are reshaped through the boom of a beauty industry directly and exclusively targeted at men in Cali, Colombia. I explore how new cultural markers of "male beauty" come into play to redefine or reshape ideals of masculinity and the male body. In addition to this, the consumption of beauty itself is considered a marker of status and class privilege. In Colombia, like many other Latin American countries, gender relations are characterized by an ideology of machismo that depicts manhood as an identity based on hyper-virility, dominance, the dismissal of emotions, and the celebration of the role of men as breadwinners or providers (Gutmann 2003; Viveros-Vigoya 2003). However, recent scholarship on masculinity has pointed out how neoliberalism has produced a "crisis of masculinity," mainly because of the increasing job instability, making such ideals of manhood harder to accomplish for some men more than others (Cornwall, Karioris, and Lindisfarne 2016). This chapter investigates how the "inclusion" of men in the beauty industry plays a major role in reshaping ideas of masculinity in Colombia.

Based on ethnographic fieldwork in Cali, Colombia, I analyze how the growth of the male beauty industry affects gender and class structures by targeting men as consumers of a "traditionally" feminine commodity: beauty. Data cited here was collected through participant observation, semi-structured interviews, and media analysis. First, I outline the ethnographic context, followed by a few remarks on how beauty is understood as an economic and cultural phenomenon for the purposes of this chapter. Then, I approach the boom of the male beauty industry, analyzing how both gender and social class classifications are reimagined.

A City of Beauty

In 1971 Cali hosted the Pan American Games, the first major international event in the city and one considered to be a milestone. This engendered the myth of Cali as Colombia's city of sports and athletes. At the same time, drug trafficking was booming in the city, which meant that the economic upturn coincided with the development and expansion of drug trafficking and narco-culture. The eruption of drug trafficking in Cali produced a crisis in governance, as political and economic elites and drug lords overlapped. However, this process also revitalized the economy of the city through the imposition of consumerism in society, and an aesthetics of excess materialized, for instance, in the boom of architecture in the 1990s (Vásquez 2001; Rincón 2009) and the arrival and rapid growth of cosmetic surgery.

In other words, drug lords' mistresses, enhanced through aesthetic surgery, and the vast houses drug lords built for themselves shared an aesthetic of excessiveness that only made sense when displayed to others as an index of power and status. This became part of the cultural ideology of the Caleño, as drug trafficking represented possibilities of social mobility and capital accumulation in a city with an impoverished population and a long history of economic stagnancy. Hence, to fully embody the role of the provider during such times of scarcity and instability, men were pushed to embrace drug trafficking as a rapid and effective solution. In addition, narco-culture engendered a dynamic where manhood encompassed both the ability to provide and consume: provide in order to be able to maintain women and mistresses as a symbol of status, and consume as an index of power according to the ethos of narco-culture. In earlier times such consumption was represented by material goods like expensive cars and mansions on the outskirts of the city in neighborhoods like El Ingenio and Ciudad Jardín.

The transition to the twenty-first century in Colombia was characterized by an economic crisis due to the opening to free global markets that affected local businesses. This was particularly disastrous in Cali, as the incipient industry and business sectors were also affected by illegal economies and the political crisis produced as the DEA (United States Drug Enforcement Administration) targeted the Cali Cartel. This was a product of the global crisis of the welfare state, which strengthened in Colombia by the end of the 1970s with the crisis of external debt. At the same time, the long-standing armed conflict in Colombia intensified, producing an extended paramilitarization of the country in the 1980s. This process was intertwined with the expansion of drug trafficking in the 1990s, which also became the target of foreign agendas and interventions, especially under the war against terrorism led by the United States.

Even though the "peace process" in Colombia started with ex-president Andrés Pastrana in 2001, guerrillas and paramilitary groups continued to strengthen, leading to the rupture of the peace talks in 2002. In 2002, Álvaro Uribe became president and was then re-elected in 2006. The years 2002–10 are characterized as the most violent period in Colombia's recent history, with large numbers of missing people, massacres, genocides, and the consolidation of urban criminal bands (Borda 2012). This political crisis occurred as neoliberal structural adjustment plans were implemented through treaties with the IMF (International Monetary Fund) in 1999, 2002, 2004, and 2005. This translated into Colombia opening its markets, privatizing public entities, cutting social welfare expenses, and granting privileges to foreign capitals to ensure the creation of new jobs. The signature of the peace agreements in 2016 by President Juan Manuel Santos and FARC (Fuerzas Armadas Revolucionarias de Colombia) leader "Timochenko" has been seen as a benefit for foreign investment, as Colombia is now perceived as a politically more stable country. However, under the administration of the recently elected president Iván Duque, protégé of former president Uribe, different initiatives to undermine the peace agreements are being implemented, putting at risk the slight economic and politic stability achieved.

After the fight against drug trafficking, the eruption of biomedicine has invigorated Cali's economy, making health, including pharmaceutical companies and laboratories, the second most dynamic economic sector in the city. This economic takeoff also modified the urban space by producing certain urban zones dedicated to beauty: cosmetic clinics, gyms, spas, public parks, and so forth. New clinics and medical schools have opened recently due to the high demand for medical services and products. This health sector encompasses beauty and wellness services, with spas, gyms, supplement shops, training boxes, and other types of businesses and venues thriving in Cali. These have reactivated the economy, as beauty and wellness commodities are seen as essential in a city where physical appearance and image are considered crucial. The beauty industry has also produced a whole new economic niche for men that grants them the possibility of displaying masculinity. By consuming beauty, men are now able to exhibit their enhanced male bodies through cosmetic surgery, aesthetic treatments, new self-care products, or dietary supplements. These reshaped male bodies reflect economic power, a feature glorified by narco-culture and ingrained ideas of masculinity in Colombia.

In a neoliberal context, the city itself works as a commodity sold for foreign investment by attracting transnational companies and tourists. What Cali has to offer now is the increasingly powerful health sector, in which cosmetic surgery is the most profitable activity. This narrative targets both foreigners and locals. The preoccupation with physical appearance is coupled with the globally increasing emphasis on wellness and healthy "lifestyles." In Cali, thus, beauty discourses are fostered at both local and global levels. This is why, among other reasons explained above, Cali is a productive place to study beauty and wellness: it is a desire of both people and the city.

Beauty as Commodity and Consumption

Beauty can be analyzed as an economic phenomenon in at least two senses: first, in terms of what people invest in it; and second, in terms of the economic dynamics it produces at a broader scale. Kaushik Sunder Rajan and Melinda Cooper have explored the relationships between biomedicine and capitalism: how they have been historically coproduced, and how these relations produce new meanings for biology and life. Sunder Rajan coins the term "biocapital" to refer to a new form of capitalism, in which biomedical knowledge intersects with globalization and neoliberalism (Sunder Rajan 2006). In this form of capital, biology is commoditized in two ways: biological materials (blood cells, tissues) and biological information (Sunder Rajan 2006). Surgical technologies, aesthetic treatments, and new beautification products can be analyzed as a commodification of biomedical knowledge. Even though beauty is *different* from health, beauty is rooted in biomedical technologies; a new discovery in biomedicine that can be applied to beauty means a new treatment or surgical procedure to be offered and thrown into the market.

The other side of this dynamic is how much and what people decide to invest in this. This topic is explored by Cooper (2008). Like Sunder Rajan, her work focuses on the political economy of biology, but Cooper is more concerned with the emergence of new biomedical technologies and the coproduction of biomedical research with neoliberal capitalism. But what is more relevant here is her concept of "financialization of the life." She refers to a shift in the "commodification" of the life: life itself becomes a matter of speculation and a sort of capital that can be financed. Cooper attaches this to the neoliberal model rooted in economic speculation and the financial deregulation that basically allows imagining any possible future (Cooper

2008). In other words, she brings to the forefront how life itself becomes a long-term project on which people "speculate." Later, Cooper argues the need to "rethink the possibilities of bodily transformation, one that needs to be read in parallel with the space-time imperatives of post-Fordist production techniques" (Cooper 2008: 101). She links this to a change in body perception: the commodification of it and its transformation into a place for economic investment and for capital extraction and accumulation.

Following this framework, the political economy of beauty can be seen as twofold process. First, it is a societal one that encompasses the production, circulation, and consumption of new technologies to increase beauty (new surgical technologies, new devices and machinery, new cosmetics and "vanity" products). As part of neoliberal capital, this "societal" dimension of the political economy of beauty is connected to global and international institutions (such as international organizations, schools and universities, and pharmaceutical companies) and to national and local governments. In this regard, beauty is a global economic and political phenomenon. The second dimension of beauty is more subjective and individual and refers to the consumption of beauty, including the strategies undertaken to obtain this commodity.

Under a financialized life scheme, to use Cooper's concept, the time and money spent on beautification hold the promise of a better future and a better life. Unlike biological materials (such as organs or tissues), when people invest in beauty, they do not invest in the prolongation or enhancement of biological life, but in the improvement of social life. Having beauty and being beautiful holds the promise of better opportunities and success in life (Edmonds 2010). Therefore, investing in beauty is investing in a better life. As a quality or skill appreciated in the social sphere, beauty is much more than the mere act of looking good, but we cannot forget that looking good is also part of the well-being that beauty offers by improving self-esteem, self-confidence, and self-trust. Put like this, beauty is almost the perfect commodity because it grants somatic health, psychological strength, mental stability, and social success (romantic, familiar, labor, sexual, and so forth). Most importantly, investments on the body through the consumption of beauty is seen by others as a symbol of prestige. Many of my interviewees ensure that they are taken more seriously by other people and desired more by romantic partners as they got a *mejor cuerpo* (better body). A *mejor cuerpo* for men is necessarily a body committed to beautification: muscular but athletic, lean, healthy (and preferably lighter) skin, good teeth and hair, and ideally taller than the average. Acquiring a better body is also an index of a healthy lifestyle, an arbitrary construction made by the beauty industry that is now broadly desired by people, but that depends mostly on the economic capital of the individual and their ability to consume beauty.

On the other hand, beauty is also a cultural force intertwined with national histories, gender, racial, and social hierarchies that acquires meaning as it circulates through society and among different societies at an international scale (Jarrín 2017). In this sense, beauty encapsulates historically constructed stereotypes and ideals, while at the same time it creates a market that offers the possibility of social upward mobility at a certain cost. In between all these, the process of achieving beauty grants or promises happiness, success in life, wellness, social acceptance, and other "therapeutic" effects (see Edmonds 2010; Jarrín 2017; Plemons 2017; Stanfield 2014). But following my interviewees' claims, it is not enough to spend money on beauty products or a gym membership. Lázaro, a 25-year-old engineer, describes his "tortuous" process for gaining muscle and the multiple dietary restrictions and choices he had to make in order to achieve such an ideal body. He told me he feels a more confident man after he put on some muscle, while he "thanked his genetics" for providing him with a decent height and dense-thick facial hair that attracts women. Emiliano, a nurse of forty-three years of age, recalls his struggle to "destroy" his *barriga de camionero* (trucker's tummy) and explained how he felt like a better man and happier in life once he attained his bodily goal. Although goals are individual and "beauty is subjective," most interviewees associate muscularity, leanness, and a strong upper body with the ideal male body. To them, this type of body reflects strength and the ability to safeguard, features acclaimed and desired by women, allegedly. More broadly, these two qualities are also glorified in a context under constant threat of conflict and violence: the ability to fight and protect the nation works as an illusion of a stronger and more stable state, echoing Foucault's arguments on biopower and governmentality regarding the organization and regulation of the citizens' bodies (Foucault 1988, 2007).

Another important point of analyzing the economy of beauty is considering the amount of money that people spend on it. In a certified clinic, surgical procedures oscillate between 2 million and 10 million Colombian pesos (*El País* 2015), roughly between US$700 and US$3,500. This amount makes sense only when compared to the minimum monthly wage (SMLV for short) in the country for 2016, which is about 700,000 Colombian pesos or US$200. This means that the cheapest surgical procedure in Colombia in a certified/legal clinic is about three times the minimum monthly wage. Thus, although beauty is portrayed as something anybody can pursue, this is not the case. As a consequence, the emergence of illegal, clandestine, and informal clinics that offer cosmetic procedures at very low cost has skyrocketed. It is important to comprehend the actual affordability of beauty for middle and lower classes, to understand whether beauty actually promotes social upward mobility (via the social benefits it produces) or whether it reproduces social hierarchies by reifying the stigma of the poor as ugly. This is an idea that has an old history in Western models of beauty, particularly since the medieval age, when society began to emphasize the differences between "the rich and the powerful, and the poor and the underprivileged" through beauty (Eco 2004).

Reshaping Male Bodies and Masculinities

New clinics and other beauty establishments (e.g., salons, spas, barbershops, wellness shops) and the growing number of cosmetic plastic surgeons account for an increasing relevance of beauty in Cali in the last ten to fifteen years. It has become a considerable source of capital in the city. This is particularly evident with plastic surgery, as these are both the most popular and most expensive procedures. According to the local newspaper *El País*, a clinic specialized in plastic surgery makes about 5,000 million Colombian pesos a year (*El País* 2011), about US$1.7 million. A single surgeon can perform three breast implants surgeries in a day (*El País* 2011), meaning at least 30 million Colombian pesos of revenue for the clinic. The market of plastic surgery is so dynamic in the city that at least two thousand surgical procedures are performed per month, and for each ten thousand residents in the city, there are more than five plastic surgeons (*El País* 2011). By 2011 there were thirty certified centers for aesthetic surgery (*El País* 2011); this number has almost certainly increased in the last decade. According to some surgeons interviewed by *El País*, although Cali does not have the largest number of establishments for plastic surgery, no other city in Colombia has a similar volume of procedures performed (*El País* 2011). The quoted surgeons add that cosmetic procedures in Cali are world-renowned because of their superb quality (*El País* 2011).

All these profits, however, were not necessarily connected to ideas of the city until health tourism appeared on the scene. An estimated 2.2 percent of people visiting from other countries go to Colombia for health tourism, which represents between four thousand and seven thousand cosmetic surgeries per year from tourists alone (*El País* 2011). Health tourism is an important component of beauty as an economic phenomenon that articulates its markets with city marketing. Health tourism evokes ideas about the history of narratives in Cali and the ideas about the city promoted to visitors. Cali is "the" city for entertainment, plastic surgery, and beauty. In an advertisement published by *Revista Imagen* in 2016, the connections between city and beauty become even more evident. The ad sponsors the plastic surgeon, his clinic, and Cali as the "world destination" for cosmetic surgery (*Revista Imagen* 2016). It states, "En Cali se están fabricando princesas" (In Cali, princesses are being manufactured), highlighting the prowess and dexterity of plastic surgeons in the city and presents this as a feature of Cali. Then, the advertisement adds, "Cali ... destino mundial para el turismo de salud y cirugía plástica" (Cali ... world destination for health tourism and plastic surgery), reinforcing the idea that people go to Cali to get medical and aesthetic procedures. The high quality of the surgeries performed in the city are marketed as one of its main attractions.

In Colombia, beauty has traditionally been associated with women and femininity. While men took care of the public and political life, women took care of private life and the body. This dichotomy is not really that accurate, as male beauty is not new. Beauty for Colombian men in the twentieth century included apparel, hairstyle, and some beautification practices such as shaving and teeth care. For men, athleticism, vitality, and virility were core components of masculine beauty. Mass media, the fashion industry, and marketing have hyper-sexualized the female body and have reinforced the idea that beauty is a feminine domain. This association has been questioned recently by people's demands for plastic surgery, another phenomenon strongly associated with the feminine body. Plastic surgery has specialized in procedures to correct, enhance, improve, or eliminate some somatic features of the feminine body specifically. However, more recently, men have started to undergo some surgical procedures, especially those that are not necessarily connected to a particular sexuality or gender (e.g., rhinoplasty, abdominoplasty).

It is difficult to tell whether patients' demands for new biomedical technologies came first or whether the market created the demand, but the point is that new surgical procedures that address a male human body have emerged and are becoming steadily popular. The two processes might be more connected than they appear at first glance, but the result is the same: the reconfiguration of male beauty. In Cali, the increase of plastic surgery performed on men has been documented in the news for the past ten to fifteen years, although reports continue to be scattered and written with the tone of a "shocking revelation." This does not mean that men did not get plastic surgery before then, but that it is now becoming a socially recognizable phenomenon. With this recognition (though not total social acceptance), not only do new biomedical technologies come into the scene, but also a whole new market of procedures and services that address a different sector of the population. In other words, this "new" male beauty implies an expansion of beauty as a business and the creation of a male beauty consumer.

According to an article by *El País* (2014b), the most common procedures among men are liposuctions (49 percent), nose jobs (26 percent), and Botox (18 percent). Aesthetics (46 percent), aging (27 percent), and vanity

(19 percent) are cited as the main reasons why men look for cosmetic procedures, followed by pressures from their partners (6 percent) and health-related reasons (2 percent) (*El País* 2014b). Intrigued by these numbers, I asked at various clinics about the percentage of men versus women who were looking for cosmetic surgery. Surprisingly, I was told that about 30–40 percent of clients were men, sometimes even more. However, during my interviews, very few men admitted having had any sort of cosmetic surgery, although all pointed out that it was becoming much more common among men and that they knew friends who were getting "some help" with their abs in the "operating room."

If cosmetic surgery among men is becoming increasingly common, why isn't this reflected in conversations with men? Most men have no issues with talking about wanting a nose job or minor aesthetic treatments for hair loss or skin cleansing, but when it comes to liposuctions or implants, the conversation gets muddy. In my interviews and conversations with men, the issue appeared not to be about getting a cosmetic procedure but about how and where one might get it. Most men agreed, for example, that getting buttocks implants is effeminizing or *de gays* (a habit of gay men). Liposuctions were less of a gendered issue, but more of an ethical issue, as most men considered liposuction a shortcut for hard work. In the words of Pedro, a fifty-year-old personal gym trainer, liposuction is an "easy and fast" solution for "lazy people who are not aware of their bodies, have no awareness of their health, and have no intentions of transforming their bad habits."

This suggests that although male cosmetic surgery is becoming increasingly popular among men, values associated with the "traditional" macho role (Gutmann 2003) remain celebrated and glorified. The expansion of the male beauty industry is producing a man who is a consumer of beauty but who also embodies the figure of the warrior or the athlete, recalling ideas of hyper-virility and hypermasculinity (Connell 2005). One might argue that the gendered ideology of machismo produces the situation in which men seek cosmetic surgery, but it is still considered a taboo among men because beauty remains perceived as feminine and effeminizing. In other words, beauty is profoundly gendered. Most men did say that cosmetic surgery was a "women's thing, although some men are starting to do it." A younger interviewee who was twenty-three years of age, Daniel, had no issue telling me that he has already gotten three cosmetic surgical procedures (nose job, cheek fat reduction, and liposuction). Other men, like Óscar, a personal fitness coach, admitted to me that he wanted a nose job and some tissue removed from his stomach. He, like many other interviewees, considered cosmetic procedures and aesthetic treatments as an "extra help" aside from rigorous fitness regimes. Some others, like Máximo, a forty-year-old doctor, considered that cosmetic surgery was the perfect complement to a healthy diet and a proper exercise program if you wanted to be beautiful, happier, and more successful in social life. Such success is also reflected in Jorge's view, quoted at the beginning of the chapter, about getting a liposuction: it would help him to attract younger and more beautiful women because, in his eyes, when women embrace cosmetic surgery and fitness, they become more demanding regarding the looks of their male counterparts.

In order to contribute to the expansion of this new market, ideas of male beauty needed to be discursively reworked. In *Revista Imagen*, some articles that covered surgical procedures for men used narratives about successful life: "Nowadays, many successful men take care of their physical image by working out, having healthy diets, set trends with their apparel, looking 'important' when sealing a deal, or when they go out with their partners, and they increasingly choose more surgical and non-surgical procedures" (*Revista Imagen* 2015a). An assertion like this one puts together all the components of the social value of beauty: successful sexual and romantic life, successful job, and a top-class lifestyle. In other words, beauty works as an index for success in life, prestige, and status. The pivot of these three things is beauty itself: looking good, but mostly taking care of one's appearance. Once again, the promise of a better life is what makes beauty such a coveted "commodity." Consuming beauty contributes to the achievement of this elusive condition. To achieve it, people need to invest money; now men can be involved in this business as much as women.

As with women, the magazine addresses the "problems" men have as time passes by, justifying the need for aesthetic interventions. For instance, aging, time, climate, bad foods, and lack of exercise are described as producing wrinkles, stress, depression, and loss of muscle tone (*Revista Imagen* 2015b: 16). The lack of beauty is discursively marketed as a health issue or as a triggering factor for future health complications. These signs of a "lack of beauty" are connected to a loss of self-confidence and therefore might produce problems with clients, partners, and life in general (*Revista Imagen* 2015b). Worrying about beauty is, in fact, taking care of the future of one's social life. This is the argument through which entering the business of beauty acquires a whole new dimension. Additionally, aesthetics for women and men are somatically different, and thus two models of bodies emerge; the more the differences between these two bodies are found, the more aesthetic procedures can be performed, and thus more profits can be extracted.

Reifying gender differences between the male and the female body allows the increase of profits from beautification; therefore, more procedures, treatments, and products exclusively for men are put into circulation as time goes on. In Cali, the distribution of patients who had plastic surgery went from 80 percent women and 20 percent men to 70 percent women and 30 percent men by 2012 (*El País* 2012). Implants in the calves, cheeks, chin, and pectorals appear now as cosmetic surgeries *for* men (*El País* 2012). According to *El País*, these surgical interventions are the supplement for "executive men who also work out frequently to keep in shape" (*El País* 2014b). As with any other surgical procedures, the cost of these medical interventions in a certified clinic oscillates between 5 and 9 million Colombian pesos (US$1,700–$3,300) (*El País* 2014b).

The prices and the idea of the "executive men" used in the article shows that this male beauty is not really affordable to all men; it is clearly addressed to upper-class men who can afford the procedures and the time involved and can afford associated activities such as frequent exercising and good dieting. Working-class men or middle-class men, by definition, do not have easy access to beauty, which means not only "not looking good" but also having fewer chances of life success. This form of masculinity, based more on consumption than on production, is described by Connell (2001) as a global/entrepreneurial masculinity where access to luxurious commodities and services sets the definition of what a "successful man" is. Such type of masculinity intertwines with an ethos of narco-culture prevalent in Cali, which glorifies conspicuous consumption and a particular type of male body that reflects hyper-virility, respect, and authority.

According to a survey quoted by *El País*, men who decide to get plastic surgery do it for the following reasons: aesthetics (45.83 percent), they feel old (27.08 percent), vanity (18.75 percent), request by their partner (6.25 percent), and health (2.08 percent) (*El País* 2014b). The publication does not clarify what it means by "aesthetics," but it is likely something that men do not like about their bodies and want to "fix." These reasons for getting plastic surgery are, however, similar to those of women, including health, recalling the ambivalent relation between beauty and health. To function, the market needs to produce the awareness of beauty in men, but this awareness is also part of a broader cultural and historical phenomenon in Cali. Colombian daily newspaper *El Tiempo* (2014) reported an overall increase of 20 percent on cosmetic surgical treatments among men in Colombia by the end of 2014.

In this publication, a specific word is used to name the men who became interested in their appearance and invest on it: "yummy," a word used to describe both something "delicious" or "succulent" to eat, but also someone "pretty" or "attractive." This word also has a sexual connotation related to the double entendre of "eating" someone who looks "yummy." The publication states that the search for aesthetics is more common among single and widowed men who want to keep themselves in a good shape

(*El Tiempo* 2014). It also mentions the most common surgical procedures and aesthetic treatments (e.g., hair removal through laser, which describes men's hair as thicker than women's, yoga, massages, hair implants, vitamin injections for wrinkles) and the most common beautification practices (e.g., exfoliation, moisturizing, beard care, hair care) (*El Tiempo* 2014). The "yummy," a synonym for "metrosexual," depicts a type of man whose *manly* body can only be achieved through the consumption of beauty. The consumption of beauty by men translates into better opportunities in their romantic, sexual, emotional, and social lives. Neoliberal ideologies have produced a masculinity that requires them to consume in order to be consumed. In a context where social class and racial hierarchies overlap, such type of masculinity reinforces inequalities, as only whiter/upper-class men are able to consume more beauty, while darker/lower-class men are pushed either to embrace a "weaker," "less successful" masculinity or to pursue cheaper but riskier options in order to remain "competitive" in the market of success and desire.

The expansion of beauty *for men* occurs in three beautification techniques: cosmetic surgery, aesthetic treatments, and self-care beautification practices. Some of these are not necessarily exclusively for women or men, such as liposuction or abdominoplasty; but others are specifically designed and created for men, for example, pectoral implants (the male version of breast implants) and "sun-bathing ritual massages" (women get "moon-bathing ritual massages"). This indicates the emergence of a new economic niche of beauty industry, one that needs to clearly differentiate from female beauty in order to fully appeal to the male public as consumers. Intertwined with these new economic niches are new biomedical findings and technologies, such as body soaps made for the pH of male skin specifically and shampoos that take into account men's hair thickness. As Cooper (2008) points out, biomedical science and neoliberal capitalism are part of the same history. Without these sorts of biomedical findings, these new markets could have not developed; without capital invested in biotechnical research, these discoveries would not have been possible. Beauty intermingles in these two spheres, neither just biomedicine nor neoliberalism, but embedded in both.

An article in *Revista Imagen* addresses "masculine vanity" and the market for beautification products, pointing out that "an attractive appearance and having good health have become a social obligation" (*Revista Imagen* 2015a). The article states that men are becoming more boastful with beauty routines and almost as strict as those of women (*Revista Imagen* 2015a), indicating the increasing market of cosmetic products for men to the extent that some companies have developed their own brands exclusively for this public (*Revista Imagen* 2015a). Developing treatments and products exclusively for men has certain consequences in terms of beauty: first, it implies that men will need to acquire new knowledge about their bodies and the appropriate products they might need; second, it will create new markets for these new consumers; and third, it will create new relations to these new commodities, as they will become necessary goods under a discourse that equates beauty with individual happiness and social success.

By being designed specifically for men, these new products and treatments acquire a particular symbolic efficacy: as they are designed for men's bodies, they will have better therapeutic effects and results than any regular version of the product. Van der Geest, Reynolds White, and Hardon refer to the efficacy of pharmaceuticals and argue that this efficacy goes beyond physical and mental health and includes social, psychological, and cultural factors (1996: 167). Thus efficacy is connected to the "thinginess" of pharmaceuticals and the fact that they hold the promise of healing and work as therapy (van der Geest et al. 1996: 155). Beautification products are clearly different from medicines, as they do not grant health but beauty, and yet again, is not beauty a synonym of health? The relation between pharmaceuticals (medicines) and beautification products is, once again, one of ambiguity. Beautification products are designed, produced, and thrown into markets by pharmaceutical companies and laboratories, and they are based on biomedical knowledge and research.

The difference between medicines and beautification products is more about their final objective and less about their composition. Medicines address health, while beautification products address beauty; they both carry meaning and have a form of efficacy, as van der Geest et al. (1996) and Appadurai (1986) argue. Their meanings are, however, different. Medicines hold the promise of healing sickness and represent a prolongation, enhancement, or improvement of biological life. Beautification products hold the promise of social success through psychological and physical individual well-being; in this case, biological life is not necessarily prolonged or improved, but the quality of life is ameliorated. In such a way, health and beauty would be complementary dimensions of life: while good health grants the basic "biological" conditions for good living, beauty would grant more and better possibilities for a better life. For instance, taking a pill for a migraine attack will let the body function at its full capacity at work; getting a treatment for facial rejuvenation will give the subject a better chance to succeed at work and improve performance.

I have described beauty as a coveted commodity, but also a luxury one, not affordable by all people. Surgical procedures, spas, and beautification products are expensive for most of the population, with Cali being a city where distribution and access to resources are unequal. In a social context in which beauty has become a social obligation, class hierarchies work as obstacles for obtaining it, and people will undertake any alternatives to achieve some beauty, even when these alternatives might mean higher risks and even death. With the increasing demand for cosmetic procedures, new institutions offering these services have also appeared, but not everybody, as noted, can afford the high costs of the procedures. In response, special offers for plastic surgery and aesthetic treatments have appeared across the city. These "special offers" are cheaper prices for, supposedly, the same sort of procedures. For instance, a breast implant intervention could cost 4 million Colombian pesos, instead of 10 million (*El Tiempo* 2016), that is, less than half the price.

This is not the lowest price that a person can get for a cosmetic procedure. Colombian daily newspapers *El Tiempo* and *El País* refer to informal establishments—or clandestine clinics—as an increasing and worrying phenomenon. *El País* mentions some advertisements that offer liposuction procedures for 1 million Colombian pesos, while this same procedure would cost 7 million Colombian pesos in an authorized clinic (*El País* 2015). Stories about cheap procedures in clandestine clinics are remarkably frequent, and the stories focus on denouncing the risks that people might incur by trying to save some money through informal interventions.

In a clandestine clinic, a silicon injection can cost 400,000 thousand Colombian pesos (about US$135) (*El País* 2015). This amount of money might still be a lot for certain people in Cali, but it is certainly much more affordable than a regular surgery in an authorized clinic. In short, beauty can potentially be pursued by everybody, but those who cannot afford expensive (safer) procedures must put their lives at greater risk. As Edmonds (2010) argues, beauty works as a societal force that pushes people to pursue beautification at all costs, while strong and structured class inequality also pushes people to pursue "alternative" methods for social upward mobility. Socially, we have seen, beauty is an index for success and more and better opportunities in life; besides this, the symbolic efficacy of beauty at a subjective level (looking good translates into feeling good) makes the pursuit of beauty meaningful and worthy. Neither class inequalities nor cultural expectations can explain on their own the significance of beauty in Cali; it is both an economic and cultural phenomenon, on both an individual and a social scale.

The "public concern" with clandestine clinics has become so prevalent in Cali that health officials have begun having formal meetings to deal with such establishments and to propose regulations for cosmetic surgery. People are also very aware of this phenomenon, and some interviewees, like Miguel, state that it makes no sense to get a cosmetic procedure if you are going to die. Miguel, a 22-year-old recent college graduate, wants to get a nose job, as he is positive it will make him feel better about himself and be more successful with women. However, he, like Jorge, lacks the money and prefers to wait and save, rather than risk his life in a *clínica de garaje* ("garage clinic," an informal/clandestine clinic). Jorge was very emphatic about this as he briefly told me the story of a friend of his who died after her breast implants procedure went wrong in a "cheap clinic."

Beauty is connected to narratives of the city and works as a social obligation for the individual. As a "commodity," beauty presents itself as accessible to everybody, but in reality it is a luxury good that only a few individuals can afford without high risks. As an economic activity, beauty articulates and creates new markets based on biomedical technologies but at the same time utilizes discourses about Cali to promote new economic niches, such as men's self-care brands and health tourism. Class inequality and social pressure for beauty have engendered a parallel informal economy, in which cheap but much riskier procedures are available to people who cannot afford standard prices of surgical intervention or aesthetic treatments. Those who cannot afford expensive procedures are portrayed as irresponsible and blamed for being poor, unmasking the fact that beauty is not for everybody. Under these circumstances, some lives and bodies become more valued and valuable as they can purchase it. Male bodies are measured by how much they are enhanced, improved, and refined through the consumption of beauty. A man who takes care of his body is assumed to be a more responsible man, concerned with his health and wellness, hence a better man. At the same time, as the consumption of beauty can be read through the body, beauty itself works as an index of status and prestige.

Final Remarks

I began by considering how beauty acts as both a societal force and a subjective pursuit that shapes and re-creates ideas of masculinity. Its connections to the history of the city, the physical aspect of people, psychological well-being of the individual, its qualification as a social obligation, its connections to individual, local, national, and international economies, its relations to health and biomedicine, its codification as a public health issue, make us think that beauty, more than a category for social analysis, can be understood as a total social fact (Mauss 1990), as proposed by Edmonds (2010). Pursuing beauty is a lifelong quest that holds the promise of a better and more successful life. To achieve this, people must engage with beautification techniques today, tomorrow, and always. The payoffs of beauty take the form of self-efficacy through strong self-esteem and confidence. Seen like this, beauty is therapeutic for the body, the mind, and the soul.

Beauty is also a matter of political economy. It prescribes certain economic behaviors (investment of money) for individuals, but it also affects city and national economy. Beauty has been defined as an economic boom that is making massive profits for Cali. By reproducing narratives about the social value of beauty in Cali, the city has created a city brand to market Cali as a beautiful place, in which nonresidents can also become beautiful through "scalpel tourism." On the other hand, class inequalities have shown that beauty is accessible only to a small portion of the citizens, excluding the larger part of the population from the benefits of beauty. This, together with the social pressure of beauty, has created an informal aesthetic economy, in which more people can have access to beauty at the cost of higher risks for life. And yet, people still recognize how important beauty is in life: if taking care of health grants a better biological life, taking care of beauty grants a better social and economic life.

Cosmetic surgery offers the possibility of reshaping the body. Compared to other "paths," it seems to be the quickest yet the riskiest. While some consider cosmetic surgery to be an easy solution for lazy people, it is more widely accepted to think of all of these technologies as complementary. When it comes to getting cosmetic surgery, a practice considered to be feminine, men seem to be a bit more open or accepting of it. However, this has actually helped to perpetuate masculine stereotypes by coding certain procedures or body parts as effeminizing. In the words of some of them, cosmetic surgery in men is okay "as long as it still looks masculine." "Looking masculine" evokes for them a built, muscular, athletic body, well-groomed face and hair, and a matching flat stomach or, ideally, a hard six-pack. Hyper-dominance, authority, virility, and economic power become the perfect match for such a masculine look. The beauty industry in this sense has fostered a masculinity based on consumption, reifying old gender and class structures, although with a different language. Achieving beauty is faster and more effective the more money you have. In this sense, while technologies for reshaping the body are thrown into the market, class hierarchies among men determine the access to such self-improvement opportunities. By reshaping the male body, neoliberal ideologies, through the consumption of beauty, reinforce gender and class hierarchies where being a "good and successful man" depends on how much men can spend and show off their new and improved (cosmetic) self.

Alejandro Arango-Londoño is a Colombian anthropologist interested in critical medical anthropology, gender, and political economy. For his doctoral dissertation, he explored the expanding economy around male beautification in Cali, Colombia. He focuses on how the emphasis on male beauty has emerged in a context that is deeply marked by the cultural legacy of narco-violence, entrenched class and racial hierarchies, and contemporary neoliberalism.

References

Appadurai, Arjun. 1986. "Introduction: Commodities and the Politics of Value." In *The Social Life of Things: Commodities in Cultural Perspective*, edited by Arjun Appadurai, 3–63. Cambridge: Cambridge University Press.

Borda, Sandra. 2012. "La Administración de Álvaro Uribe y su Política Exterior en Materia de Derechos Humanos: de la Negación a la Contención Estratégica." *Análisis Político* 75: 111–37.

Connell, Raewyn W. 2001. "Masculinities and Globalization." In Michael Kimmel and Michael Messner (eds.), *Men's Lives*, 5th ed. Needham Heights, MA: Allyn and Bacon, pp. 56–70.

———. 2005. *Masculinities*. 2nd ed. Berkeley: University of California Press.

Cooper, Melinda. 2008. *Life as Surplus: Biotechnology and Capitalism in the Neoliberal Era*. Seattle: University of Washington Press.

Cornwall, Andrea, Frank G. Karioris, and Nancy Lindisfarne (eds.). 2016. *Masculinities under Neoliberalism*. London: Zed Books.

Eco, Umberto. 2004. *History of Beauty*. New York: Rizzoli.

Edmonds, Alexander. 2010. *Pretty Modern: Beauty, Sex, and Plastic Surgery in Brazil*. Durham, NC: Duke University Press.

El País. 2011. "La cirugía plástica, un negocio que sigue creciendo y dejando muchas ganancias." *El País* website. Retrieved January 2016 from http://www.elpais.com.co/elpais/cali/noticias/negocio-cirugia-plastica-sigue-creciendo-en-cali.

———. 2012. "Conozca porqué Cali sigue siendo la capital de la silicona en Colombia." *El País* website. Retrieved January 2016 from http://www.elpais.com.co/elpais/cali/noticias/conozca-porque-cali-sigue-siendo-silicona-en-colombia.

———. 2014a. "El 'boom' de las cirugías plásticas continúa en aumento en Colombia." *El País* website. Retrieved January 2016 from http://www.elpais.com.co/elpais/cali/noticias/boom-cirugias-plasticas-continua-aumento-colombia.

———. 2014b. "Estas son las cirugías plásticas que más se hacen los hombres." *El País* website. Retrieved January 2016 from http://www.elpais.com.co/elpais/economia/noticias/estas-son-cirugias-plasticas-hacen-hombres.

———. 2015. "Autoridades advierten sobre los riesgos de las operaciones estéticas de bajo costo." *El País* website. Retrieved January 2016 from http://www.elpais.com.co/elpais/cali/noticias/autoridades-advierten-sobre-riesgos-operaciones-esteticas-bajo-costo.

El Tiempo. 2014. "Los 'yummy', metrosexuales que invierten en su apariencia." *El Tiempo* website. Retrieved January 2016 from http://www.eltiempo.com/estilo-de-vida/los-hombres-ahora-invierten-mas-en-su-apariencia/13966900.

Foucault, Michel. 1988. *Technologies of the Self*. Amherst: University of Massachusetts Press.

———. 2007. *History of Sexuality*. Vol. 1. México DF: Siglo XXI Editores.

Gutmann, Matthew. 2003. *Changing Men and Masculinities in Latin America*. Durham, NC: Duke University Press.

Jarrín, Alvaro. 2017. *The Biopolitics of Beauty: Cosmetic Citizenship and Affective Capital.* Oakland: California University Press.
Londoño, Alicia. 2008. *El cuerpo limpio. Higiene corporal en Medellín, 1880–1950.* Medellín, Colombia: Editorial Universidad de Antioquia.
Márquez, Jorge. 2005. *Ciudad, miasmas y microbios. La irrupción de la ciencia pasteriana en Antioquia.* Medellín, Colombia: Universidad Nacional de Colombia.
Mauss, Marcel. 1990. *The Gift: The Form and Reason for Exchange in Archaic Societies.* London: Routledge.
Noguera, Carlos. 2003. *Medicina y Política. Discurso médico y prácticas higiénicas durante la primera mitad del siglo XX en Colombia.* Medellín, Colombia: Cielos de Arena, Fondo Editorial Universidad EAFIT.
Pedraza, Zandra. 1999. *En cuerpo y alma. Visiones del progreso y de la felicidad.* Bogotá, Colombia: Universidad de Los Andes.
Plemons, Eric. 2017. *The Look of a Woman: Facial Feminization Surgery and the Aims of Trans-Medicine.* Durham, NC: Duke University Press.
Revista Imagen. 2015a. Edición no. 160 Versión Digital, Editora Estética Ltda. Retrieved January 2016 from https://revistaimagen.com.co/revista-digital/.
———. 2015b. Edición no. 162 Versión Digital, Editora Estética Ltda. Retrieved January 2016 from https://revistaimagen.com.co/revista-digital/.
———. 2016. Edición no. 172 Versión Digital, Editora Estética Ltda. Retrieved January 2016 from https://revistaimagen.com.co/revista-digital/.
Rincón, Omar. 2009. "Narco.estética y Narco.cultura en Narco.lombia." *Nueva Sociedad* 222: 147–63.
Stanfield, Michael Edward. 2014. *Of Beast and Beauty: Gender, Race, and Identity in Colombia.* Austin: University of Texas Press.
Sunder Rajan, Kaushik. 2006. *Biocapital: The Constitution of Postgenomic Life.* Durham, NC: Duke University Press.
van der Geest, Sjaak, Susan Reynolds White, and Anita Hardon. 1996. "The Anthropology of Pharmaceuticals: A Biographical Approach." *Annual Review of Anthropology* 25: 153–78.
Vásquez, Édgar. 2001. *Historia de Cali en el siglo 20. Sociedad, economía, cultura y espacio.* Cali, Colombia: Artes Gráficas del Valle.
Viveros-Vigoya, Mara. 2003. "Contemporary Latin American Perspectives on Masculinity." In Matthew Gutmann (ed.), *Changing Men and Masculinities in Latin America.* Durham, NC: Duke University Press, pp. 27–57.
Wade, Peter. 1997. *Gente Negra, Nación Mestiza. Dinámicas de las Identidades Raciales en Colombia.* Bogotá, Colombia: Universidad de Antioquia; ICANH, Siglo del Hombre Editores, Ediciones Uniandes.

CHAPTER 7

Reshaping and Hacking Gendered Bodies
Gay Bears and Pro-Independence Catalan Militants

BEGONYA ENGUIX GRAU

Bodies are a battleground and a playground. Feminism and gender politics have been aware of this for a long time; they are a battleground particularly for women because women are thought to suffer the pressure of normative ideal bodies to a greater extent than men. The public female representatives of the political group Candidatura d'Unitat Popular (CUP), a pro-independence and socialist Catalan group with members in the Catalan Parliament, are frequently attacked on the basis of their bodies: they are considered "unattractive" or unconcerned about their appearance. This battle regarding their bodies is transferred to their political ideology and to their skills and capacities for ruling a country. Their bodies are political weapons in their own hands and their opponents' hands in a game of political agency against norms, on the one hand, and the control and surveillance of body norms, on the other. In 2016 these women responded to the public attacks with a public event where they cried out all the insults they received, thus reversing the devaluing meanings they were attached to; with this action, women's appearance became an issue for public debate and an instrument for political (revolutionary) action.

The six groups included in the pro-independence Catalan Left (Esquerra Independentista, hereafter EI) define themselves as pro-independence, socialist (or communist), and feminist. Depending on the group, their anticapitalist stance is more or less strong. I will focus on two groups, CUP and Arran, because these groups are very active in campaigning against "correct" clothing sizes, manspreading,[1] beach bodies, and other gender-related questions. Pointed out by many people for their "peculiar" appearance, their militants have a distinctive relationship to body ideals, gender expectations, and politics. They shape and reshape their bodies in ways that are oppositional to social norms, to the rules, and to the ideals as a means of questioning them and as a strategy to fight for social transformation.

In contrast, Bears are thought to be a "subculture" of big, hairy, and not-always-young gay men. Through their big bodies and their beards, Bears are thought to have reversed the gendered norms of gayness. Their bodies do not correspond to the muscled and smart gym-gay; they mostly look like regular (big) guys. As pro-independence militants, they also oppose social norms, rules, and ideals through and with their bodies. However, as men within a world of men, their objectives and their position in the geometries of power differ from those of the EI. Despite these differences, both groups, Bears and EI militants, hack their bodies. Both understand gender in bodily terms and consider gendered bodies as a political weapon to fight for a different understanding of gender and politics. Both situate gendered bodies in the world through the claim for feminism (EI) or for a previously denied masculinity (Bears).

Bodies and Gender

Feminist writers and thinkers have long discussed topics that are central for our understandings of gender, the body, and the power of matter and discourse. Feminist epistemologies have situated the body at the center of the critique of dual, binary, dichotomous, and essentialist gender and sexual models and have connected these models to social inequality, hierarchy, and violence. Their materialist notion of embodiment allows new and more accurate analyses of power based on the radical critique of masculinist universalism (Braidotti 2013: 22).

Post-humanist scholars, and Rosi Braidotti in particular, aim to replace the unitary subject of humanism (a masculine subject) with a more complex and relational subject framed by embodiment, sexuality, affectivity, empathy, and desire as core qualities. Equally central to this approach is the insight on power as both a restrictive (*potestas*) and a productive force (*potentia*) (Priban 2018). Feminist epistemologies are influenced by "corporeal" feminism, which returns to the site of the body as an active participant in gender identity, subjectivity, and ideology (Grosz 1994; Hester 2004).

In this chapter I address the following issues: How are gender and bodies related? How important are bodies? What is political about gender and about bodies? Are they political, or rather they can become political through political action? What can gendered bodies do? I will explore some of the possible answers to these questions through feminist epistemologies such as new materialism and post-humanism and through ethnographic cases taken from my own recent fieldwork. I will also use two figurations derived from my fieldwork: overflown bodies and protest bodies.[2]

Bodies without limits (overflown bodies) are embedded and entangled in complex assemblages of gender, emotions, affects, ideologies, mobilizations, corporations, digitalities, activisms, and other expressions. Transcending the dichotomy between nature and culture, overflown bodies bring matter and discourse together; they do not end at our skin; they illustrate the complex entanglement of the material with the political and can be useful for addressing issues related to exclusion, domination, political emancipation, and transformation (Enguix 2012c, 2014, 2015, 2018). Protest bodies are bodies that are protest in themselves, not a support for protest. Through their presence, relations, and entanglements with other human and non-human elements (e.g., other bodies, banners, music, speech, marches), protest bodies resist some standardized and normalized ways of life (Enguix 2012a, 2012b, 2019).

But what is the understanding of gender I start from? Among the many possible definitions, let me take Teresa de Barbieri's definition and consider gender as a set of practices, symbols and representations, social norms, and values that societies construct departing from anatomic and physiologic difference (1993: 149). Gender is not an attribute nor a property or a qualification of sexed bodies. Gender is relation and a set of social practices. In the 1970s the anthropologist Gayle Rubin (1986: 54) stated that men and women are closer to each other than we are to mountains, kangaroos, or palms, to give just a few examples. Consequently, far from being the expression of a natural difference, exclusive gender identity suppresses natural similarities.

Gender is not a property that we naturally own but is the product of social relations (Connell 1987). As Rubin (1986) argued, a woman is a woman and becomes a wife in a relation, becomes oppressed in a relation. And, as a system of/for social classification, gender is intersected by other systems as ethnicity, class, sexuality, or education. Apart from being relation, gender is also a complex cluster of meanings, practices, experiences, and representations where context plays a very important role. For example, professional (male) football players who become emotional compensate and override this emotionality (a stereotypical feminine trait) through sporting prowess, competitiveness, and passion. The gendering of particular "traits" depends to some extent on the (sexed) embodiment and discursive positioning of the subject (Francis 2008: 216).

Apart from being a relation and cluster, gender is a system that connects, confronts, reproduces, and/or transgresses the relations between body, sex, gender, sexuality, and affects. Body, sex, sexuality, gender, and affects are entangled, but they are separate entities. I consider affect as the political grammar of feelings "in a twofold manner: as sensory register and mode of sensation, perception, recognition, and agency or what I call feeling politics; and on the other hand, as an instrument and means of the political or as I phrase it, a politics of feelings" (Bargetz 2014: 293).

The two cases that I examine here, EI militants and Bears, question or transcend what Paul B. Preciado (2018) called the antique sexual regime, that is, the rigid binary system rooted in nature and biology with opposed definitions of what being a male and a female means (sex) and of what being masculine and feminine means (gender). Arran and CUP militants question this system through the public presence and activity of their female militants, through their attire and behavior, and, of course, through their political discourse. Their way of embodying politics makes of body not only matter but also discourse. Bears challenge the idea that sexuality is necessarily connected to gender and that same-sex sexual, affective, and erotic relationships imply crossing genders, that is, a decrease or lack of masculinity and an increase of femininity (effeminacy) in the case of men.

Both use their bodies as a strategy to challenge the normative gender system and as a way to do politics; both reshape and hack their bodies in order to do so. By hacking, I do not mean the use of do-it-yourself cybernetic devices—such as magnetic implants—or introducing biochemicals into the body to enhance or change bodies' functionality. Any strategy to modify our body internally or externally can be considered as hacking. Dieting to lose or gain weight can be considered as biohacking. Biohacking is the practice of changing one's body chemistry and physiology through science and self-experimentation. However, the term incorporates a wide range of areas and methods. Biohacking can range from something as simple as using nutrition and lifestyle changes to enhancing body functions, DIY gene therapy, and altering one's body by implanting cybernetic devices.[3]

Cross-dressing, growing body and facial hair, wearing agender outfits, wearing certain types of clothes or hairstyles and not others can all be considered as hacking techniques. Body structure, skin color, cosmetic surgery, makeup, hair, hairstyle, clothes, and other accessories reshape and hack bodies. This shows how the body "is not a 'being,' but a variable boundary, a surface whose permeability is politically regulated, a signifying practice within a cultural field of gender hierarchy and compulsory heterosexuality" (Butler 1990: 189).

Bodies and genders are neither natural nor neutral surfaces. Although bodies have been thought of as the neutral ground of gendered/cultural impositions, bodies are not passive. They force certain consequences; they confront culture and upset and undermine cherished beliefs. They are *ac-*

tive participants in the environment of sex/gender (Domurat Dreger 1998: 6). The question is no longer (only) how we shape the body, but also how the body shapes us (Hester 2004: 223).

The generative capacity of bodies (Harrison 2010), their fluidity, mobility, and instability together with their messy connections with gender, affects, and sexuality, should turn our attention to the Deleuzian question of how bodies work and who they work for. We must focus on what a body can do rather than consider what a body is or what gender is (Buchanan 1997). In my view, bodies transcend skin, bodies are already gendered, and genders are always embodied. Bodies are active participants in social life: they are generative and already political. They are not fixed or stable. They are bodies in becoming (Coleman 2012), constantly in their making and part of complex assemblages.

The concept of assemblage is useful to think about social entities as wholes whose properties emerge from the interactions between the parts. Assemblages are characterized by relations of exteriority that imply that a component part of the assemblage may be detached from it and plugged into a different assemblage in which its interactions are different (de Landa, cited in Tamboukou 2010: 685). Assemblages are not just things, practices, and signs articulated into a formation, but also qualities, affects, speeds, and densities. They work through flows of agency rather than through specific practices of power. Like bodies and gender, flows of agency are never neutral (Ringrose and Coleman 2013: 132). Whereas articulation emphasizes the contingent connections and relations among and between elements, assemblage is also about their territorialization, expression, elements, and relations (Stivale 2005: 84).

If assemblage stresses relation, agency, and flow, the idea of becoming can help us escape the limitations of intersectionality (mainly its tendency to reify categories such as race and gender):

> Many of the cherished categories of the intersectional mantra, originally starting with race, class, gender, now including sexuality, nation, religion, age, and disability, are the product of modernist colonial agendas and regimes of epistemic violence, operative through a western/euro American epistemological formation through which the whole notion of discrete identity has emerged, for example, in terms of sexuality and empire. (Puar 2013: 376)

Becoming means in-betweenness. It is a threshold; becoming is not a transcendent process that tells difference from the same, nor relies on a stable identity (or sameness) for external comparisons and relations, as in social classifications. For Deleuze and Guattari (1994), difference does not exist in opposition to sameness; difference is immanent to sameness. Becoming, then, is immanent to (not outside of) the social field to which it applies.

Furthermore, becoming is not a linear process between two points (Jackson 2013: 115). Becoming and assemblage are important tools for posthumanist and new materialist thinking and can provide a deep understanding of how our bodies move, reshape, change, and are hacked.

My proposal of overflown bodies, when connected to assemblage and becomings, can be understood as an unstable assemblage of relations and lines of flight, that is, as pure relation and openness. Overflown bodies are different from "bodies not ending at skin," in Haraway's terms (1991). I do not refer to the DNA traces that we leave everywhere, connecting us with nonhuman animals and nature. I refer to the peculiar overflowing of matter in the process of becoming discourse: body matter becomes ideology, religion, family, sexuality, gender, stereotypes, desire, beauty, eroticism, attractiveness, success, failures, and so on.

Together, these three concepts—assembled, becoming, and overflown bodies—seem to be appropriate for dealing with the multiple ways in which we reshape and hack our bodies and all those '"bits of things"—affects, ideas, sensations, and movements—which are often disregarded under usual methods of working (Dyke 2013: 160). This understanding of bodies and genders as an ongoing overflown assemblage focuses on the patterns of relations and on the "encounters" between body, gender, and sexuality as well as other human and nonhuman agents; it provides the epistemological and methodological conditions for talking about reshaping and hacking of bodies and escapes the consideration of gender and sexuality as "simple entities and attributes of subjects" (Puar 2013: 382). It also situates the bodies as already political, that is, as protest bodies.

Assembling Bodies and Masculinities: Bears

Apparently, men are increasingly defining themselves through their bodies in the wake of social and economic changes that have eroded or displaced work as a source of identity. This is particularly so for working-class men (Gill, Henwood, and McLean 2005: 39). Both metrosexuality and spornosexuality, terms created by Mark Simpson, have provoked changes in men's bodies and also in men's subjectivities. According to Mark Simpson (2002):

> The typical metrosexual is a young man with money to spend, living in or within easy reach of a metropolis—because that's where all the best shops, clubs, gyms and hairdressers are. He might be officially gay, straight or bisexual, but this is utterly immaterial because he has clearly taken himself as his own love object and pleasure as his sexual preference.

Spornosexuals, a term derived from the connection of sport and sex, take metrosexuals a step further in bodily terms:

> With their painstakingly pumped and chiseled bodies, muscle-enhancing tattoos, piercings, adorable beards and plunging necklines it's eye-catchingly clear that second-generation metrosexuality is less about clothes than it was for the first. Eagerly self-objectifying, second-generation metrosexuality is totally tarty. Their own bodies (more than clobber and product) have become the ultimate accessories, fashioning them at the gym into a hot commodity—one that they share and compare in an online marketplace. (Simpson 2014)

Men are not just the subject of desire, they have become objects of desire. That has implied taking care of their bodies, their appearances, and their attitudes if they want to feel well and be attractive. This is something gay men (and straight women) have been aware of for a long time, as they have always been both object and subject of desire.

Masculinity is bodily conveyed and strongly representational (Rohlinger 2002: 62) and seems to be a matter of the body rather than the mind (Kimmel 1996). Despite the strong connection of masculinity to body, the discussion on hegemonic or non-hegemonic masculine bodies is scarce. Everybody seems to take for granted what a male body must look like.

Masculinity started to be theorized by anthropologists working on what was then called anthropology of the Mediterranean. David Gilmore (1990), in particular, after his fieldwork in Andalusia, considered that masculinity is defined for what it is not rather than for what it is: men are basically not gays, not women, not children. Gay men, women, and children police the borders of normative masculinity. According to Hearn (2018: 36), the concepts of masculinity and, in turn, masculinities (plural) are difficult to define because they can refer to practices, configurations of practice, assemblages of practice, identities, types, structures, institutions, processes, psychodynamics, and so on. Another complication is that masculinity is often understood as linked to men/male bodies, although sometimes there is a separation of masculinity from men/male bodies, as in female masculinity (Halberstam 1998). This is possible because masculinity is not a fixed entity embedded in the body or in personality traits of individuals. Masculinities are configurations of practice that are accomplished in social action (Connell and Messerschmidt 2005: 836): they concern the position of men in a gender order. They can be defined as the patterns of practice by which people (both men and women, though predominantly men) engage in that position. Different body techniques and practices serve the purpose to perform masculinity.

Those patterns of practice take us back to the masculine bodies and their complex hegemonies. When Carrigan, Connell, and Lee developed the concept of hegemonic masculinity in 1985, they did not anticipate how popular (and misunderstood) this concept would become. Raewyn Connell further developed it and gave it its current meaning: hegemonic masculinity is defined as a practice that legitimizes men's dominant position in society and justifies the subordination of women and other marginalized ways of being a man (gay men, for instance). Hegemonic masculinity proposes to explain how and why men maintain dominant social roles over women and other gender identities that are perceived as less masculine or even "feminine" in a given society (Connell 1987, 1995). It has multiple meanings. Men can adopt hegemonic masculinity when it is desirable, but the same men can separate themselves strategically from hegemonic masculinity at other moments. Consequently, "masculinity" does not actually represent a certain type of man, but rather the way in which men position themselves through discursive practices (Connell and Messerschmidt 2005: 841) and embodied gendered practices.

Gay men have served to police the borders of normative masculinity; they were a subordinated masculinity (position) devalued through the gendered practice of cross-gendering sexuality (that is, the cultural belief that a transgression in gender is connected with a transgression in sexuality [and vice versa] and that gay men are effeminate). They were attacked, among other things, because of their lack of masculinity, as if masculinity was a graded attribute. But masculinity cannot be weighed.

In the 1970s the gay movement reconciled (homo)sexuality with masculinity. Neoliberalism made gay sculpted bodies an ideal to follow for everyone, thus separating body care from sexuality (as for metrosexuals and spornosexuals). This double movement (separating sexuality from gender and separating body care from sexuality and gender) necessarily brought about a different conceptualization of gender in relation to body care. Years ago, normative canons of beauty stated that women had to be attractive for men, whereas men could not be attractive; if they took excessive care of themselves, they were accused and stigmatized for being gay. This is not always the case now. Bears' bodily and gender strategies run along different lines.

From 2012 until 2015, I conducted ethnographic fieldwork on masculine bodies (to analyze gender and/in the body), in which I used a gallery of photographs selected according to a pre-categorization of three masculine styles based on my previous fieldwork (hypermasculine, standard, and ambiguous). I conducted forty-five interviews to get free narratives on fourteen images. Informants had no information about the research and were just asked to comment on the photographs. This fieldwork was conducted in three waves: first with Spanish gay men, second with Spanish and Argentinian gay and heterosexual men, and third with Equatoguinean men as part of a research project on Equatorial Guinea (Enguix 2012c, 2014, 2015, 2018).

One of the happiest findings of that research was to discover how bodies overflow matter and refer to body and gender, but also to sexuality, family, morals, desire, the erotic, and other affects. There were no substantive differences among study sites. Another finding was that informants classified men's bodies primarily according to gender, as I had anticipated. They clearly distinguished three styles in relation to masculinity. The ambiguous or androgynous style was considered the least attractive style by all informants, whereas hypermasculinity was considered an exaggerated but valued performance.

All three styles use body techniques such as muscle, hair, attire, and accessories to police the borders of masculinity. Images of Bears were labeled as hypermasculine and considered to police the borders of sex, gender, and sexuality from the inside—not letting others in—and to defend strong, virile, assertive, and brave masculinities. Ambiguity or androgyny was defined through body techniques (lack of muscle or hair), feminine (effeminate) attire, and different accessories like shoes and makeup. According to my fieldwork data, androgyny still relies on the cultural assumption that gender (femininity) is related to (homo)sexuality. It polices the borders of sex, gender, and sexuality from the outside; it is used by hegemonic masculinities to keep apart those who do not fit in. "Standard" masculinity was defined by the "exact" quantity of hair and muscle, by the lack of effeminacy, and by being "natural." It was considered the most attractive style, with the "exact dose" of masculinity indexed by the exact quantity of muscle and hair.

Masculine body indexes still rely heavily on muscle, body, and facial hair (as in classical Greek sculptures), whereas feminine masculine styles are constructed through the lack of hair and muscle, but also through artifacts such as high heels, feminine dress, makeup, and so on. Both styles rely on traditional gender stereotypes but also perform gender play. In any case, masculinity today is still strongly expressed through bodies. In the context of gay male culture, where body is a priority and male body images are hyper-idealized, Bears are a "subculture" of gay men who appreciate big, hairy bodies. There are other gay body types, as the list in table 7.1 shows.

This list expresses two different impulses: the hyper-classificatory effort, based on body and age, and the use of animal terms to refer to the different gay types. Only Bears are identified in gender terms (as "very masculine") in this classification, so let us turn to them. Bears are in some ways the heirs of the gay clone. Gay clones are associated with the birth of the modern gay movement after Stonewall, and they were seen as a way of self-presentation to reconcile homosexuality with normative masculinity. As Levine (1998)

Table 7.1. Gay body types. Source: John Hollywood, "Gay Men: Are You a Jock, Otter, Bear or Wolf?," *Paired Life* (blog), 17 June 2019, retrieved 18 July 2019 from https://pairedlife.com/dating/Gay-Men-Are-you-a-Jock-Otter-Bear-or-Wolf.

Type	Build	Hair	Age	Example Celebrity	Notes
Otter	Thin or athletic	Lots	Any age	Scott Caan	Part of the extended bear community
Wolf	Lean, muscular	Semi-hairy	Any age	Joe Manganiello	Sexually aggressive; Silver or grey wolf is an older wolf
Bear	Big, often with a belly	Lots	Any	John Travolta	Very masculine
Cub	Husky	Lots	Young or younger-looking	Jack Black	Sugar-cubs and muscle-cubs are subtypes
Chub	Real big	Maybe	Any	John Goodman	Distinct from bears
Pup	Slender	No	Young	Joe Jonas	Energetic, cute and naive
Bull	Super-built	Maybe	Any	Dwayne "The Rock" Johnson	
Twink	Slender	No	Young	Justin Bieber	Self-centered, usually between 18 and the mid-20s
Twunk	Muscular but slender	No	Young	The muscular version of Bieber	A more muscular Twink
Gym Bunny	Sculpted	Maybe	Under 50	Shemar Moore	Fitness associated with gym, not sports
Jock	Muscular and athletic	Maybe	Any	David Beckham	Fitness is associated with sports
Gym Rat	Very lean and well-built	Maybe	Any		Addicted to working out

affirmed, gay clones had more to do with gender than with sexuality. The same is true about leathermen and Bears.

Bears originated in San Francisco in the 1980s and were related to the bikers and leather communities. Hennen considers the "bear culture" as a gender strategy to repudiate effeminacy; it simultaneously questions and reproduces the standards of hegemonic masculinity (2005: 25). Bears have separated effeminacy from same-sex desire and have created a style in which they seem a "bunch of regular guys" (Hennen 2008). They represent themselves as "embodied masculinity" (Connell 1995). Bears define their masculinity not only against the feminine, but more specifically against the feminized, hairless, and gym-toned body of the dominant ideal of gay masculinity. Apart from rejecting the body fascism of perfectly fit bodies, they share a gregarious interest in other Bears that extends beyond sexual interest. In this sense, they can be connected to some men's movements of the 1980s like the mythopoetic movement, which exalted masculine solidarity, myths, values, and support.

Bear bodies seem to be "resistant" to gay hegemonic models. For Hennen (2008: 97), the "bear culture was born from resistance... Bears reject the self-conscious, exaggerated masculinity of the gay leather man in favor of a more authentic masculinity." Whereas obesity is connected to lack of control over appetite and over all aspects of life (Ross 2010: 47), size in Bears is eroticized and fat bodies are turned into desirable bodies. However, within the "Bear community" we can also find a multiplicity of body types:

Bear: hairy man, more or less big
Cub: young guy, hairy or big
Chubby: big man with little or no body hair
Chaser: likes bears, cubs, daddies, or chubbies
Daddy: mature man or polar bear (gray hair)
Musclebear: must be muscled
Admirer: likes hairy men, can be big or slim[4]

Bear, cub, and chub (chubby) were listed as gay types in in table 7.1. Chaser, daddy, musclebear, and admirer are considered types within the Bear "community," whose limits have broadened up to include those who are not Bears but feel attracted to them (chasers and admirers). Not all informants agreed on how to define Bear subtypes, but they all agreed that this multiplicity resists normative hegemonic masculine bodies while it builds body-based hegemonies within the "community." The categories of "chaser" and "admirer" show how big bodies have come to be eroticized. The category of "musclebear" can be discussed as a "false" bear type, as the

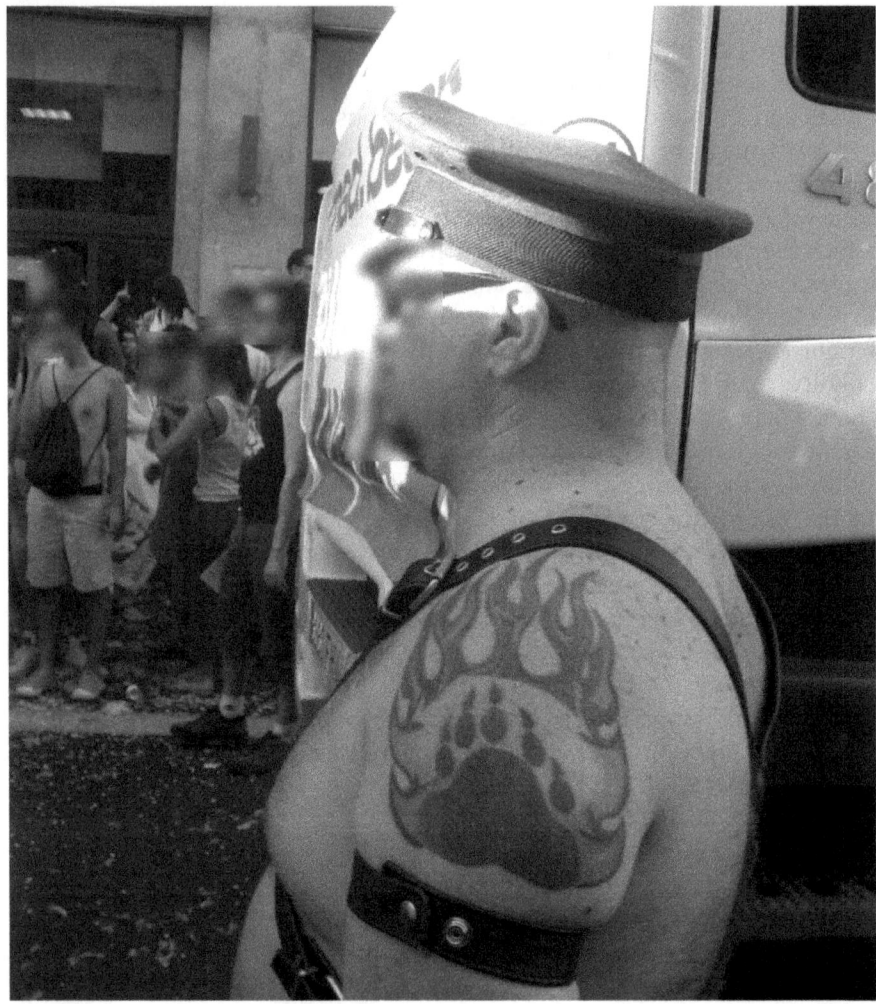

Figure 7.1. Madrid LGBT Pride State Demonstration, 2008. Photo by the author.

incorporation of standard hegemonic bodies (fit and muscled) to the bear universe or as an example of colonization of this universe characterized by nonstandard bodies by standard(ized) hegemonic bodies (Enguix and Ardèvol 2010, 2012).

Despite internal hegemonies and subordinations based on body/age relations, Bear bodies (and their subsequent subclassifications) widened the gay definitions of the attractive to men who did not fit in the homonormative ideals because of their age and/or body type. However, being a Bear does not only consist of being big, hairy, or mature; it requires an active intervention and participation of bodies. According to some interviews, being a Bear implies taking care of one's body: some of them are fat and fit; some of them are afraid of losing weight; body and facial hair are carefully looked after. Bear gendered bodies are hacked and reshaped in order to gain social and sexual value within a particular and meaningful context. With, through, and from their hacked and reshaped bodies, they prove that a gay man does not have to renounce virility; they reorganize the strategies of presentation of the culture of the closet (Levine 1998: 57); they prove that hegemonies are neither fixed nor stable processes; they show how gay men can also be hegemonic men and prove that hegemonic masculinity is not an attribute but a set of practices related to hegemonies and subordinations. They are overflown and protest bodies.

The masculinity/Bear assemblage includes ideologies about body, gender, sexuality, sexual practice, and sex liberation; technologies (tattoo, piercings, bodybuilding, hair, hormones, diet, energy drinks, drugs); the affects/effects of desiring and being desired, of the gaze, of (changing) subjectivities, of social discourses; agencies and hegemonies; body active participation; social, medical, psychiatric, and gender discourses; body techniques; respectability models of being LGTB and transnational models and homonormativity; gender meanings and the stability of the embodied and behavioral indexes of masculinity and femininity.

If we think about what is happening rather than trying to construct "meaning" (Mazzei 2014), we can say that the masculine is the instantaneous result of a messy configuration that assembles social discourses, our gaze and other people's gaze (which are both transformative for our active bodies), and one's subjectivity and body. It remains open.

Assembling Body, Gender, and Nation

One day in June 2017, I was walking to work and saw a poster on a shop window in the center of Barcelona (see figure 7.2). This all-body/embodied poster was signed by the six groups that belong to the EI. The CUP has deputies in the Catalan Parliament and is the most "institutional(ized)" organization. Coordinadora Obrera Sindical (COS) and Sindicat d'Estudiants dels Països Catalans (SEPC) are trade unions, whereas Alerta Solidària, Endavant, and Arran are political groups. Arran is a youth organization whose militants are between sixteen and twenty-six years old. They are all grassroots organizations that make all decisions as an assembly. All claim to work for an independent, socialist, and feminist Catalan Republic, and they make this evident on their webpages, campaigns, and mobilizations.

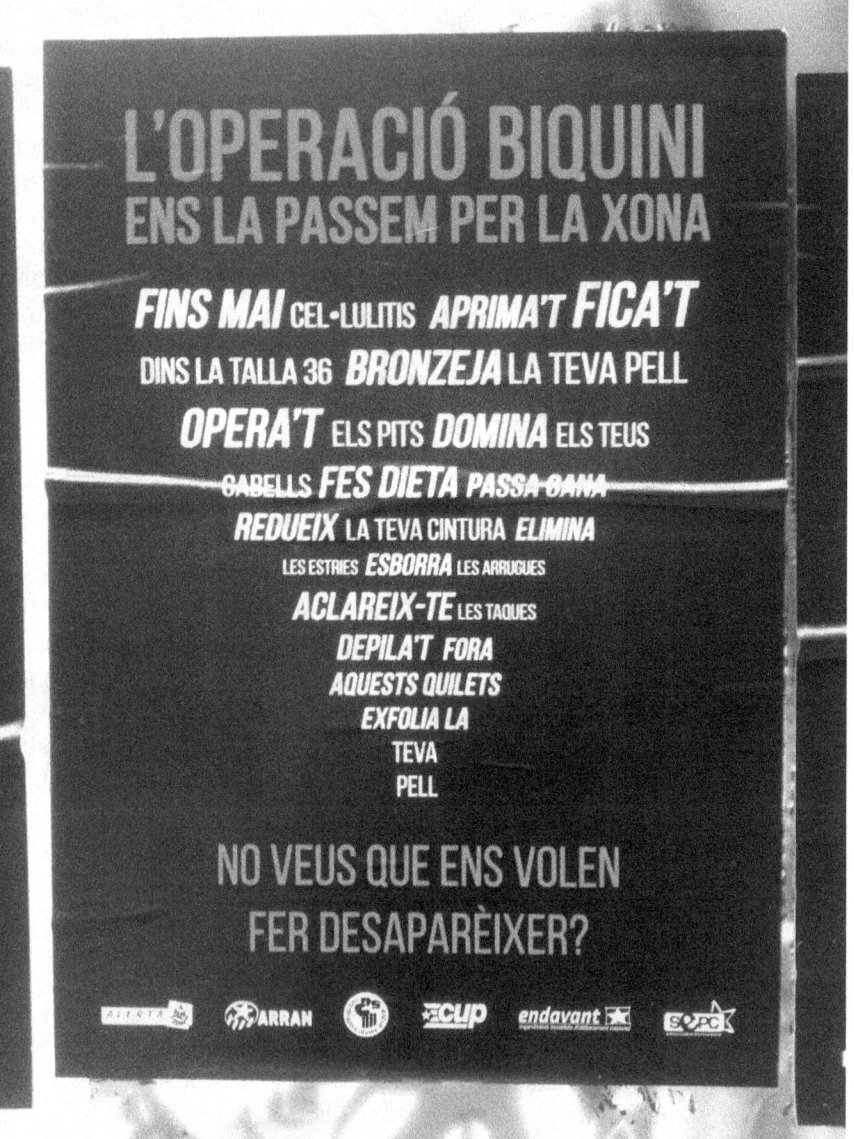

Figure 7.2. A poster on the streets of Barcelona. Photo by the author.

The text says:

> To hell with beach body plans
> Say goodbye to your cellulite
> Diet
> Become a size 36
> Get a tan
> Get cosmetic breast surgery
> Control your hair
> Get thin
> Starve
> Reduce your waist
> Erase stress
> Erase your wrinkles
> Whiten your spots
> Wax your body
> Take off those kilos
> Exfoliate your skin
> Can't you see they want to make us disappear?

According to Nira Yuval-Davis (1997), gender relations affect and are affected by national projects and processes; the constructions of nationhood involve specific notions of "manhood" and "womanhood." However, "the category 'nation' appears to be the least theorized and acknowledged of intersectional categories, rendered through a form of globalizing transparency" (Puar 2013: 377).

To serve the nation through/with one's body and dedication is a demanding task. The Spanish Legion, created in 1921 to defend Spanish borders in Africa, is known for its aggressiveness, virility, and braveness. In 2018, following orders of the army and the Spanish Ministry of Defense, legion members were put on a diet because they were becoming too fat: they did not correctly represent their country. They did not embody the nation in the correct way.[5]

As mentioned above, the EI in Catalonia defends a republic for the Catalan Countries (Catalonia, Balearic Islands, Valencian Country, and some parts of Southern France) where feminism, socialism, and independence are side by side. When asked in interviews, their members declare that none of these elements prevails over the other. However, Arran has made feminism, bodies, and gender central to their political debates and their public actions. Every time its members take part in a demonstration, their banners stress their fight for feminism.

The assemblage body-gender-nation in a particular time and space can produce rebel or traditional bodies that must meet some requirements ac-

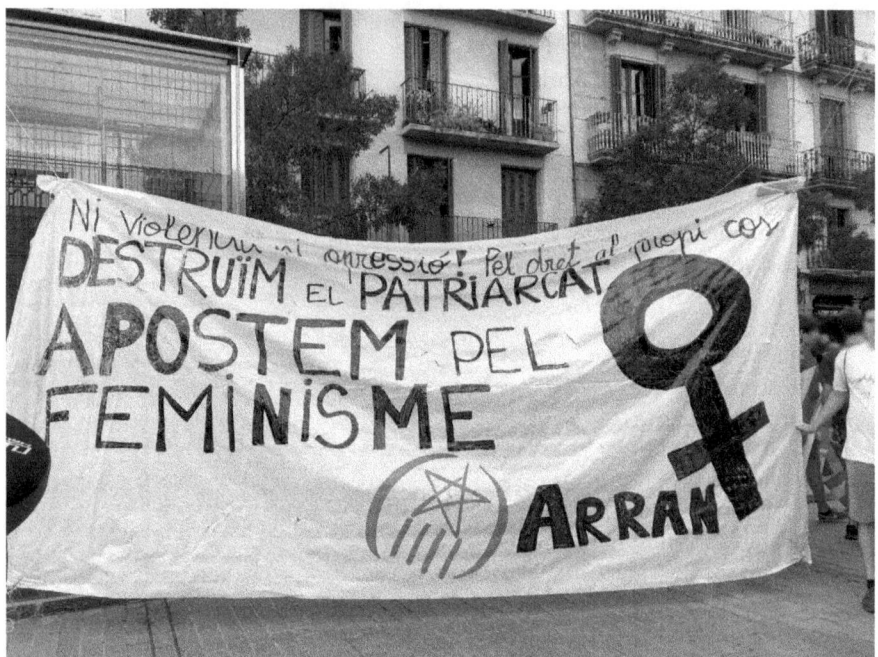

Figure 7.3. Barcelona: demonstration for Catalonia's National Day, 11 September 2018. Photo by the author.

cording to some shared meanings that are rarely expressed yet recognized by everybody. Like anti-globalization and/or anti-capitalist bodies, Arran political and protest bodies can be labeled as asexed and agendered. Agendering and asexing bodies is a political strategy related to their feminist stance. Arran is criticized for this. Some jokes are based on the fact that it is not clear whether its members are men or women. When they carry public actions, they usually dress in black bloc: black hooded sweatshirt, black trousers, black sneakers, and a black scarf covering part of the face. Piercings, hoop earrings, and partly shaved hairstyles for both young men and young women are also considered as indexes of belonging to EI. Their bodies are shaped by and shape their ideology, their experience, and their performance. As with Bears, they can be easily recognized: through, with, and within bodies, common bonds, solidarities, expectations, discourses, and objectives are constructed.

But those are not their bodies; at least, they are not their only bodies. They have others. They can wear a miniskirt and high heels. And they can do this also for political reasons, to show that they are "regular" people. Rebel bodies are not about what bodies are; they show what bodies can do as active participants in the public sphere.

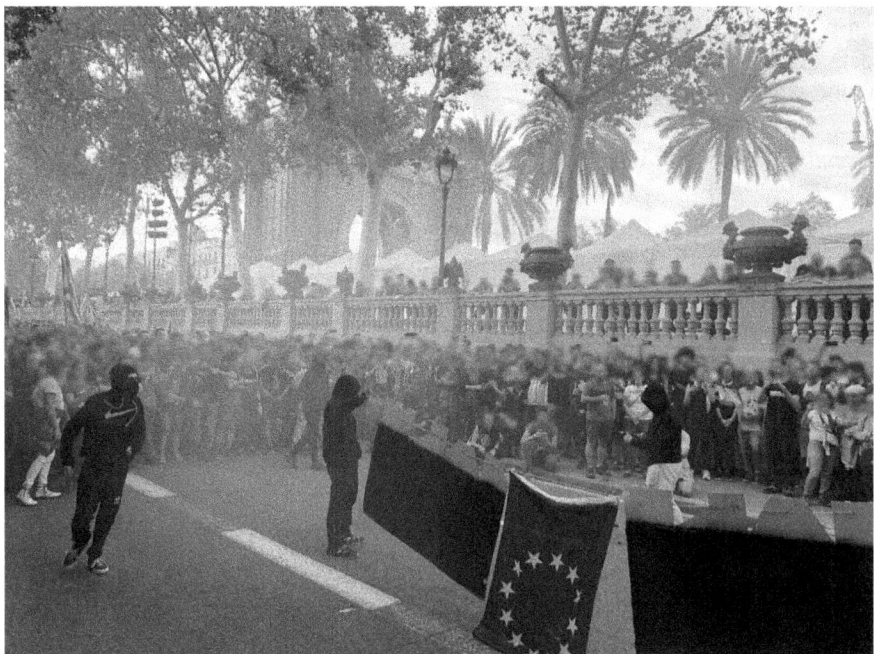

Figure 7.4. Militants in black bloc. Barcelona, 11 September 2019. Photo by the author.

Arran organized a Holi festival in October 2018 to oppose a demonstration to honor the policemen who violently repressed the Catalan Referendum conducted on 1 October 2017, which was considered illegal by the Spanish government. A Holi festival is a popular ancient Hindu free-for-all festival of colors, where people smear each other with colors. Water guns and water-filled balloons are used to play. This action covered demonstrators and police in a colored dust. Bodies were overflown into one another; vision was annihilated, smell was limited, taste was irrelevant. Touch and hearing became central. Arran militants had to bring extra clothes to change into after the action. They made and unmade their rebel bodies, shaped and hacked their flesh and bones. And everything, flesh, bones, hoods, hands, colors, blackness, black bloc, and so on, was political.

The Holi festival questioned the limits of individual bodies, like other protests or public concentrations where one becomes all. During their actions—considered violent by some people—Arran members adopt strategies to care for each other and never plan or attend actions on their own. I asked some of my Arran informants what they saw and felt when they planned and executed these actions. In protesting bodies, they see allies and companions, and the feeling of not being alone makes them "strong." In interviews, they emphasized that they are not conditioned by their sex or gender when they carry out actions that are very frequently fought by the police. On the contrary, they always try to have both men and women in the front line.

Their bodies are questioned, their gender is questioned, their sex is questioned. What is next?

We know that women in the public sphere and especially politicians are usually judged for their appearance rather than for their political performance. CUP and Arran are no exception. The difference with other contexts is that, as both CUP and Arran are pro-feminist, most of their public speakers and public figures are women, and they hack and reshape their bodies purposely to enact feminism. They always use the feminine gender when speaking in Catalan or Spanish.

What can we expect of a woman who does not "take care of herself" under the patriarchal codes or who does not assume a traditional gender role? If she cannot take care of herself, how can she pretend to rule a country? Unlike other cases in the national and international contexts, rebel bodies that contest beauty norms and canons are considered unsuitable for governance. EI women's bodies are overflown and protest bodies that embed gender and nation, but also capabilities and skills.

At some stage in the Catalan Process to Independence (as it is called in Catalonia), the Catalan government talked about the Slovenian way to independence as an example to follow. A meme comparing the photographs of Slovenian female models wearing sexy clothes and CUP female officers in municipalities and in the Catalan Parliament circulated through the internet with the following text: "Catalonia wants to be like Slovenia . . . this is not the right way."[6] The photograph of CUP female officers was taken during the public event held in 2016 when CUP deputies and counselors publicly denounced the insults they received as women politicians.

The connection between women's appearance and their capacities is a result of a patriarchal system of subordination, objectification, and hyper-sexualization of women that is profoundly embodied.

For these women and their public and political opponents, their bodies have become a battlefield. Their bodies are political weapons. Through, from, with, and within their bodies, they fight societal norms and beauty canons. That is not how their bodies are; this is about what their bodies can do. Bodies can shape and be shaped by their experiences; they can become a self-affirmative weapon in the context of their leftist stance and their feminist-socialist and pro-independence position. Bodies, then, are and become agentic, with generative capacities and political incidence. Their bodies are overflown bodies and protest bodies.

The assemblage body-gender-nation includes body; feminism; gender politics; ideology (socialism, anti-capitalism); nationalism; technologies (tattoo, piercings, hair, clothes, makeup); the affects/effects of their actions, demonstrations, and other public events; gendered and political stereotypes; agencies and hegemonies; body active participation; body techniques (strategies to talk, move, run, escape, fight, and control emotions such as fear or anxiety); public opinion; media; and supporters' and opponents' gaze. It remains open.

Final Remarks

In this chapter, I have shown how gender is relational and is connected to multiple affects and their effects, as in the assemblages I proposed. I also illustrated how gender is a malleable and complex cluster depending on the context and how gender is a system that can even affect our ideas about the way a nation must be.

In the examples I showed, gender affects bodies and produces their hacking and reshaping with the purpose of reproducing, subverting, transforming, changing, or transgressing the gendered experiences and lives of those bodies that are in/of the world. Feminist epistemologies provide us with the theoretical and the empirical tools to explore complex relations in a complex way and not in a unidirectional, simple, or deterministic way. Their feminist stance and their critical, ethical, and creative focus allow us to understand biopolitics as micropolitics and to acknowledge the embodied micropolitics of power as *potentia* (productive) and not only as *potestas* (restrictive). Recentering the body as a core element for social life, together with a materialist notion of embodiment, can provide new and more accurate analyses of the flows of power and different forms of embodied resistance suited to the polycentric and dynamic structure of contemporary power (Patton 2000). Bears and EI militants illustrate different ways of resistance through active hacked and becoming bodies.

The figuration of overflown bodies can be useful for thinking in/through assemblages because it stresses that relations and affects are more important than the different elements of the assemblage taken separately. The figuration of protest bodies situates our bodies as already political. Overflown, protest, and assembled bodies help us to understand our experience in terms of instability, process, dynamism, and change, escaping the stable identities that intersectionality requires, as Puar (2013) criticized. Overflown bodies are embedded and entangled in complex assemblages of emotions, affects, ideologies, mobilizations, activisms, and other expressions of (for) social and political action. They go well beyond their skin, and as the examples show, they are engendered and sexed, they are a playground and a battleground. They are active agents of social and political action. Overflown bodies produce bodies in becoming, and generative and open bodies. Overflown bodies make reshaping and hacking possible, thus increasing the possibilities and potentialities of bodies. Hacking and reshaping bodies are tools and processes for overflown bodies; they amplify the multiple affects of bodies.

In the two examples, gender is the driving force for hacking and reshaping bodies. Gender pushes the potential of bodies (as matter and discourse) for social critique and trans/formation because "a body affects other bodies, or is affected by other bodies; it is this capacity for affecting and being affected that ... defines a body in its individuality" (Deleuze 1988: 123). Gendered bodies are already political bodies that expand into affects, emotions, ideologies, mobilization, and other agents that affect us and affect and are affected by the world we live in.

The two cases develop two different embodied strategies for reshaping and hacking bodies in order to question, subvert, reproduce, confirm, or change social norms. Through/with/within their bodies, Bears claim the norm that was denied to them, that is, they reaffirm gay masculinity through the use of the stereotypical indexes of masculinity (body hair and size), but they also subvert the homonormative codes of the ideal gay body (muscled and fit) because of their body size, characteristics, and age. They expand the limits of attractiveness; they rewrite the lines of desire. Bears are conservative/reproductive in gender terms and revolutionary in body and age terms.

The case of EI (CUP and Arran) is related but different. Their militants subvert gender norms through embodied strategies. In their actions and in their radical outfits, Arran militants try to erase the marks of gender and sex: black bloc is not exclusive to them, it has been popularized by anti-capitalist and anti-globalization movements. But in their case, entangled with feminism, their bodies become differently both as anti-capitalist and also as feminist bodies, as matter and discourse.

CUP deputies try to undermine the patriarchal system by not adapting to the gender stereotypes on attractive, sexualized, and objectified women. Their public figures do not pretend to be passive models, but active fighters. They are criticized because of this; their subversion of the system is connected to the incapability to run the *res publica*, that is, to be in politics, let alone to hold power positions. If according to patriarchal standards, they cannot rule themselves, it is evident that they cannot rule a country.

Both examples show that bodies are always already gendered and gender still needs a body. They show how gendered bodies are matter and discourse. They are digital and physical; present and absent; present, future, and past. They are always already political. In the transformation of bodies from a "playground" into a "battleground," or vice versa, a whole set of possibilities become open to bodies; bodies actively open for those potentialities. Thinking through assemblages, relations and intra-actions, and not through the essence or the "facts," situates bodies as processes of becoming together with multiple embodied and disembodied affects. Surpassing dualistic understandings of body/mind, nature/culture, masculine/feminine, in/out, and others, we can carry out a "promiscuous analysis" (Childers 2014) that does not necessarily follow the lines, imposing logic and order to our research.

Acknowledgments

This research is a result of the research project "Genders and Postgenders: A Cartography of Meanings for Social Transformation" (I+D Programa Estatal, Ministerio de Economía y Competitividad. Gobierno de España. Referencia: FEM2016-77963-C2-2-P) (2016–21).

Begonya Enguix Grau is associate professor in the Arts and Humanities Department of the Universitat Oberta de Catalunya (UOC) and principal investigator of the research group "Medusa: Genders in Transition" (UOC). She holds a PhD in social and cultural anthropology (URV). She lectures and conducts research on masculinities and other gender expressions, bodies, and sexualities and their relationship with media, digital activism, and politics. She has participated in twenty-two research projects and has published over sixty works. Her most recent book is *Orgullo, Protesta, Negocio y otras Derivas LGTB* (2019, ed. Doce Calles). In 2019 she held the Aigner Rollett Guest Professorship in Women's and Gender Studies at Karl-Franzens Universität, Graz (Austria).

Notes

1. Manspreading refers to the masculine/masculinist practice of sitting down leaving a big space between both legs, thus exhibiting the genital area.
2. For Braidotti, figurations are politically informed images that portray the complex interaction of levels of subjectivity (Braidotti 1994: 4).
3. John Paul Power, "More Than Human: Six Body Hacks that Give You Superpowers, Kinda," 2018, retrieved 22 July 2019 from https://medium.com/threat-intel/biohacking-technology-science-2f5b5420c3de.
4. "Definitions," classification retrieved 19 July 2019 from https://www.bearwww.com/pages/faq.php?frames=no#lexique, a bear and admirers dating site.
5. *El Periódico*, "El Ejército pone a dieta a la Legión: pueden ser expulsados si no adelgazan en un año," 2018, retrieved 16 October 2019 from ttps://www.elperiodico.com/es/politica/20180105/legion-sobrepeso-adelgazar-dieta-6531759.
6. *El Cadenazo*, "Las de la CUP miran a Eslovenia . . . ," 2017, retrieved 20 October 2017 from http://elcadenazo.com/index.php/las-de-la-cup-miran-a-eslovenia/.

References

Bargetz, Brigitte. 2014. "Mapping Affect: Challenges of (un)Timely Politics." In Marie-Luise Angerer, Bernd Bösel, and Michaela Ott (eds.), *Timing of Affect: Epistemologies, Aesthetics, Politics*. Zurich: Diaphanes, pp. 289–303.

Braidotti, Rosi. 1994. *Nomadic Subjects: Embodiment and Sexual Difference in Contemporary Feminist Theory*. New York: Columbia University Press.

———. 2013. *The Posthuman*. Malden, MA: Polity Press.

Buchanan, Ian. 1997. "The Problem of the Body in Deleuze and Guattari, Or, What Can a Body Do?" *Body and Society* 3(3): 73–91.

Butler, Judith. 1990. *Gender Trouble*. New York: Routledge.

Carrigan, Tim, Bob Connell, and John Lee. 1985. "Toward a New Sociology of Masculinity." *Theory and Society* 14(5): 551–604.

Childers, Sara M. 2014. "The Promiscuous Analysis in Qualitative Research." *Qualitative Inquiry* 20(6): 819–26. https://doi.org/10.1177/1077800414530266.

Coleman, Rebecca. 2012. *The Becoming of Bodies: Girls, Images, Experience*. Manchester: Manchester University Press.

Connell, Raewyn W. 1987. *Gender and Power*. Cambridge: Polity Press.

———. 1995. *Masculinities*. Cambridge: Polity Press.

Connell, Raewyn W., and James W. Messerschmidt. 2005. "Hegemonic Masculinity. Rethinking the Concept." *Gender & Society* 19(6): 829–59.

de Barbieri, Teresita. 1993. "Sobre la Categoría Género. Una Introducción Teórico-Metodológica." *Debates en Sociología* 18: 145–169.

Deleuze, Gilles. 1988. *Spinoza: Practical Philosophy*. San Francisco: City Light Books.

Deleuze, Gilles, and Félix Guattari. 1994. *What Is Philosophy?* New York: Columbia University Press.

Domurat Dreger, Alice. 1998. *Hermaphrodites and the Medical Invention of Sex*. Cambridge, MA: Harvard University Press.

Dyke, Sarah. 2013. "Disrupting 'Anorexia Nervosa': An Ethnography of the Deleuzian Event." In Rebecca Coleman and Jessica Ringrose (eds.), *Deleuze and Research Methodologies*. Edinburgh: Edinburgh University Press, pp. 145–64.

Enguix, Begonya. 2012a. "Cuerpos, Camisetas e Identidades como Estrategias de Protesta." In Benjamin Tejerina and Ignacia Perugorría (eds.), *Global Movements, National Grievances: Mobilizing for 'Real Democracy' and Social Justice*. Bilbao: Servicio Editorial de la Universidad del País Vasco, pp. 175–200.

———. 2012b. "Cuerpos y Protesta: Estrategias Corporales en la Acción Colectiva." *Revista Brasileira de Sociologia da Emoção* 11 (33): 885–913.

———. 2012c. "Cultivando Cuerpos, Modelando Masculinidades." *Revista de Dialectología y Tradiciones Populares* 67(1): 147–80.

———. 2014. "Male Bodies and the Black Male Gaze: Is there a Cultural Interpretation of Masculinities?" In J. Martí (ed.), *African Realities: Body, Culture and Social Tensions*. Newcastle upon Tyne: Cambridge Scholars, pp. 111–46.

———. 2015. "Cuerpos Desbordados. La Construcción Corporal de la Masculinidad." *Argos* 30(59): 61–86.

———. 2018. "Cuerpos Desbordados como Ensamblaje. Habitar lo 'Masculino' de Forma 'Posthumana.'" *Quaderns de l'ICA* 34: 135–56.

———. 2019. *Orgullo, Protesta, Negocio y otras Derivas LGTB*. Madrid: Editorial Doce Calles.

Enguix, Begonya, and Elisenda Ardèvol. 2010. "Cuerpos 'hegemónicos' y cuerpos 'resistentes': el cuerpo-objeto en webs de contatos." In Josep Martí and Yolanda Aixelà (eds.), *Desvelando el Cuerpo: Perspectivas desde las Ciencias Sociales y Humanas*. Barcelona: CSIC-Altafulla, pp. 333–51.
———. 2012. "Enacting Bodies: Online Dating and New Media Practices." In K. Ross (ed.), *The Handbook of Gender, Sex and Media*. Oxford: Wiley-Blackwell, pp. 502–16.
Francis, Becky. 2008. "Engendering Debate: How to Formulate a Political Account of the Divide between Genetic Bodies and Discursive Gender?" *Journal of Gender Studies* 17(3): 211–23.
Gill, Rosalind, Karen Henwood, and Carl McLean. 2005. "Body Projects and the Regulation of Normative Masculinity." *Body & Society* 11(1): 37–62.
Gilmore, David D. 1994. *Hacerse Hombre. Concepciones Culturales de la Masculinidad*. Barcelona: Paidós.
Grosz, Elizabeth. 1994. *Volatile Bodies: Toward a Corporeal Feminism*. Bloomington: Indiana University Press.
Halberstam, Jack. 1998. *Female Masculinity*. Durham, NC: Duke University Press.
Haraway, Donna. 1991. *Simians, Cyborgs and Women: The Reinvention of Nature*. New York: Routledge.
Harrison, Katherine. 2010. *Discursive Skin: Entanglements of Gender, Discourse and Technology*. Linköping Studies in Arts and Science 513. Linköping University.
Hearn, Jeff. 2018. "Moving Men, Changing Men, Othering Men: On Politics, Care and Representation." *Quaderns de l'ICA* 24: 29–59.
Hennen, Peter. 2005. "Bear Bodies, Bear Masculinity: Recuperation, Resistance, or Retreat?" *Gender & Society* 19(1): 25–43.
———. 2008. *Faeries, Bears and Leathermen: Men in Community; Queering the Masculine*. Chicago: University of Chicago Press.
Hester, David. 2004. "Intersexes and the End of Gender: Corporeal Ethics and Postgender Bodies." *Journal of Gender Studies* 13(3): 215–25.
Jackson, Alecia Youngblood. 2013. "Data-as-Machine: A Deleuzian Becoming." In Rebecca Coleman and Jessica Ringrose (eds.), *Deleuze and Research Methodologies*. Edinburgh: Edinburgh University Press, pp. 111–25.
Kimmel M. 1996. *Manhood in America: A Cultural History*. New York: Free Press.
Levine, Martin P. 1998. *Gay Macho: The Life and Death of the Homosexual Clone*. New York: New York University Press.
Mazzei, Lisa A. 2014. "Beyond an Easy Sense: A Diffractive Analysis." *Qualitative Inquiry* 20(6): 742–46.
Patton, Paul. 2000. *Deleuze and the Political*. London: Routledge.
Preciado, Paul B. 2018. "#MeToo: Carta de un hombre trans al antiguo régimen sexual." *Diario Ara*, 26 January 2018. Retrieved 20 May 2019 from https://www.ara.cat/es/opinion/Paul-B-Preciado-Carta-hombre-trans-antiguo-regimen-sexual_0_1951605023.html.
Priban, Jiri. 2018. "Constitutional Imaginaries and Legitimation: On Potentia, Potestas, and Auctoritas in Societal Constitutionalism." *Journal of Law and Society* 45(S1): S30–S51.
Puar, Jasbir. 2013. "'I Would Rather Be a Cyborg Than a Goddess': Intersectionality, Assemblage, and Affective Politics." *Meritum–Belo Horizonte* 8(2): 371–90.

Ringrose, Jessica, and Rebecca Coleman. 2013. "Looking and Desiring Machines: A Feminist Deleuzian Mapping of Bodies and Affects." In Rebecca Coleman and Jessica Ringrose (eds.), *Deleuze and Research Methodologies*. Edinburgh: Edinburgh University Press, pp. 125–45.

Rohlinger, Deana A. 2002. "Eroticizing Men: Cultural Influences on Advertising and Male Objectification." *Sex Roles* 3(4): 61–74.

Ross, Karen. 2010. *The Handbook of Gender, Sex, and Media*. London: Wiley-Blackwell.

Rubin, Gayle. 1986. "El Tráfico de mujeres: notas sobre la economía política del sexo." Retrieved 15 May 2019 from http://www.cholonautas.edu.pe/modulo/upload/rubin.pdf.

Simpson, Mark. 2002. "Meet the Metrosexual." *Salon*. Retrieved 16 October 2019 from https://www.salon.com/2002/07/22/metrosexual.

———. 2014. "The Metrosexual Is Dead. Long Live the 'Spornosexual.'" *The Telegraph*. Retrieved 16 October 2019 from https://www.telegraph.co.uk/men/fashion-and-style/10881682/The-metrosexual-is-dead.-Long-live-the-spornosexual.html.

Stivale, Charles J. 2005. *Gilles Deleuze: Key Concepts*. Trowbridge: Cromwell Press.

Tamboukou, Maria. 2010. "Charting Cartographies of Resistance: Lines of Flight in Women Artists' Narratives." *Gender and Education* 22(6): 679–96.

Yuval-Davis, Nira. 1997. *Gender and Nation*. London: Sage.

CHAPTER 8

Remaking (Post-)Human Bodies in the Anthropocene through Bioart Practices

CHRISTINE BEAUDOIN

My aim in this chapter is to highlight the potential of some bioart practices to challenge the ways we think about living bodies—and specifically human bodies—in the context of the Anthropocene and post-humanism. The first part of this chapter briefly frames post-humanism. This is followed by an empirical discussion of the practices of biology and bioart. I first present an ethnographic account of my explorations of biology laboratories—including SymbioticA, a bioart lab run by artists and for artists at the University of Western Australia. Secondly, I discuss the work of some bioartists who have remade their own bodies into living artworks. The final part of this chapter speculates on the ways in which we can rethink human bodies in the Anthropocene. I argue that bioartistic practices can contribute to a broader remaking of humans and their relationships to the environment and may offer us productive avenues to work through the environmental crisis.

The goal of this chapter is not to present a homogenous vision of bioart practices or to generalize that every artistic work mobilizing biotechnologies concerns humans. Rather, it is to flesh out some of my experiences working in biolaboratories and to focus on some of my encounters with laboratory life and artists who used their own biomaterials to create artworks. I write of the very works that have contributed to my own questioning of what it means to be human.

Post-humanism and Going Beyond the Human

Emerging from "an urgency for the integral redefinition of the notion of the human" (Ferrando 2013: 26), post-humanism is a manifestation of the practical, ontological, and epistemological shifts and developments in the life sciences and biotechnologies. Post-humanism puts into question human hegemony by highlighting the material complexities of the world we live in and the pressures that human and nonhuman bodies face (Wamberg and Thomsen 2016). In the context of the Anthropocene and the environmental crisis, Ferrando (2016) calls for a paradigm shift toward a post-humanism that is post-anthropocentric and post-dualistic. Such post-humanism acknowledges that "humans do not live in a vacuum" (Ferrando 2016: 160) and that we must consider how we are related to the nonhumans with whom we share the planet. Ferrando (2016) calls for the environment to be considered in post-humanistic approaches, which could shift our sociocultural perceptions of what it means to be a human, with a human body.

Our very human bodies, waste, aesthetics, and technologies are always evolving with other organic and inorganic processes, which take on new meanings in the wake of the Anthropocene (Wamberg and Thomsen 2016). This geological epoch gives us a new context in which to interpret human intervention on their own bodies and the bodies of others. Though remaking human bodies has been a constant practice over time—through tattoos, piercings, ingestion of plants and mind-altering substances (Wamberg and Thomsen 2016), and more recently intrauterine contraceptive devices and mobile technologies—the emergence and accessibility of modern biotechnologies has led to a significant opening of the possibilities to practically and concretely rethink, remake, and create new human bodies.

The rise in the use of biotechnologies to control human and nonhuman bodies is related to the landscape of the Anthropocene. In this chapter, the Anthropocene and post-humanism serve as a theoretical backdrop against which I position bioart as both concrete and abstract, material and conceptual, sets of practices that contribute to the ways in which we think and rethink humans and nonhumans. Some artists literally bridge their bodies with technologies and the bodies of others, sometimes creating new living entities that are anchored in biotechnology, other times revealing unanticipated tensions and assumptions we hold as human beings. Their artworks participate in a broad rethinking and remaking of bodies that transform our conception of the human.

Biotechnologies and Bioart Practices

Recent decades have shown a massive reduction in costs associated with biotechnologies and research within the life sciences. For example, the cost of DNA sequencing dropped from $100,000 to ten cents between 2001 and 2015 (Wall 2015). This recent reduction in cost has led to the rise of people using biotechnologies in new places and in unexpected ways, within but also beyond the traditional sites of biotechnological innovation, which are academia and industry. Biohacking, citizen science, and other open source movements are recognized as a way for scientists to collaborate with new partners and give them access to research and biotechnological tools that have been kept locked behind lab doors. Do-it-yourself biology (DIYbio), which aims for public access to biotechnologies, has emerged as a global movement that articulates itself locally (Park 2013: 120). Bioart has also emerged, since the 1980s, as a field where biological and biotechnological systems or processes serve as a medium for artistic practice (Abergel 2011; Byerley and Chong 2015; Damm et al. 2013; Kac 2006; Lapworth 2015; Uhl and Dubois 2011). The proliferation of access to biology and the multiplicity of living beings involved—within industry, academic, community, and home labs—bring concrete action to theoretical post-humanistic discourse and allow us to problematize the ways in which we actively rethink and thus remake the human.

Bioart refers to using life and its processes as an artistic medium. It can be conceptualized as opening the doors to a new imaginary that moves beyond classic dualisms of mind and body, nature and culture (Uhl and Dubois 2011). It can also be seen as a transgression of the (human and nonhuman) body by technology, which leads to a blurring of many boundaries that have been so strictly established by the sciences. In this conceptualization of bioart, many notions are put in tension such as bodies, incorporation, species, animality, humanity, and ethics. In the words of Eduardo Kac, "Il s'agit ... de création littéralement basée sur la vie" (It is ... creation literally based on life) (2006: 313). The fusional character of bioart breaches disciplinary boundaries; this kind of investigation situates itself at the nexus between the arts and sciences (Abergel 2011; Catts and Zurr 2006; Kac 2006; Uhl and Dubois 2011). It is by playing with the autonomy of living things (Landecker 2007) that bioartists attempt to expose different aspects of our relationships with these life-forms and with our own human identities and bodies.

I first became aware of biohacking, DIYbio, and bioart in 2015, after joining the Pelling Lab for Augmented Biology on my home campus at the

University of Ottawa (at the time named the Pelling Lab for Biophysical Manipulation) from July 2015 to May 2016. Biohacking and DIYbio refer broadly to the use of biotechnologies by individuals or small groups to learn and experiment. I joined the laboratory as an anthropologist-in-residence, auditing a biophysics course with Andrew Pelling to familiarize myself with in vitro cell culture and cell mechanics while beginning course work as a first-year master's student. Challenging normative assumptions of what a biophysics laboratory should and could be, Pelling established his space in 2008 as an experiment to bring curious people from a broad range of disciplines together in one room (Beaudoin and Jaclin 2016; Pelling 2015). Hosting biology and physics students, Pelling also provided a space for social scientists and artists to engage directly with biotechnologies and living materials in their research. This open biolaboratory space is constituted by a multiplicity and a diversity of human and nonhuman, scientist and artistic voices. It is where I first learned the craft of mammalian tissue culture. It is the practice of growing immortal cell lines—originating from human, mice, and other species—in clear Petri dishes placed in expensive yet sensitive, sustainable yet short-lived incubators. Learning this practice involved many things: biosafety trainings and certification, theoretical knowledge acquisition, participation in lab meetings, and outreach events. Most importantly, cell culture involved the gradual development of a new skill as part of my new relationship with in vitro cells. Though this relationship leaked beyond the seemingly hermetic walls of the laboratory (which help to ensure a clean, sterile environment where cells can grow and thrive), I gained the skill of cell culture through ongoing, repeated, and practiced intimate gestures that concretely established my relationship with living cells.

In the Pelling Lab, I worked directly with C2C12 cells, which are mouse myoblasts—cells with the potential of becoming muscle fibers. I also interacted with 3T3 cells, which are mouse fibroblasts—they make up connective tissues—and green fluorescent proteins (GFP)—a protein that has been isolated from jellyfish and can be used to genetically modify in vitro cells so that they exhibit fluorescence without the need for dyes. Furthermore, I encountered a wide range of abiotic technologies and materials: incubators, water baths, centrifuges, microscopes, pipettes, tubes, Petri dishes, a saline buffer, fetal bovine serum, Dulbecco's Modified Eagle's Medium, fluorescent stains, and many more.

I encountered HeLa cells at the Pelling Lab, the first and oldest immortal human cell line. Though I did not directly work with this cell line, many of my colleagues in the Pelling Lab engaged with them. There were whispers of HeLa cells being so robust and multiplicative that they could survive out of the confines of incubators and follow us out of the sterile tissue culture rooms. Originating from the biopsy of a particularly aggressive cancer of a human body and cultivated in vitro since the 1950s, are HeLa cells still human?

Both scientific and artistic investigation was encouraged at the Pelling Lab, which hosts artists who want to engage with the life sciences. This was my first exposure to bioart practices—some of which mobilized the same biotechnological protocols I spent months learning. It is in this context that I began to recognize the power of biotechnologies not only to challenge the limits of what we thought was scientifically possible in terms of living bodies, but also to challenge the ways we conceptualize human and nonhuman bodies and the porous boundaries between them. Through art, biotechnologies can be used to raise new questions.

I came into contact with SymbioticA through the Pelling Lab. A few short weeks after my last lab session in Canada, I traveled to the University of Western Australia (UWA) in Perth. I arrived at SymbioticA Centre of Excellence in Biological Art in June 2016 and stayed until September 2016. The lab was established in the early 2000s by artists and their scientific allies in the School of Anatomy and Human Biology at UWA (SymbioticA n.d.). When the Tissue Culture and Art Project was formed in 1996 by Oron Catts and Ionat Zurr (joined by Guy Ben-Ary in 1999), the group started working with the School of Anatomy and Human Biology and UWA research centers. In 1999 Oron Catts joined forces with scientists Miranda Grounds and Stuart Bunt to open a space permanently dedicated for artists to engage with the life sciences and biological systems. SymbioticA hosted its first two residents in 2000 and has since become an official research center at the university; it runs a residency program for artists, designers, social scientists, philosophers, and pretty much anyone who is interested and willing to learn about critically, artistically, or creatively engaging with the life sciences and biotechnologies. SymbioticA has participated in numerous collaborations within Australia and beyond with artists, engineers, and scientists, among others. As the first laboratory of its kind—SymbioticA has also organized conferences and exhibitions, such as the 2018 Quite Frankly: It's a Monster Conference. Andrew Pelling himself pursued a residency at SymbioticA in 2014. At the time of my fieldwork, these two laboratories shared interests in pushing the boundaries of what we thought possible through curiosity-based research and critical thinking. The Pelling Lab tried to answer funny questions that caught their attention, while SymbioticA director Oron Catts explained his intention to raise questions in people's minds, not necessarily answer them. I took the title of anthropologist-in-residence at SymbioticA, where I pursed a three-month residency.

At SymbioticA, I continued to engage in mammalian tissue culture, performing the intimate gestures I learned at the Pelling Lab, but with the intricacies of encounters increasingly revealing themselves over time spent practicing the gestures. I kept working on staining, mounting, and microscopy techniques and worked on developing a protocol to grow cells on barks and wood. I had to complete a new set of online trainings in biosafety, lab safety, and gene technology. Through reading groups and Friday seminars, I continued to be exposed to new thoughts and ideas from artists but also from scientists and others interested. Through learning to craft with slime mold (*Physarum polycephalum*) and fungal bodies, I ended up spending some time at the Chooi Laboratory for Fungal Chemistry at UWA. Through spending much time in the SymbioticA lab and office spaces, engaging with students and other residents, I understood it as a space that provides access to biological systems for explorations that go beyond scientific research. More and more "have brought Petri dishes out of the lab and into the museum" (Wohlsen 2011: 201). At SymbioticA, I was surrounded by numerous artists, bio and other, who developed relationships with different laboratory livings—humans, bees, mammalian cell lines, yeast, fungi, amoebas, plastics, electronics, wood, glass, metals, hair,

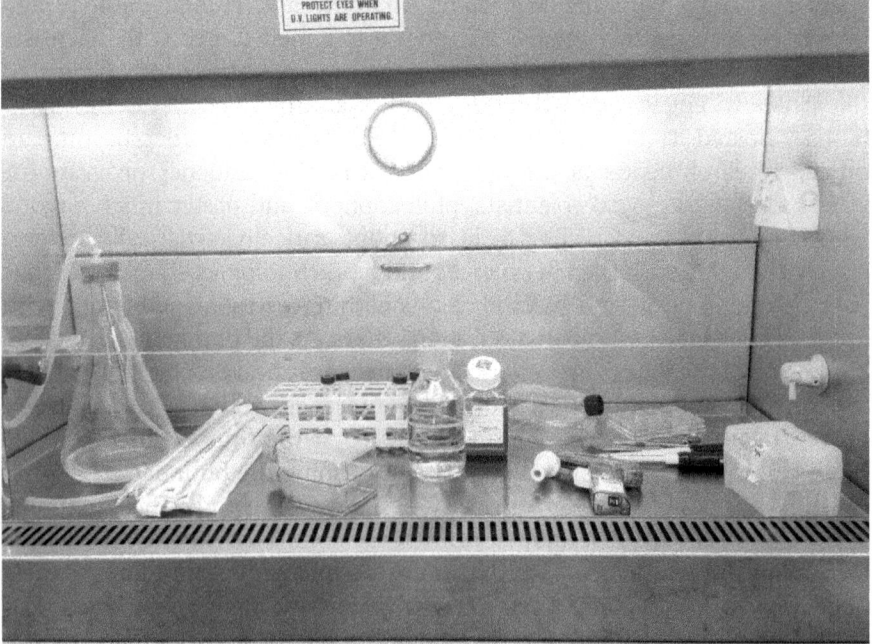

Figure 8.1. Setup for mammalian tissue culture in a biosafety cabinet at SymbioticA, 2016. Photo by the author.

liquids, solids, gases, fluids, visible, invisible. Though motivations behind—and methods of—bioartistic production vary, the unanimity of bioartists rests in the creative use of biotechnologies and "new ways of exploring the living and the partially living" (Byerley and Chong 2015: 213).

The transgenic organism, hybrids, and fragments that emerge from bioart and biohacks can pose an ontological problem, but also a great opportunity. For Lapworth (2015), the relationship that establishes itself between art piece, artists, and spectators is not one of domination but of affect, which could generate ontological (re)conceptualization. This change would emerge from artistic encounters, which lead to new ways of thinking and feeling: it is the establishment of a dialogue with our own bodies and other forms of life, a becoming together (Deleuze and Guattari 1980; Lapworth 2015). Lapworth (2015) argues that bioart could lead to a new relational ontogenesis (becoming together rather than being alone), a way of engaging the world, which relies on rhizomatic processes, not hierarchical arborescence (Deleuze and Guattari 1980; Ingold 2017).

At the center of ontogenesis emerges the question of material practice. Living entities are curious beings who love to explore and experiment in their material world, and laboratories are purely spaces of experimentation (Edwards 2010). All laboratories are positioned in larger cultural networks that lean toward utility and profit but can also be opened up to other ways of being (Zurr 2012). Spending time in various laboratories leads to cultivating different modes of attention and to the making of different world lenses. In this sense, laboratories lead to the development of various specialized sensorium, specific ways of being in the world, which manifest themselves through thinking and making.

This experimental and intimate mode of attention, inherent to work with biotechnologies, provides an opportunity for bioart practices to rethink, transform, and remake the boundaries of human bodies and conceptions. Thus, the harnessing of biotechnologies—understood as an assemblage of tools, methods, protocols, materials, and perceptions that include animate or biological processes (Beaudoin 2018; Stevens 2016)—by (bio)artists, biohackers, and the DIYbio community is seen as part of a shift in practices that holds post-humanist potential. Their activities are part of a global community promoting access to biological systems and biotechnologies and contribute pragmatically to changing the practices and norms we associate with biotechnology. Some bioartists engage with post-humanism by effectively redefining and hybridizing the boundaries of (human) lives and bodies (Abergel 2011; Uhl and Dubois 2011). This leads to radical transformations in the broader anthropocenic landscape that structures our social, political, and economic processes, but also the lived experiences of people and communities.

Rethinking and Remaking Human Bodies through Bioart

Specific practices of bioart and biohacking participate in post-anthropocentric efforts to rethink and actively remake the human. Bioartists participate in reshaping normative definitions of living bodies in part through concrete reshaping, repairing, and sometimes replacing human bodies. This part of the chapter engages the work of (bio)artists who have various ties to SymbioticA. I have met these artists during my stay at SymbioticA. I got to know Tarsh Bates and Guy Ben-Ary quite well during my three months at UWA, and I briefly met Nina Sellars, Stelarc, and Jaden A. Hastings during my stay.

Bioart practices are plural and diverse, and many artists engage with life and its extensions beyond the human at different scales. I discussed this question with Oron Catts and Ionat Zurr during my time at SymbioticA:

> Something that was apparent from the very beginning was that in that level of interaction and engagement with living systems, there's no difference between human and nonhuman cells. From the very beginning, we decided that wasn't going to be a defining criteria for us in regard to what types of cells we're using. *We often deliberately wouldn't use human cells* because of the fear that it was going to take us down the path of less resistance of existing discourses that are irrelevant. . . . What we found is when we talked about growing skin, most people would think about it in terms of human skin. Even if they were rabbits' eyes, people would still think that we grow human skin because we used the generic term, skin cells. *And we also made a very conscious decision not to work with our own tissues* [author's emphasis].

This highlights the plurality of bioart practices. Oron Catts, cofounder of SymbioticA and member of the Tissue Culture and Art Project with Ionat Zurr, consciously avoids working with human tissue to focus on life as a whole. However, artists engage with biological materials in many different ways, and this is the choice of one group of artists. I met others at SymbioticA who specifically mobilized materials of their own bodies to research, explore, create, but most importantly engage life and its processes in novel ways. It is some of their work that I argue contributes to reshaping, transforming, remaking, and in some cases replacing humanity and its bodies through complex manipulations (Uhl and Dubois 2011). A good analogy to think of the networks of artists who engage with biotechnologies and living media are cells themselves. Bioart networks remind me of cells growing on a dish: movement can go in all directions, sometimes it works, sometimes it doesn't, but it's all driven by curiosity and life with a desire to explore and engage the world in various ways.

I first discuss the work of Guy Ben-Ary, a Perth-based artist who works with SymbioticA, and his project titled *CellF* (2015–18). *CellF* began in 2012 and has progressed over many years of bioengineering explorations; it is a collaborative project also involving artists Nathan Thompson, Andrew Fitch, and Darren Moore and scientists Stuart Hodgetts, Mike Edel, and Douglas Bakkum (Ben-Ary 2019; Ben-Ary and Ben-Ary 2016). *CellF* is described by Guy as the world's first neural synthesizer (Moore et al. 2016). Its brain is biological, living tissue growing in a special Petri dish armed with electronics that can pick up the subtle voltage resulting from cell activity. Guy showed me the electrode arrays he uses for *CellF* when I was at SymbioticA. They are these little dishes sitting on top of a plaque with electrodes; they are placed in a Petri dish and in an incubator, which acts as a body for the in vitro cells that require specific living conditions to survive. The electrical activity picked up by the Petri dishes is transduced in sound to create an audio output that fills a room, thus emphasizing the agency of the cells. The custom synthesizer is a large structure, giving cells a massive body and a massive voice that comes in dialogue with other musicians. This is the core of *CellF*, a piece where human musicians, technologies, and living cells come together as a cybernetic musician (Ben-Ary and Ben-Ary 2016).

The cells that generate music in *CellF* are no standard immortal cell line. Guy had a biopsy of his arm taken in 2012, and he cultivated his own cells (Ben-Ary and Ben-Ary 2016). He reverse engineered his skin cells into stem cells, which were then differentiated into neural stem cells and grew to become neural networks. He showed me small vials containing the many different materials used for this specific protocol, which are not required

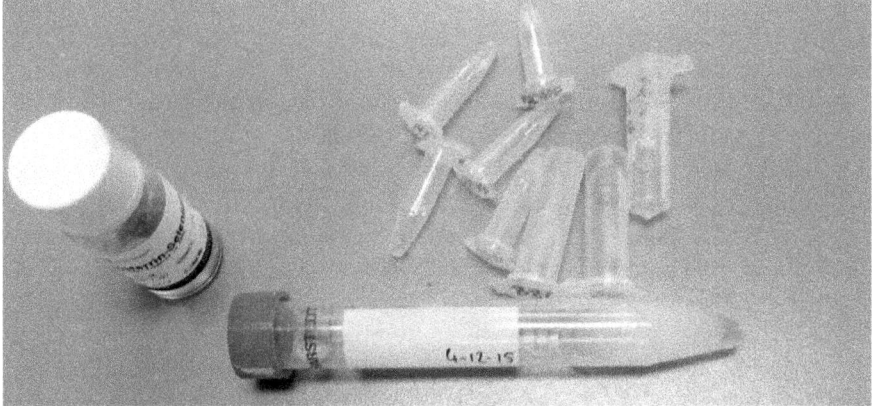

Figure 8.2. Guy Ben-Ary's vials to make the biochemical soup that allows his external brain to grow. At SymbioticA, 2016. Photo by the author.

for standard tissue culture of an established immortal cell line. This project rests in the alignment of complex biological protocols and the development of a robotic interface that helped serve as a body for the independent brain (Ben-Ary and Ben-Ary 2016). This creative endeavor resulted in new protocols that had yet to be developed by science. I looked at these cells through a microscope in one of the labs at UWA: I had a strange feeling, knowing these were Guy's cells growing and moving under my eyes, though I wondered if these cells were still Guy. In a way, Guy Ben-Ary re-embodied himself as a rock star by harvesting his cells and creating his own external brain. *CellF* has performed on many occasions with various musicians, like an electronic keyboardist and a group of drummers.

During my discussions with Guy on his work, and more broadly bioart, the question of consent arose. Guy stated that he works with human cells because humans can provide consent for their cells to be harvested and used, while other species cannot. For Guy, consent seems to extend from the original body and apply to the cells, which are perceived as an externalization of the consenting body. In the context of *CellF*, Guy took his own cells from his arm and fully consented to the procedure. Despite this action of quite drastic separation, remaking, and reshaping, Guy seemed to still have a sense of belonging with his external brain. He shared with me in conversation that he considers those cells are still part of him. This underlines some assumptions about what a human body is or could be. In Guy's case and in contrast with Oron's position, cells seemed to be an externalized extension of the human body. This new way of thinking of the human, a human that is not bound by skin but that leaks beyond and establishes relationships with technologies and other living beings, would have been impossible a hundred years ago. This work also points to the importance of respectful collaboration among humans and technologies and across the various forms that human beings can take. This is a clear example of how bioart practices actively, concretely, and pragmatically contribute to repairing, reshaping, replacing—in sum, remaking and opening up—what it means to be a human. Guy Ben-Ary has worked on many other projects with various collaborators, including "MEART," a robotic arm that created drawings under the control of living neuronal networks grown on a multielectrode array (Bakkum et al. 2007).

I turn to Tarsh Bates and her work *Surface Dynamics of Adhesion* (2016). Tarsh Bates was a PhD candidate at SymbioticA when I was there. She obtained her PhD in biological arts in 2018 and is now a postdoctoral research associate at SymbioticA supported by the Seed Box (an international environmental humanities collaboration based at Linköping University in Sweden). She works with yeast and biofilms, and as I got to know her, I discovered her deep, caring interest for *Candida albicans*, the living

Remaking (Post-)Human Bodies in the Anthropocene through Bioart Practices 175

being that is responsible for yeast infections. Tarsh referred to herself as a microbioartist, that is, she makes art in a microbiology laboratory. Whereas other artists I met at SymbioticA sometimes hesitated or outright rejected the terminology "bioart" (in favor of "performance artist" or more simply "artist"), Tarsh wanted everyone to see the kind of work she was doing, thus giving the microbiome its own voice even as she simply presented herself and her practice. Spending time with Tarsh at SymbioticA, discussing our respective works and experiments with living beings in laboratories, I came to see one of Tarsh's underlying assumption about the human body: the human body is itself a multispecies ecology that is part of a broader ecosystem (Bates 2013, 2017). Part of this discourse is the idea that the diversity of the microbiome, microbes, and fungi themselves make us human, more than the human DNA with which we traditionally identify. In a presentation at SymbioticA during my time there, Tarsh argued that human DNA represents the smallest portion of all of the DNA materials that can

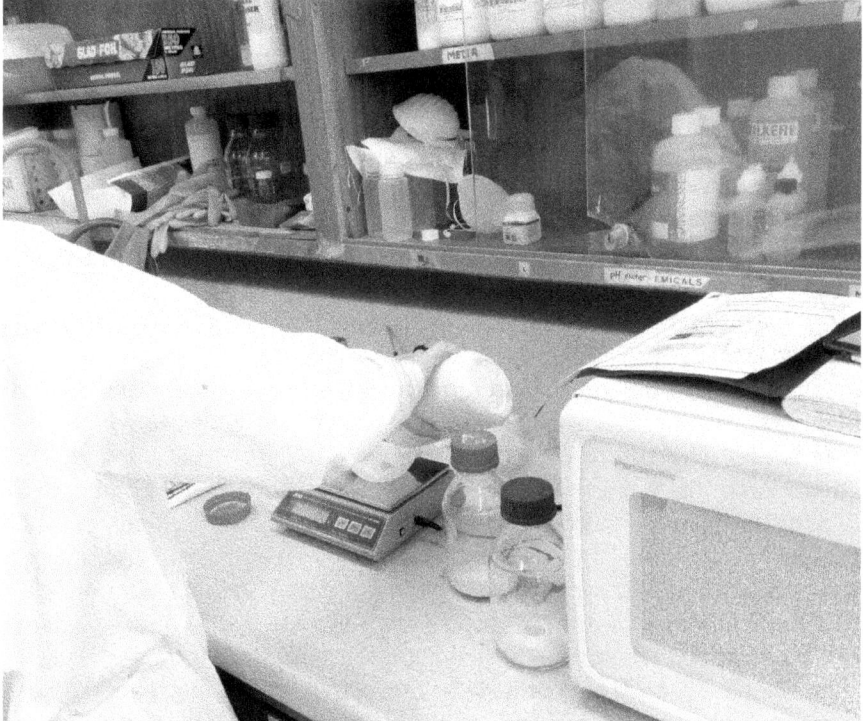

Figure 8.3. Following the recipe shared by Tarsh Bates to make agar plates that support growth of yeast, bacteria, and fungi. At the microbiology lab where she worked on her art at the University of Western Australia, 2016. Photo by the author.

be found within the boundaries of our skin, which we identify as being the human body. This is where *Candida albicans* comes into play: we intimately cohabit with this yeast that lodges itself into the mouths and cervixes of up to 80 percent of humans.

Tarsh developed a special interest in *Candida albicans* because of its gendered relationships with human societies, but she also gained an interest for their own internal societies and how they intimately interact with humans. She wanted to avoid quantification and scientification of her relationship with *Candida* to focus on story-building and storytelling. *Candida albicans* grow as a community of individual cells that are visible to the naked eye. Their filamentous bodies attach and tightly embed themselves in human tissues with which they have coevolved, physiologically responding to the human body that is their living environment. Though we generally live in balance with *Candida albicans*, unbalance can lead this yeast to build scaffolds and biofilms that fight off our immune system, resulting in infection. Tarsh has coproduced many artworks with *Candida albicans*: live and projected time lapses and animations, growth of *Candida Albicans* on film, bread making using *Candida albicans* in place of baker's yeast, and finally the creation of flocked wallpaper on custom agar plates that promotes a patterned growth.

This last work is *Surface Dynamics of Adhesion* (2016). Through this piece, Tarsh gave *Candida albicans* a new home in agar prepared from her own blood. This emphasizes a new way of seeing the human in relation to other living beings. As discussed in her presentation at SymbioticA (24 June 2016), humans are both the hosts and the guests of *Candida albicans*. The intimate coming together of human blood and *Candida albicans* as wallpaper makes us rethink the boundaries of bodies as a porous enmeshment of life, of humanness and nonhumanness all at once. Tarsh's work highlights the opportunity provided to us by (micro)bioart to rethink human bodies. This begins by acknowledging the limits of our current categorization of life forms, which continually reproduce, shift, and move. By looking at the human as not only an end in itself, but as the living grounds of the microbiome (Bates 2013), we can move forward with a post-anthropocentric post-humanism (Ferrando 2016). We can acknowledge that human bodies have never been only human and that humanity itself can be redefined when we start paying attention to the intimate relationships we have with those who share our bodies and living spaces. Moreover, we can redefine, reshape, and replace our analytical and concrete, material conceptions of human bodies when we start caring for other livings (Bates 2014, 2017, 2019). Through bioart practices, we can create new conditions of possibilities and new ways of thinking and performing what it means to be human.

Two additional works by artists related to SymbioticA contributed to my questions and thinking about how we could rethink the human body. Stelarc is a world-renowned performance artist who has spent his career remaking and extending his own body through various technological apparatus often including robotics (Jagodzinski 2012; Manderson 2016; Massumi 2002; Stelarc 2016). Nina Sellars is an artist and research fellow at Curtin University in Perth (Australia) alongside Stelarc. Our conversations of her work concerned biomaterials and her work with human fat tissue as a medium for—and an object of—artistic investigation. These two artists joined forces in 2005 to create *Blender*. For this piece, Stelarc and Sellars underwent liposuction to extract some of their subcutaneous fat and other connective tissues (Clarke 2006). These biomaterials found a new home in an automated, human-size blender. This work redefines and replaces the human body, both concretely and metaphorically, and shows how technologies can lead us to a rethink what a human could or should be. Every few minutes, *Blender* (re)circulated the biomaterials within the closed system of air pumps and pneumatics, distorting yet emphasizing the humanness of the liposuction remnants. Like Guy Ben-Ary's notion of consent on his own biomaterials, Stelarc and Sellars use of their own fat for this project enabled them to avoid ethical issues (Clarke 2006).

Jaden J. A. Hastings attended a plant tissue culture workshop held during my last week at SymbioticA. Jaden's work captured my attention, as she uses her own body and biological matter to create traditional materials. *Bennu* (2015), ash made from Hastings's own blood, highlights the power of biotechnologies to create new possibilities for human tissue and bodies. Hasting considers the human body as a "contested space, contextualized within a contemporary, expanded definition of body boundaries," and her works join others who "dissect the complexities of our modern relationship with our own biomaterials" (Jaden J. A. Hastings n.d.). She sees experimentation with one's own body, the extreme end of the biohacking spectrum, as a question of self-determination and personal autonomy (Hastings 2019). This challenges the normativity that permeates our conceptualizations of what is a human body and the ways in which we engage these bodies.

These examples show not only that bioart practices allow us to rethink our theoretical conceptions of the human, but that artistic practice concretely contributes to a material remaking of human bodies. Through externalization, extension, transduction, automation, and radical transformation, Guy Ben-Ary, Tarsh Bates, Stelarc and Nina Sellars, and Jaden J. A. Hastings join the legacy of humans who have transformed their bodies. Their work takes it a step further by actively reshaping and remaking the very boundaries of what we imagine humans to be. It allows us to see that humanness itself is but a label within a relational and ever-changing web of entanglements. Discussions on consent, embodiment, shared ecologies and bodies, storytelling, technologies, and boundaries provide us with material and conceptual tools to remake the humans in ways that could help us tackle the environmental crisis by moving towards a post-humanist Anthropocene. Human bodies can be externalized and thrive in technological apparatus, but they are also the home of many species who have evolved to survive alongside human tissue. Human bodies are part of a broad system of relationships unfolding between and across living and nonliving things. Human bodies can be used as a basic building block to create new materials and new forms of lives. These ideas—which have taken some form of materiality through art—are useful to think of what a post-anthropocentric human could be.

Anthropocenic Speculations

The Anthropocene marks the scientific acknowledgement of humans' impact on planet earth. By studying mineral deposits, atmospheric concentrations of carbon dioxide and methane, global rise in temperatures and sea levels, biological changes, and extinction rates, scientists have determined that humans have altered the planet in ways that justify the formalization of the Anthropocene as a defined geological epoch (Waters et al. 2016). These findings characterize the environmental crisis in which we find ourselves as a species, a crisis in which we play a large role and whose effects are felt by many other livings. Rapid advances in the fields of bioscience and biotechnologies have led to changes in our twenty-first century societies, especially as these tools become more accessible, normalized, and even mundane (Šlesingerová 2018).

This shift toward expanded access to the biotechnological is unfolding in an anthropocenic landscape. A new geological epoch, the Anthropocene gives us the opportunity to challenge and rethink the anthropocentric nature-culture dichotomy. However, we must remain critical of the concept, as it can also participate in the reproduction of these very dichotomies by reaffirming human dominance and power over other life forms and the environment we live in (Lecain 2015; Šlesingerová 2018). Ionat Zurr (2012) of SymbioticA writes about exploitation of life by humans—resulting from historical and contemporary advances in biotechnologies and synthetic biology—where life is seen as something to manipulate, engineer, design, and manufacture. There is both risk and potential to be found in the increasingly biotechnological character of our present epoch.

Broadly speaking, the ecological crisis and the anthropocenic context are now part of contemporary public and academic discourses. Though artistic exploration of human and nonhuman bodies predate the term "Anthropocene," its forces and discourses now contribute to shaping the ways in which thinkers, scholars, and artists (re)conceptualize humans and their bodies in relation to the environment and other inhabitants of the earth. Lecain (2015) argues that rather than proving transformative, the concept of the Anthropocene reinforces a tendency to overestimate human agency and contributes to widening the gap between humans and nonhumans. He proposes the Carbocene as an alternative to the Anthropocene to emphasize how carbon-based fuels have led humans into a particular way of living (Lecain 2015). This neo-materialist argument seeks to displace and replace what we conceptualize as human agency by recognizing the planet as "both powerful and dangerous" (Lecain 2015: 23). By acknowledging human embeddedness in our planetary ecological systems, humans can be (re)conceptualized as beings subject to material forces that are both within and beyond its control. Haraway also argues that the Anthropocene needs to be challenged, despite the evidence of human impact on the planet. By opening up the epoch of the Anthropocene and giving it multiple names—Plantationocene, Capitalocene, and Chthulucene—Haraway is giving us tools to rethink the human in the context of planetary changes that have been attributed to humans and their activities. The Chthulucene encourages us to join forces with the myriad of other species and beings across temporalities and spatialities to rethink kinship and to build relationships with others (Haraway 2015). Speaking of kin, Haraway has often argued that we have never been human. In fact, "to be one is always to become with many" as we live in assemblages with other biotic and abiotic actors (Haraway 2008: 4).

The need to rethink the human can be tackled with post-humanist thinking and (bio)art practices. Biotechnologies have traditionally been used for medical research and applications (Zurr 2012; Catts and Zurr 2014). However, engaging with biotechnologies beyond their initial applications generates new symbolic and aesthetic beings that lead to the production of new cultural meanings (Catts and Zurr 2014). Biotechnologies, and especially the techniques I engaged with in the lab—that of tissue culture—literally create new living bodies that could not survive without technology. Labs are kept sterile and incubators act as a body by providing heat to cells that grow on the plastic of Petri dishes, bathing in a liquid soup of nutrients and hormones. Catts and Zurr of SymbioticA refer to these human or nonhuman bodies that cannot survive on their own as semi-living (2008). Semi-living and biological art projects and objects actively contribute to rethinking human nature, its role in ecology, and its subjectivity and ability to create symbolic meaning by raising technical, aesthetic, and ethical questions.

Artists who engage with living bodies provide us with new aesthetics possibilities and strategies to imagine post-human worlds (Zurr 2012). This chapter discussed messy, wet, leaking artworks that go beyond their enclosures to create new imaginaries and contribute to consistently redefining what is a human. For Nina Sellars, developments in technology and art have "provided us with new ways of conceptualizing these recently discovered bodily structures and their representations." (Sellars 2015: 481). Guy-Ben Ary's CellF allows us to rethink human embodiment and intelligence by exploring the idea of a robotic and biological brain (Bakkum et al. 2007). The reshaping and remaking of bodies in bioart can also lead to exploring questions of movement and its relation to the notion of agency (Zurr 2016). Stelarc emphasizes the need to question the forms and boundaries of human bodies, recognizing its obsolescence, to redefine our roles as humans in contemporary biotechnological terrains (Stelarc 1989). For Guy Ben-Ary, "art has the potential to initiate public debate and critical reflection on a unique cultural moment" (Ben-Ary 2019: 405; Moore et al. 2016). Artistic practices that engage with human biomaterials thus provide us with artworks, questions, and reflections that help us problematize what it is to be human in the Anthropocene where biotechnologies are increasingly accessible. Art and experiential engagement with living human and nonhuman bodies allows us to critically engage with normative discourses around human bodies, exposing the futility of attempts to control biology (Zurr 2012). By acknowledging and questioning our understandings of human bodies and more-than-human entanglements, we can establish new kinds of ecological kinships and build an (aesth)ethic of care (Bates 2014, 2017, 2019).

Artists who engage biology—though their works and perspectives vary—give us leads on how to rethink our relationship to living bodies, both human and nonhuman, to technology, and to the ecology in which we are embedded. By proposing an aesthetic, empathetic, and even romantic approach to engaging human bodies and biotechnologies, we can imagine a caring and nurturing paradigm of human-environment, body-technology interactions where the focus is shifted away from exploitation and toward re-singularization and care (Zurr 2012; Zurr 2016; Guattari 1989). Guattari (1989) explores this re-singularization through an aesthetic paradigm that recognizes the interactions between mental, social, and environmental ecologies. Along with bioart practices that rethink and remake human bodies, this provides us with symbolic and concrete tools to productively imagine a post-humanistic, post-anthropocentric, and post-dualistic future. Oron Catts and Ionat Zurr, founders of SymbioticA, call for vitality instead of utilitarian technology and urge us to step away from control to embrace play and care (Catts and Zurr 2018).

Bioart is one type of human practice that pushes the boundaries between humans and nonhumans, contributing to a concrete and speculative remaking of human bodies. It can lead us to think about new materialisms in the context of the Anthropocene: how we can shift our perceptions and understandings of life, death, sentience, and materiality of the human body (Ben-Ary 2019) in an epoch characterized by (bio)technological acceleration and ecological destruction. The work of these artists brings into questions what we consider to be human bodies and suggests possibilities for a future that aligns with post-human thinking where humans go beyond the human (Ben-Ary and Ben-Ary 2016; Moore et al. 2016). The potential of (bio)art rests in the ways in which it generates questions rather than provides ready-made answers. Artists have a "different and unique role in their relationship with society" (Catts and Zurr 2018: 51). By harnessing biotechnologies in creative and transformative ways, artists establish new questions, new ideas, and new practices.

Conclusion

"One way to live and die well as mortal critters in the Chthulucene is to join forces to reconstitute refuges, to make possible partial and robust biological-cultural-political-technological recuperation and recomposition, which must include mourning irreversible losses" (Haraway 2015: 160).

In this chapter, I drew from my fieldwork incursions in the world of biotechnologies and bioart to speak of post-humanism and the Anthropocene. As humans are threatened by climate change, biodiversity loss, and other anthropocenic pressures, I argue that rethinking the human and its relationship to other livings is essential. As Haraway states, we must mourn what we have lost in this environmental crisis and join forces with others to move forward. I argue that through their concrete remaking of human and nonhuman bodies and through the deconstruction of traditional dichotomies, bioart practices gives us tools to rethink our humanity—metaphorical and embodied—in ways that could help us get through the environmental crisis. By (re)conceptualizing humans as living with other forms of life in a shared techno-ecology, opportunities arise to reshape, transform, and create new bodies that transcend and go beyond the human. Post-humanism highlights the material complexities of the Anthropocene and changes the ways we think of bodies, aesthetics, and technologies (Wamberg and Thomsen 2016). The Anthropocene calls attention to the need to transform post-humanism into an actual practice oriented toward a post-anthropocentric and post-dualistic paradigm shift (Ferrando 2016). Participating in this shift is the harnessing of biotechnologies by bioartists, biohackers, and the DIYbio community. Their activities are part of a global community promoting access to biological systems and biotechnologies and contribute pragmatically to challenging the practices and norms we associate with biotechnology. Some bioartists engage with post-humanism by effectively redefining and hybridizing the boundaries of (human) lives and bodies (Abergel 2011; Uhl and Dubois 2011).

I have explored laboratory practices and the work of artists who harness the practices of bio(techno)logy, using living things and/or processes as a medium to create artworks (Kac 2006). More specifically, I discussed the works of artists who have taken parts of their own bodies to create art. Their work highlights a radical remaking of human bodies that goes beyond the traditional boundaries of our skin in ways that mobilize a distinct aesthetic of beyond-the-body modifications. This provides us with concrete examples on how to remake the human. I argue that bioart practices provide us with new conditions of possibilities to effectively move toward a post-humanism that takes into account all others with whom we share and live with on this planet (Ferrando 2016). We have much to learn from the questions raised by bioartists.

Christine Beaudoin is a PhD candidate in sociology at the University of Ottawa and has a master's in anthropology. Her research focuses on interactions between humans and the environment. She takes a relational approach to include nonhumans in social science research. She has done fieldwork with scientists and artists. She is currently working with stakeholders and ecologists to better understand historic waterways in Ontario (Canada). Christine is a member of the HumAnimaLab, a research group on the Anthropocene at the University of Ottawa. She joined the board of the Environmental Studies Association of Canada in 2020.

Artworks

Guy Ben-Ary. 2015–18. *CellF*. http://guybenary.com/work/cellf/.
Tarsh Bates. 2016. *Surface Dynamics of Adhesion*. https://tarshbates.com/portfolio/surface-dynamics-of-adhesion-2016.
Nina Sellars and Stelarc. 2005. *Blender*. http://stelarc.org/?catID=20245; http://www.ninasellars.com/?catID=8.
Jaden J. A. Hastings. 2015. *Bennu*. http://jadenhastings.com/#home.

References

Abergel, Élisabeth. 2011. "La Connaissance Scientifique aux Frontières du Bio-art: le Vivant à l'Ère du Post-naturel." *Cahiers de recherche sociologique* 50: 97–120.

Bakkum, Douglas J., Philip M. Gamblen, Guy Ben-Ary, Zenas C. Chao, and Steve M. Potter. 2007. "MEART: The Semi-living Artist." *Frontiers in Neurorobotics* 1: 5.
Bates, Tarsh. 2013. "HumanThrush Entanglements: *Homo sapiens* as a Multi-species Ecology." *PAN: Philosophy, Activism, Nature* 10: 36–45.
———. 2014. "Performance, Bioscience, Care: Exploring Interspecies Alterity." *International Journal of Performance Arts and Digital Media* 10(2): 216–31.
———. 2017. "Queer Affordances: The Human as a Transecology." *Journal of the Theoretical Humanities* 22(2): 151–54.
———. 2019. "The Queer Temporality of *CandidaHomo* Biotechnocultures." *Australian Feminist Studies* 34(99): 25–45.
Beaudoin, Christine. 2018. "Crafting with Livings: An Inquiry of Cellular Anthropology through Laboratory Gestures." Unpublished master's thesis, University of Ottawa.
Beaudoin, Christine, and David Jaclin. 2016. "Repurposing Emergence Theories: An Interview with Andrew Pelling." *Social Science Information* 55(3): 357–68.
Ben-Ary, Guy. 2019. "Questioning Life." *Nature Nanotechnology* 14: 405.
Ben-Ary, Guy, and Gemma Ben-Ary. 2016. "Bio-engineered Brains and Robotic Bodies: From Embodiment to Self-Portraiture." In Damith Herath, Christian Kroos, and Stelarc (eds.), *Robots and Art: Exploring an Unlikely Symbiosis*. Singapore: Springer, pp. 307–25.
Byerley, Anne, and Derrick Chong. 2015. "Biotech Aesthetics: Exploring the Practice of Bio Art." *Culture and Organization* 21(3): 197–216.
Catts, Oron, and Ionat Zurr. 2006. "Towards a New Class of Being: The Extended Body." *Artnodes* 6: 1–9.
———. 2008. "Growing Semi-living Structures: Concepts and Practices for the Use of Tissue Technologies for Non-medical Purposes." *Architectural Design* 78(6): 30–35.
———. 2014. "Growing for Different Ends." *International Journal of Biochemistry and Cell Biology* 56: 20–29.
———. 2018. "Artists Working with Life (Sciences) in Contestable Settings." *Interdisciplinary Science Reviews* 43(1): 40–53.
Clarke, Julia. 2006. "Corporeal Mélange: Aesthetics and Ethics of Biomaterials in Stelarc and Nina Sellars's *Blender*." *Leonardo* 39(5): 410–16.
Damm, Ursula, Bernhard Hopfengärtner, Dominik Niopek, and Philipp Bayer. 2013. "Are Artists and Engineers Inventing the Culture of Tomorrow?" *Futures* 48: 55–64
Deleuze, Gilles, and Félix Guattari. 1980. *Capitalisme et Schizophrénie: Mille Plateaux*. Paris: Éditions de Minuit.
Edwards, David. 2010. *The Lab: Creativity and Culture*. Cambridge, MA: Harvard University Press.
Ferrando, Francesca. 2013. "Posthumanism, Transhumanism, Antihumanism, Metahumanism, and New Materialisms: Differences and Relations." *Existenz* 8(2): 26–32.
———. 2016. "The Party of the Anthropocene: Post-humanism, Environmentalism and the Post-anthropocentric Paradigm Shift." *Relations* 4(2): 159–73.
Guattari, Félix. 1989. *Les trois écologies*. Paris: Éditions Galilée.
Haraway, Donna J. 2008. *When Species Meet*. Minneapolis: University of Minnesota Press.

———. 2015. "Anthropocene, Capitalocene, Plantationocene, Chthulucene: Making Kin." *Environmental Humanities* 6(1): 159–65.
Hastings, Jaden J. A. 2019. "When Citizens Do Science." *Narrative Inquiry in Bioethics* 9(1): 33–34.
SymbioticA. n.d. "History." SymbioticA website. Retrieved June 2019 from http://www.symbiotica.uwa.edu.au/home/history.
Jaden J. A. Hastings. n.d. "[I'M]MORTAL." Jaden J. A. Hastings website. Retrieved June 2019 from http://jadenhastings.com/immortal#bennu.
Ingold, Tim. 2017. *Correspondences.* Aberdeen: University of Aberdeen.
Jagodzinski, Jan. 2012. "The Affective Turn or Getting Under the Skin Nerves: Revisiting Stelarc." *Medienimpulse* 50(2): 1–20.
Kac, Eduardo. 2006. "Bio Art." *Information sur les Sciences Sociales* 45(2): 311–16.
Landecker, Hannah. 2007. *Culturing Life: How Cells Became Technologies.* Cambridge, MA: Harvard University Press.
Lapworth, Andrew. 2015. "Habit, Art, and the Plasticity of the Subject: The Ontogenetic Shock of the Bioart Encounter." *Cultural Geographies* 22(1): 85–102.
Lecain, Timothy J. 2015. "Against the Anthropocene: A Neo-materialist Perspective." *International Journal for History, Culture and Modernity* 3(1): 1–28.
Manderson, Lenore. 2016. *Surface Tensions: Surgery, Bodily Boundaries and the Social Self.* London: Routledge.
Massumi, Brian. 2002. *Parables for the Virtual: Movement, Affect, Sensation.* Durham, NC: Duke University Press.
Moore, Darren, Guy Ben-Ary, Andrew Fitch, Nathan Thompson, Douglas Bakkum, Stuart Hodgetts, and Amanda Morris. 2016. "*CellF*: A Neuron-driven Music Synthesiser for Real-Time Performance." *International Journal of Performance Arts and Digital Media* 12(1): 31–43.
Park, Simon. 2013. "DIY Biology: Bio-inspired or Bio-hazard?" *Microbiology Today* 40(3): 120–22.
Pelling, Andrew E. 2015. "Re-purposing Life in an Anti-disciplinary and Curiosity-Driven Context." *Leonardo* 48(3): 274–75.
Sellars, Nina. 2015. "The Optics of Anatomy and Light: A Studio-Based Investigation of the Construction of Anatomical Images." *Leonardo* 48(5): 481.
Šlesingerová, Eva. 2018. "Biopower Imagined: Biotechnological Art and Life Engineering." *Social Science Information* 57(1): 59–76.
Stelarc. 1989. "Redesigning the Body—Redefining What Is Human." *Whole Earth Review* 63: 18.
———. 2016. "Encounters, Anecdotes and Insights—Prosthetics, Robotics and Art." In Damith Herath, Christian Kroos, and Stelarc (eds.), *Robots and Art: Exploring an Unlikely Symbiosis.* Singapore: Springer, pp. 427–56.
Stevens, Hallam. 2016. *Biotechnology and Society: An Introduction.* Chicago: University of Chicago Press.
Uhl, Magali, and Dominic Dubois. 2011. "Réécrire le Corps : l'Art Biotech ou l'Expression d'une Genèse Technique de l'Hominisation." *Cahiers de Recherche Sociologique* 50: 33–54.
Wall, Kim. 2015. "Biohackers Push Life to the Limits with DIY Biology." *The Guardian*, 18 November. Retrieved June 2019 from http://www.theguardian.com/science/2015/nov/18/biohackers-strange-world-diy-biology.

Wamberg, Jacob, and Mads Rosendahl Thomsen. 2016. "The Posthuman in the Anthropocene: A Look through the Aesthetic Field." *European Review* 25(1): 150–65.

Waters, Colin N., Jan Zalasiewicz, Colin Summerhayes, Anthony D. Barnosky, Clément Poirier, Agnieszka Gałuszka, and Alejandro Cearreta, et al. 2016. "The Anthropocene Is Functionally and Stratigraphically Distinct from the Holocene." *Science* 351(6269): aad2622.

Wohlsen, Marcus. 2011. *Biopunk: DIY Scientists Hack the Software of Life*. New York: Current.

Zurr, Ionat. 2012. "Of Instrumentalisation of Life and the Vitality of Matter: Aesthetics of Creation and Control for Post-human Worlds." *Dialogues in Human Geography* 2(3): 288–91.

———. 2016. "Futile Labor." *GeoHumanities* 2(1): 188–202.

PART III
REPLACEMENT

CHAPTER 9

Can You See the Real Me?
Cyborg, Supercrip, or Simply a Lover of Sport?

P. DAVID HOWE AND CARLA FILOMENA SILVA

Movement technologies such as the wheelchair and prosthetic limbs have functioned as the ubiquitous signs of disability in various cultural contexts for well over fifty years. One can travel all over the globe and see parking spaces reserved for people with mobility impairments with the universal symbol of a wheelchair. This symbol represents a greater diversity of bodies than those who simply use a wheelchair, but the symbolic reference to a wheelchair has somehow become a default signifier for people who experience disability. Because disability is such a generalized qualifier, the technology used by bodies that need to either be replaced or repaired to be functional impacts upon all people experiencing disability, even those whose bodies cannot use this type of technology.

In this chapter, we ethnographically explore the image of the cyborg athlete. Performances of these bodies may be seen as a way of manipulating and transforming stereotypes (Sandahl and Auslander 2005). Certainly, the sporting prowess of Oscar Pistorius came to the attention of the international media, in part because he was able to compete against the most able athletes on the Olympic stage. For sport fans, the "blade runner" imagery attested the inclusion and capabilities of people with impairments within the realm of high-performance sport. The reality surrounding the inclusion debate is not so simple, and such giant leaps in understanding can be problematic (Howe and Silva 2018; Silva and Howe 2018). Here, we draw upon the first author's lifetime experience in the world surrounding parasport track-and-field athletics as both an athlete and anthropologist (see Howe 2018). Parasport entails all sporting activities that follow the rules and regulations of the International Paralympic Committee (IPC), which includes hosting summer and winter Paralympic Games. Perhaps more importantly this chapter is the culmination of a productive working relationship that centers on debates regarding how society can be more accepting of diverse embodiments. At regular intervals these debates have centered on the significance of bodily replacement movement technologies and their use as both representational and empowering to all parasport participants (Silva and Howe 2012, 2018; Howe and Silva 2018).

The utilization of bodily replacement technology such as wheelchairs and prosthetic limbs by parasport athletes embodies Haraway's (1991) concept of cyborg bodies, that is, hybridized entities resulting from the fusion of a live organism and manufactured technology. Regardless of whether these "sporting cyborgs" use a wheelchair or prosthetic limbs as their preferred mode of movement, their performances are always celebrated. These technologies replace "faulty" or missing body parts so that they can actively engage in disability sport and other physical activity cultures. Because these movement technologies often enhance sporting performance beyond those of most non-cyborg competitors, athletes with disabilities who achieve at this level transcend the ableist assumptions entrenched within Western society. Before we expand this debate further, it is important to highlight the distinctiveness of parasport culture for those unfamiliar with it.

Parasport Culture

The IPC is the international federation that administers both the Paralympic Games and World Championships for individual Paralympic sports such as athletics and swimming. Using the resources of the International Organisations of Sport for the Disabled (IOSD) (Jones and Howe 2005)[1] (including athletes, volunteer administrators, and classification systems), the IPC has made the Paralympic Games into the most recognizable and influential vehicle for the promotion of disability sport globally.

Given the broad diversity of "disabled" bodies involved in parasport, the competition is structured upon a complex classification system, comparable to the systems used in the sports of boxing and tae kwon do where competitors perform in distinctive weight categories (Jones and Howe 2005; Howe and Jones 2006). Within parasport, competitors are classified by their body's degree of performative functionality within their chosen sport. Classification takes the form of a series of functional tests that determine the appropriate category in which to place a competitor so that equitable sporting contests can be achieved (Sherrill 1999). Classification consequently is a fundamental component of Paralympic culture (Howe

2008), conducted by a group of qualified classifiers who combine expertise in physical and/or sensory impairments and the sporting practice in which they are classifying athletes (Tweedy and Vanlandewijck 2009). If this process is successful, athletes in each class should have an equal chance of accumulating physical capital (Jones and Howe 2005) from their competition category. In reality, however, a number of factors impact upon the accumulation of capital (both physical and cultural), the most salient of which is whether the athlete uses mobility technologies while they perform. Previous research noted the existence of a hierarchy of "acceptable" impairment within the community of Paralympic athletes (Sherrill and Williams 1996; Schell and Rodriguez 2001), with wheelchair athletes on the top of a hierarchy of disabilities that locates athletes with less socially acceptable disability categories, such as cerebral palsy or individuals who do not rely on replacement technologies, as marginal (Kama 2004; Haller 2000; Mastro et al. 1996).

As an increasing number of athletes with different impairments aspired to get involved in parasport International Wheelchair and Amputee Sport Association (IWAS), the first IOSD established a broad class known as *les autres*.[2] Some *les autres* athletes who used wheelchairs, including those with spina bifida and polio, were able to be slotted into the IWAS system. However, many *les autres* were ineligible to compete in parasport because they did not need to use a wheelchair. This exclusion eventually led to the development of the remaining IOSDs (e.g., CP-ISRA and IBSA) and, ultimately, the development of the IPC. In this way, the classification system that led to the development of parasport was never politically or culturally neutral. In other words, the classification systems developed within the cultural context of parasport are the product of the history of this sporting movement (see Howe 2008). One of the most significant changes in sporting practices happened when the technology for lower leg prosthesis entailed the creation of sporting prosthesis for particular sports (e.g., running, cycling, long jump); many of the bodies previously classified into wheelchair sports became standing athletes as replacement technologies became more available (Howe 2008, 2011).

Observations since the late 1980s highlight the development of blade technologies and the move from four-wheeled chairs to three as significant. There has been a marked improvement in the technology, particularly in Western nations, associated with leg prosthetics. The materials from which prostheses are made have changed markedly from wood to fiberglass to all manner of carbon fiber and lightweight metals used in advanced scientific design (Howe 2008). Reducing the number of wheels on a racing chair and making it more aerodynamic and lighter is also a development over the last thirty years. These mobility replacement aids have been a product of state-of-the-art technologies, and as a result, the athletes who are the vanguards of the deployment of this new technology are delivering performances that would have been considered impossible twenty years ago.

A track-and-field athlete who has been involved in parasport since the late 1980s and worked as a journalist covering the 2016 Paralympic Games in Rio stated:

> In my lifetime I have gone from wearing a wooden leg, to a fiberglass one to this current carbon fiber contraption that I currently wear. Each time there is a change in technology I feel more liberated in the way I can navigate the world. The key thing for me is the manner in which my stump connects to the prosthesis as this join used to cause a great deal of pain and discomfort. It is really good that young amputees do not have to go through the same and can simply get on with enjoying your sport.

Prosthetic sporting technology has advanced with three aims in mind: to produce better performances; to increase the comfort for an individual, athlete or otherwise; and to enhance the efficiency of movement. Such advancements are most evident on the track, but also in field events, where athletes with amputations have the option of competing as standing athletes or as athletes who use throwing frames.

In contemporary terms, the technological sophistication of both prosthetic limbs and wheelchairs extends the performativity capabilities of one's body, producing a new corporeal entity: what Haraway terms a hybrid body (Haraway 1991: 178) over time. This process is laborious:

> Because my disability is above the knee, I use a wheelchair regularly for getting around daily. I am comfortable in it and this technology does not change, but almost every year there is some change, they call it an enhancement, that occurs to my prosthetic limb—while 90 percent of the time these things are improvement, they do take time to get used to—which can have a negative impact upon my training.

All athletes who can make use of replacement technologies are individuals who take time to get accustomed to using these technologies for moving in sport and daily life. New movement patterns take time to develop and become habitual, but the ultimate aim is to foster a hybridization of their bodies. The goal is that the biological body and machine become one in the pursuit of embodied excellence. Yet, even small changes in one of the segments of such symbiotic structure (for instance, in the technological apparatus) always require laborious adjustment of the biological body and a reconfiguration of their hybrid bodies (DesGroseillers et al. 1978).

Cyborg to Supercrip

The cultural fascination with these hybrid, cyborg bodies goes some way to explaining that their presence in the sporting arena often elevates them to "supercrips" (Howe 2011; Silva and Howe 2012). At the same time, the advancing of movement technologies has had a profound impact on how this sporting world is perceived by those outside parasport culture. We now turn to explore how the embodiment of the cyborg body in the context of parasport has led to the contemporary manifestation of the supercrip. In the context of parasport, the most successful cyborg athletes may be seen as supercrips (Howe 2011; Silva and Howe 2012):

> "Supercrips" are those individuals whose inspirational stories of courage dedication, and hard work prove that it can be done, that one can defy the odds and accomplish the impossible. The concern is that these stories of success will foster unrealistic expectations about what people with disabilities can achieve, what they *should* be able to achieve if only they tried hard enough. Society does not need to change. It is the myth of the self-made man. (Berger 2004: 798)

The label of supercrip can be negatively bestowed upon impaired individuals who simply manage to live "an ordinary" life (Kama 2004). But specifically, in the context of parasport and for this chapter, the supercrip is the athlete who succeeds (despite and because of their disability) and is celebrated with relatively high-profile media exposure (Grue 2015). Those athletes who win but do not receive recognition in mainstream media are not supercrips in the context of the Paralympics; on the contrary they are often marginalized by the degree or nature of their impairment (Howe 2011; Silva and Howe 2018). The following quote is from an athlete who competed in the 2005 IPC European athletic championships in Finland:

> As an athlete who does not use a [wheel]chair [or prosthetic] I am not seen as a "serious" Paralympian—I win most of my races and have set world records, but the media does not seem to care. If I were racing in a chair or with a prosthesis and getting the same results, I am certain I would be a Para-celebrity back home.

This type of comment is commonplace in parasport. The use of movement technologies sells parasport to a wider audience, mesmerized and positively inspired by the restorative and even enhancing potential of technological apparatus. Yet, for most athletes, the technologies that cyborgify their bodies are simply tools required to compete on a level playing field in the sports they love (Howe 2013).

The process of making a cyborg we articulate as cyborgification (Howe 2008, 2011). Rather than rare, this is an insidious process in our contemporary world, since most of our bodies in some way use technology to augment or replace capability. Our bodies can be placed along a continuum from those that require very little technological aid (eyeglasses, for example) to those whose lives depend greatly upon technology to participate in society or even to survive. Perhaps the epitome of the promise of cyborgification for human advancement, Paralympian wheelchair racers and prosthetic-wearing athletes are the most celebrated bodies in parasport cultures (Howe and Parker 2012). We now turn to the notion that such cyborgified athletes and their celebration are the result of the hegemony of a "technocratic ideology" (Charles 1998), that is, the elevated importance and hope that society places upon technology and its role in shaping Western ways of thinking. Such technocratic ideology is becoming increasingly pervasive within parasport.

Parasport and Technology

Movement technologies used in parasport like wheelchairs and prosthetic limbs have to be purchased, and therefore the Paralympic movement represents a developing market for the sale of technologically advanced mobility apparatus. Many of the most up-to-date replacement technologies central to this chapter are inaccessible to athletes from much of the "developing" world, where costs are prohibitive. In this context, parasport athletics may be seen as technologically advanced on the one hand, but isolationist and exclusionary on the other. This of course is not unique to the culture of parasport, but it is something that we need to be mindful of. State-of-the-art technologies are expensive, and in the world of parasport (reflecting the world outside it), there will be the haves and the have-nots.

The move to hi-tech mobility devices specifically designed for sport stems from the general push for more technological advancement in society, but it also responds to the desires of the athletes to perform with greater proficiency:

> I am lucky in that I am able to get a new racing chair every year. The technology keeps improving and the "fit" to my body seems to get better every year. It feels like a well-worked-in glove from the first couple of training sessions. It helps that I have been with the same company for a decade now—if I had to pay for this technology, I could not afford to be in the sport.

As highlighted by the quote above, from an athlete taken during the IPC World Athletic Championships in London in 2017, today many elite athletes work with leading wheelchair and prosthesis suppliers to ensure their future success is based on the technologies they use as much as it is the training regimes they follow. As a result, the top cyborg athletes also receive commercial reward for their involvement in the development and manufacture of state-of-the-art technology at the heart of technocratic ideology. In other words, technology is literally as well as figuratively pushing parasport forward. As Charles suggests:

> Technology and kinesiology are symbiotically linked. They have a mutually beneficial relationship. As technology advances, so does the quality of scientific research and information accessible in the field. As kinesiology progresses and gains academic acceptance and credibility, technology assumes a more central role in our field. The more scientific the subdiscipline, the more we can see technology at play. (1998: 379)

The field of high-performance parasport has clearly benefited from an increase in technologies developed to harness the power of the human body (Burkett 2010). *Able-bodied*[5] high-performance athletes rely on technology in their day-to-day training (Hoberman 1992; Shogan 1998), yet when these athletes perform in sports like track-and-field athletics, the technology that has allowed them to train and compete in the sporting arena may be completely obscured from view. Able-bodied athletes take technology with them to the start of an Olympic final, as their clothing and footwear are highly technological products. Butryn (2002, 2003) has highlighted that high-performance (able-bodied) track-and-field athletics is surrounded by technology that enables athletes to become cyborgs. However, in comparison to racing wheelchairs and prosthetic limbs, specialist clothing and shoes appear less advanced, as they do not explicitly, visibly, and "unnaturally" replace part of the biological body and aid performance.

> When persons with disabilities use technologies to adjust the participation in "normal" physical activity, the use of these technologies constructs this person as unnatural in contrast to a natural, nondisabled participant, even though both nondisabled participants and those with disabilities utilize technologies to participate. (Shogan 1998: 272)

Technologies such as racing wheelchairs and prostheses have enhanced the performances of athletes for whom the loss of function deriving from specific impairments can be restored by the use of a replacement technology. The perception of success in their hybridization depends upon the extent to which their performances are seen as close to "normal." This normalization is always underpinned by an "overcoming" of disability.

> A winning wheelchair athlete is seen as the epitome of rehabilitative success. The vision of strong male bodies competing for honours on the sports field is an image that has currency in the able-bodied world. Bravery in overcoming the catastrophe of a damaged body is a quality everyone can admire. (Seymour 1998: 119)

This image extends to amputee athletes who have also suffered traumatic injuries and use performance-enhancing prosthetic limbs. The use of these mobility replacement technologies provides an opportunity for re-embodiment, the emergence of a new hybrid body (Seymour 1998), a process that is not available to most congenitally impaired individuals. That is, users of both wheelchairs and prosthetic limbs who have acquired their impairment have the opportunity to establish a distinctive identity with their new *cyborg* bodies. These bodies are the hallmark of IWAS and central to the public understanding of the parasport movement.

(Re)Embodiment

In order to explain the idea of re-embodiment, we draw upon Merleau-Ponty's conceptualization of embodiment as "a grouping of lived-through meanings which moves towards its equilibrium" ([1945] 1962: 288). Merleau-Ponty sought to reject the dichotomization and fragmentation of Western scientific thought that broke down reality into zones of mutual exclusivity: nature/nurture, body/soul/, subject/object, etc. (Iwakuma 2002). Following Csordas, who suggests that embodiment is "an indeterminate methodological field defined by perceptual experience and mode of presence and engagement in the world" (1994: 12), inanimate and handmade objects can become incorporated into a person's body image, such as the cane for a visually impaired person moving through spaces (Iwakuma 2002). Furthermore, objects can become an integral part of someone's identity, something that is illuminated by "people's peculiarities, obsessions and mixed feelings towards their aids [which] cannot be explained satisfactorily if they are seen as mere instruments" (Iwakuma 2002: 79). This can clearly be seen in the attachment that some athletes have to their mobility aids/sporting equipment (Howe 2011).

Iwakuma suggests this "embodiment cannot be complete as long as s/he is conscious of, for example, pushing a wheelchair for transportation or is making an effort to flip a page while using a prosthetic arm" (2002: 81). In other words, time and training are required for bodily replacement technologies to become hybridized. The quote below was collected during a "training camp" before the London 2012 Paralympic Games that gave developing athletes the opportunity to train alongside those who would be competing in the forthcoming Paralympics and highlights this issue:

> Because I am just on the parasport pathway (development program) I am not able to afford to get a new chair every season. But at nineteen I am still growing a bit—I bought my last chair with a bit of extra room to grow into. Last year I

felt like I was "swimming" in it. As I have grown it feels more a part of me—I am beginning to feel more like a racer.

Every time an athlete needs to "break in" new replacement body parts, this transition will impact upon their identity. As Seymour (1998) signifies, re-embodiment takes time.

Haraway writes that her cyborg theory is "about transgressed boundaries, potent fusions, and dangerous possibilities" (1991: 154) and that "a cyborg world might be about lived social and bodily realities in which people are not afraid of permanently partial identities and contradictory standpoints" (1991: 154). She sees the image of the cyborg as a means of overcoming divisions between people. This position is somewhat ironic when we think of re-embodiment of cyborgs in the context of parasport. The cyborg body is celebrated, yes, but at the expense of those whose impairments make a cyborg identity improbable, as in the case of many athletes with acquired impairments. This exclusion is in clear opposition to Haraway's vision regarding transgressing the boundaries between perceptual divisions of us and them. This is nicely articulated by an athlete with mild cerebral palsy:

> I feel like an outcast on my own Paralympic track team because 85 percent of the athletes are using fancy technologies when they are performing, and this somehow makes me inferior—surely it should be the other way around—I am almost normal—and can directly compete in mainstream sport.

The assumption here regarding normality is an interesting one. Parasport has always celebrated wheelchair movement as part of its culture because IWAS was the founding federation (Howe 2008). Over time, as previously mentioned, the ubiquitous symbol of the wheelchair emblematic of "disability" has helped those in the parasport movement who use this replacement technology to gain wider acceptance. Internally, within parasport, wheelchair users are celebrated for their greater (though by no mean complete) acceptance within mainstream able-bodied society. They are, along with prosthetic-wearing amputees, the face of parasport. They can be accepted as disabled sportspeople.

The lack of acceptance of disability, though somewhat dated, was nicely articulated by Murphy (1990). In an anthropological account of slowly become paralyzed from a tumor growing on his spine, Murphy wrote that he could feel his social standing slip as he became disabled: "A serious disability inundates all other claims to social standing, relegating to secondary status all the attainments of life, all other social roles, even sexuality. It is not a role; it is an identity, a dominant characteristic to which all social roles must be adjusted" (Murphy 1990: 106). Most parasport athletes can never simply be athletes; they are always "disabled" athletes, and this identity marker remains attached to them throughout their lives, inside and outside the boundaries of competition. As Seymour writes, "Success in disabled sport, unlike success in able-bodied sport, is not associated with mastery in other dimensions of life. Achievement in wheelchair sport does not have the power to transform the primary status, that of patient. Disabled sport remains sport for people with damaged bodies" (1998: 115). In other words, because of the way that disability is viewed in wider society, the accumulation of capital, both physical and cultural, is possible through participation in the Paralympic Games, but only to a certain extent and for a particular kind of body. As a competitor at the 2015 World Athletics Championships in Doha Qatar commented, sometimes the type of impairment matters if you are to be accepted.

> I am so fortunate. As a bi-lateral below the knee amputee I have the "same" body as Oscar Pistorius—it makes people think I am a serious athlete without them ever seeing me race. It does get me a lot of media attention compared to other impairment groups—but people get surprised when I can't beat world-class abled runners like Oscar can—the public really have no idea regarding the abilities of Paralympians—other than a few marquee names.

Coming to terms with one's re-embodiment can be a problematic. Parasport athletes do not live in isolation and can be celebrated and shunned at one and the same time. Within the parasport movement, hybridized bodies are celebrated, but often outside the privileged position within parasport, they are shunned by able-bodied society. Unfortunately, ideals of masculinity and femininity conspire against women in rehabilitation and make their task more difficult (Seymour 1998). Because men are more likely to suffer spinal injuries, they outnumber women in rehabilitation centers, and the culture of rehabilitation is "dominated by masculine ideas and values ... and rehabilitation projections reflect fixed and static views of men's and women's roles" (Seymour 1998: 113). This is culturally significant to parasport, as women with impairments are less likely to engage in the practice of sport because of these barriers (DePauw 1997). We must be mindful moving forward that the hybridized bodies that are central to this discussion entail more than disability as part of their identity.

Celebrated Parasport Hybrid Bodies

The bodies that are celebrated within the Paralympic movement—highly functioning wheelchair racers (Howe and Parker 2012) or those who use technologically advanced prosthetics (Howe 2011)—have increasingly become high profile because the technology they use enhances their "normality." Those bodies who do not use movement technologies to compete in disability parasport still benefit from advances in sport science support, such as biomechanical and physiological analysis, but are still marginalized. For people who are vision impaired, have ambulant cerebral palsy, or have intellectual impairments who are able to compete in sport without the use of special technologies of mobility, relative or apparent normality can be detrimental to how they are treated both inside and outside parasport. Athletes with vision impairment are relatively easily understood by the public, given that a high percentage of the world's population use either eyeglasses or contact lenses. As our eyesight deteriorates as a result of spending too much time at the computer or through the passage of time and aging, we can understand and appreciate the difficulties associated with poor sight. As a result, athletes with vision impairment are not treated as marginal to the same extent as those who have cerebral palsy or an intellectual impairment (Sherrill and Williams 1996). A medalist at both the Paralympic and IPC World Athletics Championships in the 2000s highlighted the marginality related to their impairment:

> Because my CP [cerebral palsy] looks different, to some offensively so, and it impacts my ability to speak fluently and the fact that I am a runner with CP in both my legs—means that I will never be a "media darling." My classification gets little to no attention—I think it is because we don't appear to be athletes—try as we might—even I can see that.

Neurological disabilities are usually more difficult to understand than others. An individual with the uncontrollable spasticity of cerebral palsy or an athlete with an intellectual disability is seldom celebrated by the media in the way in which cyborgs are. Mobility technological intervention has a minimal role to play in managing these types of bodies to a norm that is thought of as acceptable to mainstream sporting practices. As a result, it is rather difficult for the general public to see ability in some of the performances of individuals with these types of impairment.

Following Shogan (1998), it could be argued that the mobility technology used in sport for the disabled is unnatural because it makes athletes less than human. In fact, in the lead-up to the London 2012 Paralympic Games, a television station in the United Kingdom ran an awareness campaign entitled "Freaks of Nature" (Silva and Howe 2012). This campaign was designed to highlight "supercrip" in parasport, but it did not translate well. For those whose bodies are explicitly cyborgs, the "superhuman" results achieved through the use of either state-of-the-art wheelchairs or prosthetic limbs within Paralympic track-and-field athletics have become the new norm and accepted currency over the last two decades within the public understanding of ability within parasport. Replacement technology allows for exceptional sporting performances celebrated by the able-bodied public, but such performances are unlikely to be achieved by athletes who compete without these mobility aids. This use of what Butryn (2003) coined "implement technology" has transformed parasport into a significant sporting spectacle.

Discussion

In an increasingly commercial world, the technocratic ideology (Charles 1998) surrounding track-and-field athletics at the Paralympics Games and parasport more generally will be hard to challenge. The athletes who use wheelchairs and prostheses are at the center of the Paralympic movement and will be better consumers simply because they have specialist materials to purchase if they wish to compete at the highest level. The body policing on what is acceptably human and what is not (Cole 1993, 1998), evident in mainstream high-performance sport, has been reversed in parasport world.

In Paralympic track-and-field athletics, the closer a body is to a cyborg, the more capital it holds, in opposition to the world articulated by Haraway (1991) in relation to the boundaries between humans and nonhumans. Wheelchair users and amputees who use prostheses are explicitly tied to sport technologies and therefore blur the lines between "natural" and "artificial." They are perhaps the best example of the cyborg in contemporary society. Butryn sees the nexus between the natural and legal and the artificial and illegal as hegemonic humanness (2003: 28). Hegemonic humanism can be seen to have been practiced when Oscar Pistorius was initially excluded from competing in able-bodied athletics (Howe 2008, 2011). The restoration of his right to compete on his prosthesis was restored because he had no other option but to run on man-made legs and by the fact they were not advantaging him in the context of competition. In a sense, parasport celebrates "transgressing the taboo boundary between blood, sweat, and tears, and blood, sweat and gears" (Butryn 2003: 28). Here, the cyborg wheelchair user and the prosthetic limb wearer are the role models, and the supercrips parasport movement triumphs in a way that the Olympics and other mainstream sport cultures have failed to achieve. This is largely because the Paralympics Games was designed to celebrate a corporeal entity that is distinct from the able-bodied norm. Yet, today it appears that Paralympic distinctiveness must increasingly take on a cyborg form.

Where does this leave *les autres*, the athletes whose bodies do not fit neatly in discrete categories? They certainly have a part to play in the

Paralympic movement, but the more marginal the physicality of the body, the further away it is from the potential of cyborgification and the more likely that a tragic rather a heroic allegory will follow them. This analysis tells us a great deal about the politics of disablement. While it is considered an infringement for the able to become too cyborg, for the disabled it is highly advantageous because technology can normalize their "inferior" bodies to the point where they can produce superhuman results. Of course, there is a tension here. MacIntyre (1999) tells us that vulnerability and affliction and the related quality of dependence are central to the human condition. The susceptibility to injury and misery, distress and pain is likely to befall us all at some point in our existence. We all will be reliant on others from time to time. It begs the question why impaired bodies are so harshly disabled by society and, at least in the context of Paralympic sport, only those who are cyborgs are celebrated at length. Of these cyborgs, the winners are held up on a pedestal as supercrips.

Conclusion

In the last thirty years, the associated development of biomechanically and ergonomically responsive prostheses has meant that many athletes who in the past would have competed from a wheelchair are now able to compete from a standing position. While the development of replacement mobility technology that enhances sport performance is understandably beneficial for those who can go through the process of cyborgification, it marginalizes further those athletes who do not use technologies directly in their competitive performance. Because the high-end wheelchair athlete is able to perform at the same level or better than an able-bodied athlete, the abilities of these athletes are obvious to the public. On the other hand, it might be difficult to see the ability of an athlete whose cerebral palsy affects both legs and runs one hundred meters much slower than an able-bodied counterpart.

The possibility of a re-embodiment for certain athletes with disabilities is provided through acquiring expensive sporting technologies central to the process of cyborgification, while excluding many others through lack of financial means. In parasport, there are increasing numbers of athletes with mechanical, artificially designed, hybrid bodies creating new sporting potential. The technology they use has the capacity to "normalize" their bodies and in so doing produces "sporting cyborgs," who are celebrated both inside and outside the parasport movement, because they increase its marketability and the public's awareness of the ability of certain impairment groups. A technocentric ideology underpins the cyborgification process celebrated within Paralympic parasport and has made celebrities of the athletes who are successful in using the state-of-the-art replacement technologies to achieve super performances (Howe 2008, 2011). Regrettably, such elevated status of handpicked cyborgs can be problematic for the communities of impaired individuals who can never achieve such a position. As Kama argues:

> Well-known, successful disabled people are put on a pedestal for their demonstrated ability to triumph. This triumph is used to validate the disabled individual and to alter societal perceptions. Consequently, the wish to see disabled who "have done it" is particularly intense while the pitiful disabled trigger antipathy because they reproduce and reinforce disabled people's inferior positionality and exclusion. (2004: 447)

Ultimately, the Paralympics risk becoming a replacement technology showcase, rather than a contest of athleticism, leaving behind those who cannot either afford or use performance-enhancing technology. In short, technological advancement in relation to parasport is not dissimilar to other changes in society; it is clearly a mixed blessing:

> Prosthetic medicine is dedicated to physical normalisation and is devoted to the artificial alteration of both function and appearance, but it enters the realm of biopolitics because it uses the "normal" body as its tribunal and blueprint for action, and treats the impaired body as a spoilt entity that must be hidden and corrected. (Hughes 2000: 561)

Technology empowers some while leaving the status of others at best unaltered or, at worst, increasing their liminality. While Haraway (1991) believes that cyborgization can bring more people into the fold of the "humanist subject," maybe the whole notion of what constitutes a humanist subject has to be reformulated. A long-serving administrator in parasport commented at the London 2017 IPC World Athletics Championships:

> All too often we expect the Paralympic movement to help transform social attitudes toward disability over night. It has changed some attitudes but very slowly. The wheelies and the amputees are now being celebrated a bit more in public, but the process for those athletes who don't have cyborg bodies will take much longer. Not every Paralympian should be seen as a supercrip—most should simply engage in the pursuit of higher, faster, and stronger for their own personal growth and love of the sport.

P. David Howe holds the Dr. Frank J. Hayden Endowed Chair in Sport and Social Impact in the School of Kinesiology at Western University, Canada. His ethnographic research focuses on unpacking the embodied sociocultural milieu surrounding inclusive physical activity and disability sport. He is also editor of the Routledge book series Disability, Sport and Physical Activity Cultures and holds a guest professorship at Katholieke Universiteit Leuven, Belgium.

Carla Filomena Silva is an assistant professor in the School of Health Studies, at Western University, Canada. Before starting at Western, she worked at Nottingham Trent University, UK, and for the UNESCO chair in Inclusive PE, Sport, Fitness and Recreation, in the Institute of Technology, Tralee, Ireland. She has for the past few years contributed in the area of disability studies and sport on the Erasmus Mundus Master in Adapted Physical Activity, Katholieke Universiteit of Leuven, Belgium.

Notes

1. The federations, namely the Cerebral Palsy International Sport and Recreation Association (CP-ISRA), International Blind Sport Association (IBSA), International Sports Federation for Persons with Intellectual Disability (INAS-FID), and the International Wheelchair and Amputee Sport Association (IWAS). This is a federation that was launched in September 2004 at the Athens Paralympic Games. It is the result of a merger of two federations, the International Stoke Mandeville Wheelchair Sports Federation (ISMWSF) and the International Sport Organisation for the Disabled (ISOD), which have been part of the IPC since its inception.
2. *Les autres* is a French phrase used within disability sport circles meaning "the others." Originally the term refers to athletes with a disability who did not directly fit into the classification system established by IWAS. Today *les autres* is used to highlight any athlete who is not specifically referred to in the classification systems of the IOSDs and who is able to be slotted into an existing classification system. I use the term here specifically to refer to athletes with a disability who do not use either a wheelchair or prosthesis while competing in athletics.
3. We use the term "able-bodied" here because it is the term used by athletes within the cultural context of the Paralympic movement.

References

Berger, Ronald. 2004. "Pushing Forward: Disability, Basketball, and Me." *Qualitative Inquiry* 10: 794–810.
———. 2008. "Disability and the Dedicated Wheelchair Athlete: Beyond the 'Supercrip' Critique." *Journal of Contemporary Ethnography* 37(6): 647–78.
Burkett, Brendan. 2010. "Technology in Paralympic Sport: Performance Enhancement or Essential for Performance." *British Journal of Sports Medicine* 44: 215–20.

Butryn, Ted. 2002. "Cyborg Horizons: Sport and the Ethics of Self-Technologization." In Andy Miah and Simon Easson (eds.), *Sport, Technology: History, Philosophy, and Policy*. Oxford: Elsevier Science, pp. 111–34.
———. 2003. "Posthuman Podiums: Cyborg Narratives of Elite Track and Field Athletes." *Sociology of Sport Journal* 20: 17–39.
Charles, John. 1998. "Technology and the Body of Knowledge." *Quest* 50: 379–88.
Cole, Cheryl. 1993. "Resisting the Canon: Feminist Cultural Studies, Sport, and Technologies of the Body." *Journal of Sport and Social Issues* 17: 77–97.
———. 1998. "Addiction, Exercise, and Cyborgs: Technologies and Deviant Bodies." In Geneviève Rail (ed.), *Sport and Postmodern Times*. Albany: State University of New York Press, pp. 261–75.
Csordas, Thomas. 1994. *Embodiment and Experience: The Existential Ground of Culture and Self*. Cambridge: Cambridge University Press.
DePauw, Karen. 1997. "The (In)visibility of Disability: Cultural Contexts and "Sporting Bodies." *Quest* 49(4): 416–30.
DesGroseillers, Jean-Pierre, J. P. Desjardins, J. P. Germain, and Alfons Krol. 1978. "Dermatologic Problems in Amputees." *Canadian Medical Association Journal* 118: 535–37.
Grue, Jan. 2015. "The Problem of the Supercrip: Representation and Misrepresentation of Disability." In Tom Shakespeare (ed.), *Disability Research Today: International Perspectives*. London: Routledge, pp. 204–18.
Haller, Beth. 2000. "If They Limp, They Lead? News Representations and the Hierarchy of Disability Images." In Dawn Braithwaite and Teresa Thompson (eds.), *Handbook of Communication and People with Disabilities: Research and Application*. Mahwah, NJ: Lawrence Erlbaum, pp. 273–88.
Haraway, Donna. 1991. *Simians, Cyborgs, and Women: The Reinvention of Nature*. London: Routledge.
Hoberman, John. 1992. *Mortal Engines: The Science of Human Performance and the Dehumanization of Sport*. Oxford: Free Press.
Howe, P. David. 2006. "The Role of Injury in the Organization of Paralympic Sport. In S. Loland, B. Skirstad, and I. Waddington (eds.), *Pain and Injury in Sport: Social and Ethical Analysis*. London: Routledge, pp. 211–25.
———. 2007. "Integration of Paralympic Athletes into Athletics Canada." *International Journal of Canadian Studies* 35: 134–50.
———. 2008. *The Cultural Politics of the Paralympic Movement: Through the Anthropological Lens*. London: Routledge.
———. 2011. "Cyborg and Supercrip: The Paralympics Technology and the (Dis)empowerment of Disabled Athletes." *Sociology* 45(5): 868–82.
———. 2013. "Supercrips, Cyborgs and the Unreal Paralympian." In M. Perryman (ed.), *London 2012: How Was It for Us?* London: Lawrence & Wishart, pp. 130–41.
———. 2018. "Athlete, Anthropologist and Advocate: Moving toward a Lifeworld Where Difference Is Celebrated." *Sport and Society: Culture, Commerce, Media, Politics* 21(4): 678–88.
Howe, P. David, and Carwyn Jones. 2006. "Classification of Disabled Athletes: (Dis) empowering the Paralympic Practice Community." *Sociology of Sport Journal* 23: 29–46.
Howe, P. David, and Andrew Parker. 2012. "Celebrating Imperfection: Sport, Disability and Celebrity Culture." *Celebrity Studies* 3(3): 270–82.

Howe, P. David, and Carla Silva. 2018. "The Fiddle of Using the Paralympic Games as a Vehicle for Expanding [Dis]ability Sport Participation." *Sport and Society: Culture, Commerce, Media, Politics* 21(1): 125–36.

Hudson, Elizabeth. 2016. "Should 'Blade Jumper' Markus Rehm Be Allowed in the Olympics?" *BBC Sport*, 17 February. Retrieved 20 November 2020 from http://www.bbc.co.uk/sport/athletics/35568770.

Hughes, Bill. 2000. "Medicine and the Aesthetic Invalidation of Disabled People." *Disability and Society* 15(4): 555–68.

Hunt-Grubbe, Charlotte. 2007. "The Blade Runner Generation." *Sunday Times* (London). Retrieved 20 November 2020 from https://www.thetimes.co.uk/article/the-blade-runner-generation-k8pf9v667dp.

Iwakuma, Miho. 2002. "The Body as Embodiment: An Investigation of the Body by Merleau-Ponty." In Mairian Corker and Tom Shakespeare (eds.), *Disability/Postmodernity: Embodying Disability Theory*. London: Continuum, pp. 76–87.

Jones, Carwyn, and P. David Howe. 2005. "Conceptual Boundaries of Sport for the Disabled: Classification and Athletic Performance." *Journal of Philosophy of Sport* 32: 133–46.

Jönsson, Kutte. 2010. "Sport beyond Gender and the Emergence of Cyborg Athletes." *Sport in Society* 13(2): 249–59.

Kama, Amit. 2004. "Supercrips versus the Pitiful Handicapped: Reception of Disabling Images by Disabled Audience Members." *Communications* 29(4): 447–66.

Kelso, Paul. 2012. "Oscar Pistorius Knocked Out of London 2012 Olympics But His Achievements Will Resound for Years to Come." *The Telegraph*, 6 August. Retrieved 20 November 2020 from http://www.telegraph.co.uk/sport/olympics/athletics/9454624/Oscar-Pistorius-knocked-out-of-London-2012-Olympics-but-his-achievements-will-resound-for-years-to-come.html.

Keogh, Justin. 2011. "Paralympic Sport: An Emerging Area for Research and Consultancy in Sports Biomechanics." *Sports Biomechanics* 10(3): 234–53.

MacIntyre, Alasdair. 1999. *Dependent Rational Animals: Why Human Beings Need the Virtues*. Chicago: Open Court.

Mastro, James, Allen W. Burton, Marjorie Rosendahl, and Claudine Sherrill. 1996. "Attitudes of Elite Athletes with Impairments toward One Another: A Hierarchy of Preference." *Adapted Physical Activity Quarterly* 13(2): 197–210.

Merleau-Ponty, Maurice. (1945) 1962. *Phenomenology of Perception*. Translated by Colin Smith. London: Routledge.

Mott, Sue. 2000. "Impaired Logic Keeps Heroes Off the Stage." *Daily Telegraph*, retrieved 21 November 2020 from https://www.telegraph.co.uk/sport/2994384/On-Monday-Impaired-logic-keeps-heroes-off-the-stage.html.

Murphy, Robert. 1990. *The Body Silent*. New York: W. W. Norton.

Rossi, L. F. A. 1974. "Rehabilitation following Below-Knee Amputation." *Proceeds of the Royal Society of Medicine* 67: 37–38.

Sandahl, Carrie, and Phillip Auslander. 2005. "Introduction: Disability Studies in Commotion with Performance Studies." In Carrie Sandahl and Philip Auslander (eds.), *Bodies in Commotion: Disability and Performance*. Ann Arbor: University of Michigan Press, pp. 1–12.

Schell, Leah Anne, and Stephanie Rodriguez. 2001. "Subverting Bodies/Ambivalent Representations: Media Analysis of Paralympian, Hope Lewellen." *Sociology of Sport Journal* 18: 127–35.

Seymour, Wendy. 1998. *Remaking the Body: Rehabilitation and Change*. London: Routledge.
Sherrill, Claudine. 1999. "Disability Sport and Classification Theory: A New Era." *Adapted Physical Activity Quarterly* 16: 206–15.
Sherrill, Claudine, and Trevor Williams. 1996. "Disability and Sport: Psychosocial Perspectives on Inclusion, Integration and Participation." *Sport Science Review* 5(1): 42–64.
Shogan, Debra. 1998. "The Social Construction of Disability: The Impact of Statistics and Technology." *Adapted Physical Activity Quarterly* 15: 269–77.
Silva, Carla F., and P. David Howe. 2018. "The Social Empowerment of Difference: The Potential Influence of Parasport." *Physical Medicine and Rehabilitation Clinics of North America* 29(2): 397–408.
———. 2012. "The (In)validity of *Supercrip* Representation of Paralympic Athletes." *Journal for Sport and Social Issues* 36(2): 174–94.
Swartz, Leslie, and Brian Watermayer. 2008. "Cyborg Anxiety: Oscar Pistorius and the Boundaries of What It Means to Be Human." *Disability and Society* 23(2): 187–90.
Tuscher, Amy. 2016. "Paralympic Champion Hopes Taking on Greg Rutherford Leads to Olympic Ticket." *The Guardian*, 19 January. Retrieved 20 November 2020 from http://www.theguardian.com/sport/2016/jan/19/markus-rehm-greg-rutherford-paralympics-olympics-rio.
Tweedy, Sean, and Yves Vanlandewijck. 2009. "International Paralympic Committee Position Stand—Background and Scientific Rationale for Classification in Paralympic Sport." *British Journal of Sports Medicine* 45(4): 259–69.

CHAPTER 10

Unfixing Blindness
Retinal Implants and Negotiations of Ability in Postsocialist Russia

SVETLANA BORODINA

For Russian ophthalmology, 2017 was a big year. Two people who were deafblind underwent successful retinal prosthesis implantation surgeries. Russian media reports—mainly on pro-governmental federal media outlets—presented these surgeries as remarkable achievements in "the fight against blindness." The reports' tone was triumphant—the circulated narratives transmitted the sentiments of wonder, awe, and enthusiasm about what seemed to be Russia's participation in the inevitably coming technoscientific progress. Although for different stakeholders, the progress came at different costs and generated different values, they were all generally united by their interpretation of what happened—a team of Russian clinicians made two patients see again. Through various platforms, clinical and governmental spokespersons presented these procedures as a complexly coordinated benevolent solution to the "problem of blindness." They counted that already today there are fifty thousand individuals with retinitis pigmentosa in Russia who may benefit from this procedure (So-Edinenie 2017b). But this was only the beginning—it felt as if tomorrow with the help of science blindness would be eradicated altogether. Thus, the retinal prosthetic system implanted into the eyes of both patients emerged not only as a token of technoscientific power to cure but also as an ableist artifact of public desire and hope to erase blindness from the spectrum of available human experiences.

I do not argue against needed and wanted medical interventions; neither do I understand biomedicine as an institution that gathers unempathetic and self-interested actors. I do, however, challenge the unquestioned benefit of these procedures and the presented simplicity of the choices that the patients—Grigoriy Uliyanov and Antonina Zakharchenko—made. Moreover, I question whether it was actually a choice at all. I reject the dominant framework that defines blindness through one's inability to see as much as a "normal" individual does. My hesitation to accept the globalized biomedical understanding of blindness comes from eighteen months of fieldwork in urban Russia, where I collaborated with a group of blind professionals in carefully nurturing and promoting the cultures of inclusivity. Their distinct interpretation of blindness highlighted the abilities and unique experiences that blindness affords and helps to develop. Such a conceptualization of blindness stands close to the concept of deaf gain that captures the unique opportunities and experiences that deafness delivers to people (Bauman and Murray 2014). With this model in mind, I turned to my blind interlocutors for their insight on the significance of the two retinal implantations.

In this chapter, I engage with the experiences of eight blind individuals from Russia, whom I invited to comment on the public discourse surrounding these surgeries. Four of them identify as men; the other four as women. Their lives unfold in urbanized and secularized environments—somewhere in between socializing, work, and social activism. Two are students; the others are young and middle-aged professionals. All qualified for the Group I disability status,[1] through which they received a monthly pension; this ensured they had income—modest yet reliable—regardless of their employment status. All are adept users of white canes and for several years have navigated familiar and new urban environments on their own. None is deafblind. And none of them occupies a position of precarity due to their disability status and their form of embodiment.

Their critical insights enable me to challenge the often unquestioned epistemic authority of clinicians and medical professionals concerning blindness and the well-being of blind people. I also would like to acknowledge the unequal distribution of social investment in various forms of knowledge about blindness: biomedical knowledge, experiential knowledge of disabled experts and their family members, knowledge of rehabilitation workers, and knowledge produced and circulated by popular media. The dominant medicalized understanding of blindness (for a discussion of medicalization, see Conrad 1992; Rose 2007) poses the risk of uncritical reproduction of ableist social attitudes that, at their core, ignore the complexity and richness of blind people's lives and devalue past and present contributions of blind individuals, thus rendering them permanent societal burdens. As disability studies scholars argue, ableist social structures and attitudes become internalized and acted upon by both disabled and nondisabled people, resulting in exacerbated inequalities along the lines of abilities (Campbell 2009).

On a broader scale, my interlocutors' critiques challenge the widespread assumption that a world experienced from a position of a blind person or their allies is replaceable and *should be* replaced by one derived from and centered around sightedness. They problematize the logic that aligns blindness with incapacitation and disregards individual agency and other structural forces that shape the lives and experiences of blind people and their allies. In place of imbuing seeing, taken outside of the specifics of a particular context, with unquestioned value, they suggest considering the scope of associated abilities as a significant factor in choosing between blindness and the form of embodiment granted as a result of the surgery. For them, replacing their blind bodies with a body with a retinal implant means *losing* something of value—their sensory experiences, unique skills and abilities they developed qua blind individuals, acquired patterns of sociality, and relatedness to others. It also means facing the challenges of having to lose even more, through the time- and labor-consuming process of rehabilitation. For them, this replacement incurs losses.

My ultimate goal in this chapter is to show the sheer complexity of these cases and to contest the constructed obviousness of the decision to replace blindness with sightedness. By holding opposing views together—those of the operated individuals and those of my interlocutors—I hope to highlight the internal diversity of the blind population often ignored by the sighted. Additionally, an analysis of the Russian cases of the retinal prostheticization shows how divergent agendas work together to achieve a common goal. This account will help to develop a more nuanced understanding of the ambivalent ways in which medicalization works (Mauldin 2016) in postsocialist and other states that rely on the authority of biomedicine to advance agendas of a broad spectrum of stakeholders.

The Story and the Prosthesis

In 2017 Russian medical collectives conducted two implantation surgeries of bionic eyes to Russian individuals: one on 30 June and the other on 4 December. Both procedures consisted of implanting Argus II, a US device, to senior deafblind patients who lost their sight to retinitis pigmentosa. Both patients were chosen from the pool of patrons of the foundation for the support of the deafblind So-Edinenie. Both surgeries were sponsored by a charity foundation and supported by the Ministry of Healthcare.

Argus II is a complex prosthetic system that is made of several networked elements: a pair of glasses with a camera (to capture images) and a microcomputer (to render them into an appropriate format), a transmitter, and a set of sixty electrodes to be implanted onto the retina (to stimulate the remaining retinal photoreceptor cells and send the signal to the brain through the optic nerve). The brain then has to (learn to) decipher the signal and convert it into meaningful visual information that would further be of use to the patient in navigating their everyday life. In practice this means that in addition to the post-surgery period of healing, operated patients have to go through rigorous rehabilitation, during which they have to train their brain to make sense of this artificial signal. Argus II, thus, is not merely an optical device. Instead, it is a complex neuro-optical system that intervenes in the work of the individual's eye and neural system (see also Cartwright and Goldfarb 2005).

As the operating surgeon Dr. Khristo Takhchidi mentioned at a press conference (So-Edinenie 2017a, 40:43), the device was developed as a *model* for solutions to remedy blindness. In practice, this meant that the developers chose a condition (retinitis pigmentosa) that encapsulated key problems that contemporary bioscience has with blindness, that is, problems that are relatively common and rarely associated with other impairments. They chose retinitis pigmentosa because it is an approximated *version* of blindness; it ostensibly captures the essence of what blindness is for biomedicine. By substituting the biomedical term "retinitis pigmentosa" with "blindness"—which was done in the majority of popular publications—authorized spokespersons not only aggrandized the scale of achievement but also enabled the use of affectively charged references that would mobilize spectators' and readers' emotions to support the surgeries. In practice, only a fraction of blind people in Russia would be eligible for this procedure; in 2017 only sixty-seven could potentially qualify (Kuznetsov, Demchinskiy, and Kuleshov 2018). The limitation of the target group is significant, for it excludes populations whose involvement tends to dramatically affect public perception of such proedures. In effect, their target group was senior individuals with stable health and normative family arrangements. Such a selection excluded children (candidates must be older than twenty-five)—culturally hypervalued and universalized figures associated with the very possibility of having a future (Edelman 2004; Malkki 2015). It also excluded congenitally blind people who have neither a neurological nor a social skill of seeing and using vision as their primary source of information. Thus, the eligibility criteria ensured that the recruited patients would crave sight and have a potential to become protagonists of narratives of a happy homecoming. Here, home would signify sight and home in the literal sense—a dwelling of a normative family waiting for the operated person to return to normative functioning and division of labor.

What these patients acquired is eyesight as understood "narrowly" (Orlova 2017). Sixty electrodes implanted on their retinas transmit sixty signals that are further interpreted by their brains and shaped into images. The patients say they see flashes; an object for them appears like a white field with black surroundings—they see in black and white; the angle of vision is about thirty degrees (Burlakova and Chirkov 2018). The implanted system opened up an opportunity to identify large objects, track movement, and navigate the street (still with the help of a white cane [Chinyonova, Kurenkov, and Takhchidi 2017]) once they train their brain to "see again," that is, convert sixty flashing signals into meaningful information about their environment. The president of the charity foundation that organized the surgeries and the patients' subsequent rehabilitation characterized the vision that the patient acquired not as the vision that "we" have, as it is not full-colored, but, for "a person who hasn't seen, it is a substantial progress in terms of their socialization and their return to active life" (So-Edinenie 2017a, 22:36).

As we learn from the anthropology of the senses (Classen 1993; Geurts 2003; Howes 2003; Seremetakis 1994), sensory regimes differ from one context to the next. Vision is a powerful—although not the only—sensory channel through which meaning and power are negotiated, memories are created and reanimated, values are materialized, and social relations are lived (see also Garland-Thomson 2009). Vision is selective and contextual: in everyday life, what counts as seeing varies, which sometimes provides opportunities for legally blind people to pass as sighted (Kleege 1999; Michalko 1998; Omansky 2011). The patterns of this contextuality can be understood as a sensory culture. Campbell (2005) notes with regard to sound:

> "Sound" is not a value-neutral or mere audiological concept; rather it is possible to speak of cultures of sound and hearing. Some sounds and hearing are deemed pathological—*hearing voices* being a case in point, while other formulations such as *seeing sound*—invoke the strange and unknown. CI [cochlear implants] adherents could be accused of proposing a moral quality to sounds, not unlike the ways that advertisers attempt to seduce customers with certain sounds identified as highly desirable and pleasurable.

Like sound, vision is not value-neutral. Instead, one's fluency in visual cues and visual references enables access to multiple social arenas and resources of this ocularcentric world (Omansky 2011); it manifests one's belonging and willingness to belong to the community of the sighted. One's ability to participate in visual culture, comprehend visual metaphors, use visual cues, and share the taken for grantedness of visual perspectives increases one's chances to be recognized as an equal fellow citizen. Such an arrangement is deeply exclusionary in its nature. And yet, the question remains: Does one have to be able to see and to see well to participate visually in a community?

With these particular cases, the answer was ambivalent—yes, one has to be able to see, but how well remains unclear. The developer of the implant claims that patients who have been operated on have a prospect of forming valuable social skills: they will be able to identify paved walkways, detect where the sidewalk ends, perceive doorway entrances and windows, use porch lights for orientation and tell if someone is in front of them (SecondSight n.d.). Among improved social abilities, the provider offers differentiation between low- and high-contrast objects and edges, sorting laundry/socks, noticing doorways, street curbs, and buildings, detecting their dinner plate, the moon at night, fireworks, Christmas tree lights, knowing when someone has left the table or room, feeling more comfortable in social settings now that they know if someone walked away or changed position so they are not talking into empty space, and participating in hobbies they thought they couldn't, like darts or bowling. This is close to 5 percent of what counts as normal eyesight. In practice, these abilities can be restored as a result of rehabilitation. One of my interviewees confirmed:

> What for do you need a surrogate that doesn't even remind you of the original function? What can you do with it? Orient yourself on the streets? I can do it without it: without sight altogether or with my remaining sight. Read? With the contemporary development of technologies, reading and accessing information is not a problem at all. Drive? So not worth it. And you won't become a painter with this vision. Ten years ago, I had this thought that now is more well-shaped: one can and should live a full and interesting life with and without sight.

A white cane enables my interlocutors to identify paved walkways through touch, detect where the sidewalk ends, perceive doorway entrances and windows (they often also detect these through sound), and identify if there is someone in front of them. The majority cannot use porch lights for orientation, although some of them do. Those more visual elements listed by SecondSight—identifying the moon or Christmas tree lights—exemplify the ocularcentric framework that the developers use to appeal to the sighted audience. Noticing Christmas tree lights and the moon are instances of visualist modes of intimacy. I do not mean to imply that blind and sighted people do not bond over Christmas or that it is hard to find other ways to connect. Instead, I am suggesting that the rhetoric offered by SecondSight and uncritically adopted by Russian media and spokespersons framed blindness as an aspirationally sighted form of embodiment and not as a unique and worthy sensory mode. This narrative targets those who mourn sight and are unwilling to develop and value nonvisual ways of bonding and being with others.

The excitement with which the patients speak about the procedure (So-Edinenie 2018a, 2018b) does not serve as evidence of how great a solution this is. Neither does it offer evidence to label the patients irresponsible as they have not developed sufficient living skills to enjoy their lives with blindness. It does, however, serve as evidence to the fact that there are two blind individuals who have not been provided with adequate resources to enable an enjoyable and valuable life as a blind person. Their preference for sightedness is cultivated in a context where living with blindness is socially punished through exclusion, social distancing, and stigmatization. My interlocutors—privileged enough to access quality rehabilitation and an alternative discourse about blindness—are a minority among a much larger population of blind people.

Public Presentation

Dr. Khristo Takhchidi, the supervising surgeon, pithily presented the major framework through which these surgeries had been conceptualized:

> The most important is done: we have established a connection [between the prosthetic device and the brain]. Now we have to develop it. It's analogous to what we had with mobile phones. Remember the first mobile phone which was half a kilo heavy, with which you had to run around the field to catch [the signal] where possible, and take the contemporary model—it is almost a full computer. How quickly everything advanced. Because we had solved the most important thing—we have the connection. Here we have it . . . we need to improve it. (Chinyonova et al. 2017)

These surgical interventions became interpreted as milestones in the linear progress of technoscience. Dmitriy Polikanov, the president of the foundation that organized the surgeries and the subsequent rehabilitation, compared the first patient to cosmonaut Yuri Gagarin—the first man to fly to outer space (So-Edinenie 2017a, 21:25). This comparison drew parallels between the procedure of surgically inserting the retinal implant system into humans and outer-space human travel in terms of their significance for humanity—colonialist in spirit, conquering and subjugating what previously had been out of reach. Finally, the involved scientist also promised that in the future, it would only get better, "just like with cell phones" (Lebbekh and Takhchidi 2017).

I would like to juxtapose this narrative with the popular meme about Russia's technological power that was gaining momentum at the time. This meme—"Kak tebe takoe, Ilon Mask?" (How do you like that, Elon Musk?)—derives its humorous momentum from the comparison of Russian makeshift solutions to infrastructural breakdowns and Elon Musk, who in this context signifies the power of well-funded advanced technological progress (see also Hartblay 2017). The popularity of this meme pays tribute to individual savviness in generating solutions from the scrap materials at hand, in the context where better, more quality solutions remain out of reach. In other words, "Kak tebe takoe, Ilon Mask?" highlights the fantastic and almost insurmountable gap between the advertised prowess of Russian technoscience and the everyday experiences of Russia's broader population.

In this fantastic tale of technoscientific progress, much is left out. The flows of capital, negotiations across the borders of Russia and the United States, and the work and effort of those who labor to sustain the image of this progress escape public attention. There is little information about the benefits of the stakeholders involved in orchestrating these surgeries. All authorized spokespersons—medical experts, governmental representatives, NGO staff, operated patients and their family members—frame their participation as guided by the same value: the well-being of blind people. The reports uncritically present clinicians as the ultimate experts in issues that blind people encounter. Ophthalmologist Vyacheslav Kurenkov, MD, professor at the Department of Eye Diseases at the Federal Medico-Biological Agency of Russia, exemplifies this:

> Blindness is a major cause of vision disability that *prevents one from living a normal life. One cannot socialize, cannot get socially rehabilitated, one has limited capacities, one doesn't have a profession.* Of course, there are homes for the partially sighted and blind, there are some opportunities, but, we, as ophthalmologists, have a golden dream for our patients and us, to return a capacity to see to such patients. (Chinyonova et al. 2017; my emphasis)

The paradox here is that ophthalmologists' engagement with blind people usually ends once blindness manifests itself. There is virtually no communication between rehabilitation professionals, organizations of blind people, and ophthalmologists. Because ophthalmologists mostly work with sighted individuals and those with curable eye-related issues, they develop little expertise in the capabilities and functioning of blind people. All of my blind interlocutors who commented on the retinal implantation surgeries identify as well rehabilitated and fully socialized, despite Dr. Kurenkov's beliefs. In this sense, the choice of soliciting advice from clinical professionals on matters of blind people's well-being becomes controversial (see also Michalko 1998).

The materials about the surgeries that circulated on the country's main media outlets and the voices authorized to speak about the procedures materialize the medical model of disability that does not provide discursive and conceptual tools for imagining blindness other than as a lack and a tragedy (Devlieger, Rusch, and Pfeiffer 2003). Blind bodies configured within the framework of the medical model are configured as broken, suspended in the waiting for technoscientific progress to deliver a solution to "fix them." Regardless of one's disability status, stakeholders and protagonists of the publicized story of the retinal implantation surgeries in Russia reproduced the "the value system of ablenormativity which privileges the supposedly neurotypical and ablebodied" (Lydia X. Z. Brown's definition of ableism, in Scuro 2018: 48) at the expense of disabled individuals.

In *The Normal and the Pathological*, George Canguilhem (1991) describes the positivist interpretation of disease as quantitative, but not qualitative, differences in bodies. In this ontology, he claims, biomedicine justifies practices of treatment and rehabilitation that aspire to reduce the quantity of pathology in a given body. This logic often instantiates itself as increasing devaluation of multiply and complexly impaired bodies. When this argument is applied to the cases at hand, it becomes evident that the medical model of disability configures blind people as sighted people who do not see well. The sighted body remains the reference, and blind bodies emerge as their "weaker" versions. If taken seriously, this critique may help to unpack the constructed "derivativeness" of blindness and critique the binary damaged = blind and undamaged = sighted (Davis 1995: 14) upon which the medical model of blindness relies. To counterbalance the discourse based on the medicalized ideas of disability, I offer my blind interlocutors' reading of the retinal implantation surgeries.

Blind Interlocutors' Comments

For all eight interviewees, blindness is a fact of their life, a feature of their body that demands specific procedures and manners of action but that is not a barrier in itself. Three were born blind; five became blind later in life. In 2018, when I interviewed them, all had been trained and were experienced in urban navigation, everyday living skills, the use of technology and assistive devices, and profession-specific skills. In other words, all spoke from the position of a blind person with developed functional routines and rituals to navigate ocularcentric urban environments.

My first interviewee, Ilya,[2] shared the following:

> Everybody assumes that the loss of sight robs one's life of some purpose, that it diminishes the quality of life. With my own example, I can say that I do not see any problem with the quality of my life. It is just a different life; to claim that I'd live better were I not blind is simply stupid and arrogant. We cannot know what affects a person's development.... It is impossible to determine with certainty what affected the quality of my life and how.

Ilya critiques the foundational idea that drove the decision to operate on the patients in the cases at hand—the idea that blindness inevitably impoverishes one's life. His perspective is nuanced and intersectional; he suggests that there are different experiences of blindness and different ways in which blindness may affect and shape one's life. This impact cannot be predicted and determined a priori. Hence, Ilya states that the uncritical attribution of the responsibility for one's quality of life to their vision impairment is "stupid and arrogant." His response challenges the idea that blind people need their sighted peers to save them from blindness. Instead, if we treat blindness as just one factor in the broader spectrum of other factors shaping the individual's life, we come to question the presumed value attributed to these procedures as devices of life improvement.

Another respondent, Viktor, expressed concern about the public effects of this discourse:

> [The retinal implant system] is a good innovation, but I am not ready to use it, because I am happy without it. I leave it to those who seek fame or those who genuinely believe that this can change their blind life, to wait for [bionic eyes]. For me and others, it's better to act now. . . . You see, when this information [about bionic eyes] goes public, it gives people futile hope. And they start waiting, and their life passes by.

Viktor claims that the assumption that blindness is definitionally an inferior form of life is both ungrounded and detrimental; it robs blind people of their ability to live in the present, accept their body, and enjoy their life. In his opinion, it is not blindness itself but this line of thinking that disables the individual. The futuristic orientation fueled by the compulsive hopes for technoscientific invention and cure—what Alison Kafer (2013) calls the curative imagination—prevents a person from exploring their agency as a social participant and provokes withdrawal from social life as it unfolds here and now. Eli Clare states that the ideology of cure is about the temporal dislocation as it "grounds itself in an original state of being, relying on a belief that what existed before is superior to what exists currently. . . . It seeks to return what is damaged to that former state of being" (2017: 15). The ideology of cure does not leave disabled bodies in the present moment. Instead, it channels the lives, efforts, and preoccupations of people with disabilities to the past—pre-disability times—or the future—allegedly, the post-disability era. This effect of waiting and the refusal to act—here, as a blind person—works as another way in which internalized ableism harms disabled bodies and precludes their flourishing (Campbell 2009).

Viktor urged me to acknowledge the importance of losing hope, which he qualified as "futile." Anthropological research shows that sometimes hope "involves the practice of creating, or trying to create, lives worth living even in the midst of suffering, even with no happy ending in sight" (Mattingly 2010: 6). But other times, hope for a medical fix and a medical solution encourages inaction and prevents one from learning how to use their environment in new ways and develop new modes of relating to themselves and their physical and social environment. Thus, the problem here is not the solutions offered by biomedicine but the presentation of them as the *only* thinkable solutions to the problem of exclusion of people with disabilities. Two other of my interlocutors, Yulia and Vika, commented:

> New eyes will not help an isolated, asocial, angry, and offended person to become the center of social life. It requires substantial work on oneself, and sight has nothing to do with it. . . . I mean it is not about physical limitations. They cannot affect the person's generosity, energy level, charisma, and sense of humor.
>
> Who says that if a person acquires sight, this will change their quality of life? [With sight] the person will not stop isolating themselves because they are used to complaining about how bad everything is. [Sighted] eyes will help see more but will not change your character. It will not help one become a socially significant person either.

Like Ilya, Yulia and Vika offered their interpretations of what constitutes a "problem" for blind people. This relates not to their inability to see or the physical or psychological barriers that blind people experience. Instead, they configure the problem with blindness as a problem of exclusion. My interlocutors find opportunities for inclusion in one's character and one's motivation to pursue ways to be an active member of society (for a discussion of the value of being active and the imperative to live an active life, see Robbins 2013). As exemplified in this individualizing rhetoric, my blind interlocutors do not seek a collective identity around blindness as rights bearers and political subjects who make claims to the state (as was the case with disability rights activists [Charlton 2000]). Rather, their aspirational and chosen identity becomes that of contributing members of society.

Such individualizing logic of reframing blindness from an incapacitating condition to a condition of unique productivity has long roots in Russia. Throughout the Soviet era, blind people self-organized and developed a vast network of factories and plants, libraries, and cultural and social centers united under the umbrella of the All-Russia Society for the Blind (the Russian acronym for which is VOS). The stories of blind soldiers' heroism during World War II—in then-Leningrad, blind citizens served as *slukhachi* (listeners)—rendered them socially revered protagonists in national narratives of victorious triumph (informal conversation with a member of the Saint Petersburg branch of VOS, July 2015). Especially in the later Soviet period (1960s–1980s) VOS flourished. Exempt from paying taxes, VOS enterprises provided employment opportunities to its members and invested their funds in social programs. VOS configured blind people as *historically productive individuals* in Russia. Despite the economic failure of VOS enterprises today, new businesses have emerged that hire blind professionals in such services as business coaching in the dark, restaurants in the dark, exhibitions in the dark, and escape-room quests in the dark. Private and public funding provides opportunities for social projects designed and executed by blind activists and engaged volunteers. Despite changes in economic and political regimes, some blind individuals have consistently found ways to demonstrate their productivity and social contributions. Although scholars of disability have critiqued the unquestioned value of productivity and addressed its profoundly harmful effects on those who fail to qualify as a normatively productive subject (Aho 2017; Hartblay 2014; Taylor 2004), my blind interlocutors invest substantial efforts to experience and demonstrate their contributions and forms of social participation. Becoming a responsible and "socially significant person" through working on the self does not have a strong connection with one's ability to see. Yet it determines one's ability to generate self-worth and social appreciation, according to my interlocutors. In concert with this line of thinking, Lina commented:

> I'm curious to see how [the implant] works. But as any unnecessary but trendy gadget, soon it will become boring. Once people get bored with it, it will be abandoned on a shelf or sold on Yula [a seller platform analogous to Craigslist]. This hype around bionic eyes proves that humans aspire to the new and unknown. It is excellent and worthy of respect. But it's also essential to keep in mind that this is just a tool.

My interlocutors consider themselves social innovators: they work to change cultures of inclusivity and promote the idea that disability is not a tragedy but a different form of life that offers unique ideas and experiences. They live comfortably in their bodies, but they do not occupy a militant position against technology per se. Lina treats such innovations and the work that goes into producing and delivering these solutions to their target population with respect. But she cautions others—blind and sighted people alike—against fetishizing these solutions and attributing all responsibility for the quality of life to these tools. She references a phenomenon common among blind people in Russia—the general curiosity about new consumer goods designed for blind users and the quick loss of interest in these gadgets—as a potential risk. My interlocutors are already sufficiently prosthesized through their use of white canes, smartphones, computers, and other body enhancement and supplemental technologies. Their lack of interest in this new device emerges in response to the unending supply of other gadgets—of good and bad quality—that end up in their balconies and closets, underused or unusable.

The central concerns for my respondents were if the new technology enabled them to achieve their desired goals, if it activated existing skills, and if it helped them develop new abilities. Their metric of effectiveness differed from the one introduced by the state-medical complex. The latter configured blind people as patients, and the surgeries' effectiveness was spoken about in terms of the number of recognized objects, the duration of the recovery period, and acquired percentage of eyesight. My interlocutors' tool kit for measuring this device's worth was organized differently: around new abilities to do something previously inaccessible to them as well as the abilities to perform better socially. This difference in assessing the procedures raises the question of whether adopting an identity of a patient versus a position of a social innovator is a choice and to whom this choice is available.

This story is not a unique or unprecedented occurrence. Its significance comes from the fact that it repeats itself in multiple forms and iterations. Despite Russia's ratification of the United Nations Convention on the Rights of Persons with Disabilities, despite the rich history of blind self-organization in Russia, and despite the present-day emergence of new forms of blind people's social participation, the current system still invests substantial resources into maintaining the idea that blindness is a condition of sickness or deferred sightedness, not of a different mode of social participation and bodily being. The new alliances are formed—symbiotic arrangements of the state, private foundations, media platforms, biomedical experts, health-care bureaucrats, people with disabilities—to reproduce the model that does not offer solutions to the problem it creates, that is, the problem of the exclusion of people with disabilities and their further marginalization. The emergence of the retinal prostheses—with the trumpeting of this occurrence on federal media channels—is part of a longer biopolitical history in which people with sensory differences have served as the token subjects of state care.

Conclusion

Interventionist forms of care such as retinal implantation surgeries for patients with retinitis pigmentosa are made impressive and fantastic in contemporary Russian contexts: impressive because they create an impactful object of admiration—the sighted-blind persons—and the idea about the potency of domestic biomedical technoscience; fantastic because they promise desirable but improbable futures where the forms and shapes of embodiment of those future residents are carefully curated and, if necessary, "fixed." Expensive and technologically complex, they become publicized as a result of a successful alliance of the state, businesses, and the civil society, in their quest of taking care of the marginalized group of blind people. These occurrences are instances of care, as defined by Lisa Stevenson: a series of events and activities of attending to those who matter, even though that sometimes these forms of attending may be harmful (Stevenson 2014: 3).

Are such interventions as vitally *needed* as have been presented? Does this system eliminate or supply deficiencies, "in the sense of instigating the needs for the consumption of technologies" (Jain 1999: 50)? If the operated persons still use white canes, if they still use the sighted body as the reference and thus derive little value from their current mode of experiencing the world, and if they still have not achieved a sought-after ability to pass as sighted, what justifies the labors and challenges of learning to live with a prosthesis (Cartwright and Goldfarb 2005)? In researching these cases, I did not have access to the patients themselves. Yet Sharon Kaufman's concept of the chain of dense connections between the state, businesses, technoscience, and experts that shape the ethical field of contemporary medical settings helps to illustrate how "patients and families (and sometimes doctors) actually do not *decide* about treatments as much as they yield to procedures that the chain has made normal and ordinary" (Kaufman 2015: 7). Similarly, in present-day Russia, blind people are rarely given a chance to choose between equally appealing options: a life qua a blind individual and a life qua a sighted (yet still blind) individual. The access to the former is often hard to secure, and it generally comes down to the individual's ability to mobilize enough resources to connect to those blind persons who have had a chance to learn from exceptional role models.

Surgery is not necessarily *needed*. But it is framed and perceived as a need in the cultural field that does not support forms of disability culture and public presence. Those who choose not to undergo procedures that have a potential of improving one's eyesight even a little are viewed as not willing to participate in their own recovery and thus not caring enough to lift the burden for their care from others. This individual responsibilization and moralization of choices over one's bodily and mental condition is the present-day reverberation of biological forms of citizenship where individuals become responsible for the well-being of themselves as members of the broader collective (Rose 2006).

Acknowledgments

I thank my eight interlocutors for their comments. This research received the generous support of the Mellon/ACLS Dissertation Completion Fellowship, the Social Science Research Council, the Wenner-Gren Foundation, the Social Sciences Research Institute, and the Department of Anthropology at Rice University.

Svetlana Borodina is a postdoctoral research scholar in the Harriman Institute at Columbia University. Her research interests include cultural, socioeconomic, and political configurations of inclusion outside of the liberal contexts, blindness, and the shifting dynamics of bodily and mental vulnerability in Russia. She received her PhD in anthropology from Rice University. She also holds graduate certificates in critical and cultural theory as well as in the study of women, gender, and sexuality.

Notes

1. Group I disability status is attributed to people with severe functional limitations that require permanent assistance and care.
2. To protect my interlocutors' privacy, I use aliases instead of real names.

References

Aho, Tanja N. 2017. "Active Citizenship, Liberalism, and Labor-Normativity: Queer-crip Resistance, Sanist Anxiety, and Racialized Ableism in Viewer Responses to *Here Comes Honey Boo Boo*." *Journal of Literary & Cultural Disability Studies* 11: 321–37.

Bauman, H.-Dirksen L., and Joseph J. Murray (eds.). 2014. *Deaf Gain: Raising the Stakes for Human Diversity*. Minneapolis: University of Minnesota Press.

Burlakova, Dariya, and Aleksandr Chirkov. 2018. "Kontury budushchego: kak sovremennye tehnologii vozvrashchayut zrenie absolutno slepym" [The contours of the future: How modern technology returns vision completely blind]. *TASS*, 30 January.

Campbell, Fiona Kumari. 2005. "Selling the Cochlear Implant." *Disability Studies Quarterly* 25(3). Retrieved 5 July 2019 from https://dsq-sds.org/article/view/588/765.

———. 2009. *Contours of Ableism: The Production of Disability and Ableness*. New York: Palgrave Macmillan.

Canguilhem, Georges. 1991. *The Normal and the Pathological*. Cambridge: Zone Books.

Cartwright, Lisa, and Brian Goldfarb. 2005. "On the Subject of Neural Prosthesis." In Joanne Morra and Marquard Smith (eds.), *The Prosthetic Impulse: From a Posthuman Present to a Biocultural Future*. Cambridge, MA: MIT Press, pp. 125–54.

Charlton, James. 2000. *Nothing About Us Without Us: Disability Oppression and Empowerment*. Berkeley: University of California Press.

Chinyonova, Kseniya, Vyacheslav Kurenkov, and Khristo Takhchidi. 2017. "Bionicheskiy glaz. Budushchee proiskhodit segodnya" [Bionic eye: The future takes place today]. Doctor.Ru website. Retrieved 1 July 2019 from https://doctor.ru/view/53738/.

Clare, Eli. 2017. *Brilliant Imperfection: Grappling with Cure*. Durham, NC: Duke University Press.
Classen, Constance. 1993. *Worlds of Sense: Exploring the Senses in History and across Cultures*. New York: Routledge.
Conrad, Peter. 1992. "Medicalization and Social Control." *Annual Review of Sociology* 18: 209–32.
Davis, Lennard. 1995. *Enforcing Normalcy: Disability, Deafness, and the Body*. New York: Verso.
Devlieger, Patrick, Frank Rusch, and David Pfeiffer. 2003. *Rethinking Disability: The Emergence of New Definitions, Concepts and Communities*. Antwerp: Garant.
Edelman, Lee. 2004. *No Future: Queer Theory and the Death Drive*. Durham, NC: Duke University Press.
Garland-Thomson, Rosemarie. 2009. *Staring: How We Look*. Oxford: Oxford University Press.
Geurts, Kathryn. 2003. *Culture and the Senses: Bodily Ways of Knowing in an African Community*. Berkeley: University of California Press.
Hartblay, Cassandra, 2014. "A Genealogy of (post-)Soviet Dependency: Disabling Productivity." *Disability Studies Quarterly* 34(1). Retrieved 1 July 2019 from https://dsq-sds.org/article/view/4015/3538.
———. 2017. "Good Ramps, Bad Ramps: Centralized Design Standards and Disability Access in Urban Russian Infrastructure." *American Ethnologist* 44(1): 9–22.
Howes, David. 2003. *Sensual Relations: Engaging the Senses in Culture and Social Theory*. Ann Arbor: University of Michigan Press.
Jain, Sarah S. 1999. "The Prosthetic Imagination: Enabling and Disabling the Prosthesis Trope." *Science, Technology & Human Values* 24(1): 31–54.
Kafer, Alison. 2013. *Feminist, Queer, Crip*. Bloomington: Indiana University Press.
Kaufman, Sharon R. 2015. *Ordinary Medicine: Extraordinary Treatments, Longer Lives, and Where to Draw the Line*. Durham, NC: Duke University Press.
Kleege, Georgina. 1999. *Sight Unseen*. New Haven, CT: Yale University Press.
Kuznetsov, Daniil, Andrey Demchinskiy, and Denis Kuleshov. 2018. "Novoe 'bionicheskoe zrenie' dlya slephykh" [New "bionic vision" for the blind]. *Osobyi Vzglyad* [Special view]. Retrieved 1 July 2019 from http://specialview.org/article/post46.
Lebbekh, Inessa, and Khristo Takhchidi. 2017. "Vykhod iz temnoty. Slepota i implantatsiya setchatki" [Exit from the dark: Blindness and implantation of the retina]. Doctor.Ru website. Retrieved 1 July 2019 from https://doctor.ru/view/51525/.
Malkki, Liisa H. 2015. *The Need to Help: The Domestic Arts of International Humanitarianism*. Durham, NC: Duke University Press.
Mattingly, Cheryl. 2010. *The Paradox of Hope: Journeys Through a Clinical Borderland*. Berkeley: University of California Press.
Mauldin, Laura. 2016. *Made to Hear: Cochlear Implants and Raising Deaf Children*. Minneapolis: University of Minnesota Press.
Michalko, Rod. 1998. *The Mystery of the Eye and the Shadow of Blindness*. Toronto: University of Toronto Press.
Omansky, Beth. 2011. *Borderlands of Blindness*. Boulder: Lynne Rienner.
Orlova, A., 2017. "'Ya vizhu, no ne tak, kak vy': kak zhivet pervyi rossiyskiy patsient s bionicheskim glazom" ["I see, but not like you": How the first russian patient lives with a bionic eye]. Agentstvo Sotsialnoy Informatsii website [Agency of

Social Information]. Retrieved 1 July 2019 from https://www.asi.org.ru/article/2017/11/13/pervyj-patsient-s-bionicheskim-glazom/.

Robbins, Jessica C. 2013. "Understanding Aktywność in Ethnographic Contexts: Aging, Memory, and Personhood in Poland." *Forum Oświatowe* 1(48): 103–19. Retreived 1 July 2019 from http://forumoswiatowe.pl/index.php/czasopismo/article/view/78.

Rose, Nikolas. 2006. *The Politics of Life Itself: Biomedicine, Power, and Subjectivity in the Twenty-First Century*. Princeton, NJ: Princeton University Press.

———. 2007. "Beyond Medicalisation." *Lancet* 369(9562): 700–702.

Scuro, J., 2018. *Addressing Ableism: Philosophical Questions via Disability Studies*. New York: Lexington Books.

SecondSight. n.d. "Frequently Asked Questions." SecondSight website. Retrieved 1 July 2019 from https://secondsight.com/faq/#.

Seremetakis, C. Nadia (ed.). 1994. *The Senses Still: Perception and Memory as Material Culture in Modernity*. Chicago: University of Chicago Press.

So-Edinenie, 2017a. "Vernut' Zrenie: v Rossii Ustanovili Retinal'nyie Implanty Sleupoglukhomu Patsientu" [To restore vision: Retinal implants have been installed in russia for a deafblind patient]. YouTube video. Retrieved 1 July 2019 from https://youtu.be/uqp1zhx9vhk.

———. 2017b. "Vtoroy rossiyskiy patsient s bionicheskim glazom" [The second Russian patient with a bionic eye]. YouTube video, Moscow. Retrieved 1 July 2019 from https://www.youtube.com/watch?v=zscfhQs4HI4.

———. 2018a. "Ne odin v temnote. Grigoriy" [Not alone in the dark: Grigoriy]. YouTube video, Moscow. Retrieved 1 July 2019 from https://www.youtube.com/watch?v=_wV19faDv0E.

———. 2018b. "Ne odna v temnote. Antonina" [Not alone in the dark: Antonina]. YouTube video, Moscow. Retrieved 1 July 2019 from https://www.youtube.com/watch?v=0tIdsshB9LU.

Stevenson, Lisa. 2014. *Life Beside Itself: Imagining Care in the Canadian Arctic*. Oakland: University of California Press.

Taylor, Sunny. 2004. "The Right Not to Work: Power and Disability." *Monthly Review*, 1 March. Retrieved 1 July 2019 from https://monthlyreview.org/2004/03/01/the-right-not-to-work-power-and-disability/.

CHAPTER 11

Learning through Apps
The Replacement of Offline Cis-Female Bodies with Digital Pregnancies and Menstruations

DANIELA TONELLI MANICA, MARINA FISHER NUCCI,
AND GABRIELA CABRAL PALETTA

Fertility and reproduction have long been strategic targets for biopolitical and medical interventions (Foucault [1976] 1988; Oudshoorn 1994; Clarke et al. 2010; Sanabria 2016). In this chapter, we discuss the impact of the emergence and dissemination of information and communication technologies (ICTs) on practices related to reproduction.

This text is based on research about apps that monitor the reproductive system in cis-female bodies, specifically pregnancy and menstrual cycle apps currently being used in Brazil. We describe the different interfaces involved in the process and discuss issues related to medicalization, gender normativity, surveillance, and health data production. We examine some of the entanglements between bodies, health, technologies, and gender present in menstrual cycle and pregnancy apps to ask some key questions: What kinds of bodies are enacted at these interfaces? What kinds of data are being produced by these devices? And finally, how can the huge amount of information being produced through ICTs be capitalized?

We take a critical perspective on the relations between bodies, codes, and information. The ironic myth of the cyborg (Haraway 1991) formulated some of the first important criticisms around this topic, and this was followed by rereadings from contemporary gender techno-politics, which comment on the articulations between biomedicine, the pharmaceutical and pornography industries, and digital technologies (Preciado 2008). Given the current radical threats to women's rights in Brazil, especially regarding sexual and reproductive rights, we align our critical stance to feminist activism when formulating our analysis of these apps. According to this perspective, health-related information technologies are a form of self-tracking technology (Lupton 2014) focused on body monitoring.

In what follows, we consider "remaking the human" by addressing menstrual cycle and pregnancy apps as forms of more affordable and less invasive biopolitical interventions. Such interventions help reshape bodies and notions of fertility and reproduction by replacing previous bodily perceptions and practices with new and ever-changing technological assemblages, where digital information and potentially capitalizable data acquire an important, if not central, place.

Departing from a preliminary analysis of these apps (Paletta 2019), we noticed the importance of accessing the users' perceptions about gender, fertility, and reproduction when inquiring about their motivations, uses, and engagements with the apps and the data they produce and circulate. Below, we show how these apps have been mobilized to reshape understandings of pregnancy, the menstrual cycle, fertility, and reproduction and explore contemporary aspects of information and communication technologies related to bodies, gender, and health. We illustrate how novel digital practices of mastering fertility and bodily functions (such as menstruation) and monitoring pregnancy and fetal development replace the existing "offline" practices, renewing the scope of activities and procedures used to monitor and manage the body and reproductive functioning.

Pregnancy and Menstrual Cycle Apps: Engaging with Health Data Production

For this research, we selected four of the most downloaded pregnancy and menstrual cycle apps, both in iOS and Android operating systems.[1] The two pregnancy apps selected were Pregnancy+ (Gravidez+), with more than 10,000 downloads at Apple Store and 10 million downloads at Google Play Store, and BabyCenter, with almost 5,000 downloads at Apple Store and 10 million at Google Play Store. Both apps are free and with interfaces available in Portuguese.

Pregnancy+ was launched in January 2013 by the American companies Health & Parenting Ltd. and Philips Consumer Lifestyle CV. It is available in ten different languages. BabyCenter was created in March 2011 by the American company BabyCenter, L.L.C. It is available in six different languages and nine different versions. Besides the app, there is also a website with the same name and an online forum accessible through both the website and the app, where users can exchange various information about fertility, pregnancy, and parenting.

At the time of first access, the user is solicited to register by inserting data such as name, country, date of birth, and date of last menstrual period. Using this last piece of information, the apps calculate the probable date of the baby's birth (usually forty weeks after the date of the last period) and the gestational week. Both apps have informational texts about pregnancy and fetal development, and these change on a weekly basis throughout the pregnancy.

The selected pregnancy apps provide numerous stylized fetal images, 3D simulations of fetuses inside the belly, and resources that compare the fetus's size in that specific gestational week with fruits or vegetables. As an example, if you access the app at the thirtieth week of pregnancy, BabyCenter will inform that the fetus is "the approximate size of a cabbage."

Among the most downloaded health and fitness free apps in this research, we also analyzed two "menstruapps" (Paletta 2019):[2] Menstrual Calendar (Calendário Menstrual), launched in March 2012 by the Chinese company Simple Design, and Clue, Calendário do ciclo menstrual e ovulação, developed in October 2014 by the German BioWink GmbH. They have, respectively, more than 50 million and 10 million downloads at Apple and Google Play Stores.

In slightly different ways, the menstrual cycle monitoring apps offer tools to record information about the cycle, such as a notepad, emoticons that index a diverse array of moods and symptoms (physical, emotional, social, and sexual), graphics with weight and basal temperature variation, and reminders indicating the arrival of one's fertile period and imminent menstruation. Although this information may be associated with becoming aware of one's fertility cycles, it may also exceed this purpose.

At the time of first access, for both menstrual cycle apps, it is necessary to answer questions about the duration of the menstrual cycle and the specific dates the last menstruation has begun and ended, among other pieces of information. The app Clue allows you to save the data in a cell phone device, and not in an online account. Menstrual Calendar has a "forum" where different chat rooms with different debate topics are available for the users should they wish.[3] Menstrual Calendar is available in forty different languages. Clue is offered in thirteen languages and explores more intensely the offline habits of users by providing the option of recording physical activities, sleep quality, party days, skin characteristics, and so on.

In this text we present data from twenty semi-structured interviews with women using these apps, ten from menstrual cycle apps and ten from pregnancy apps. The interviews were conducted by us, with Brazilian users of these selected apps, in person when possible, but most of the times (eighteen of twenty) via online conference software. Ethical procedures like informed consent were followed, and the interviews were recorded and transcribed. Participants were contacted through our personal networks and through specific calls for participants published in menstruation and pregnancy discussion groups in digital social networks. All participants lived in medium to large cities or state capitals and come from the middle class, with access to education (almost all had completed college by the time of the interview). We enlisted participants from five different states in three different regions of Brazil: Northeast, Midwest, and Southeast.

Participants using menstrual cycle apps were aged eighteen to thirty-six years old. The majority (seven women) self-declared as nonwhite (black or *parda*), three as white. Six self-declared as heterosexual, three as bisexual, and one as a lesbian. Only two had children (one child each, under two years old). The pregnancy app users were aged thirty to forty-one, and most self-declared as white (eight) and heterosexual (nine). Eight of the ten users were pregnant with their second child; the age of the first child varied from six months to seven years.

They were invited to talk about their understandings of pregnancy and the menstrual cycle and relate them to their experiences with the apps. We asked about the frequency of access, motivations, and preferences of use regarding the apps, how long they have used the app, how they got to know about the app, and whether they had previous techniques for monitoring the menstrual cycle and pregnancy. They were asked about the kind of data they insert, the things they learn about through the app, if they trust the information shared by the app, and whether they sought other sources and opinions about the menstrual cycle and pregnancy. We also inquired about data circulation: whether they make "prints" of the app's interfaces and share them or other pieces of information with other people and with whom. We usually ended the interview by asking them if they had read the privacy policies before/during the app installation and if they worry about data security.

Monitoring Menstruation and Fertility: Temporalities and the Menstrual Cycle Apps

Menstrual cycle apps are downloaded more often than pregnancy apps. And the type and amount of data women provide to menstruapps is very different; there is a much broader array of elements that can be monitored and a larger set of information about the body and a user's emotions available for input in these interfaces.

For menstrual cycle apps to operate well, the user must engage with them on a regular basis, making it a habit to feed them information, at least during three full menstrual cycles. All apps advertise that the more information you insert, the "smarter" the app gets. The app's "artificial intelligence" sustains its ability to predict the cycle duration and to share this information with the user, focusing on aspects such as fertility period and the imminent arrival of menstruation.

Women are asked to insert basic data such as the dates when the bleeding started and ended, but these apps open the possibility of monitoring other aspects of women's lives. The information collected is linked to biomedical understandings of the "menstrual cycle," such as ovulation, fertility, and contraception (sexual relations, orgasms, and libido) and "premenstrual symptoms" (headaches, swelling, breast pain, irritation, or depression). It also includes more general data about humor and disposition, bowel functioning, skin, hair, and weight.

When asked about how they perceived their menstrual cycle, many of our interlocutors said they understand it as something "natural," a part of life, connected to femininity and to fertility, and other natural cycles, such as the lunar cycle. Some also referred to menstruation as a moment of discomfort and pain, and that is why they considered it important to monitor its onset.

For others, the connection of the menstrual cycle to fertility is important, and the app is seen as an informational overlay to better situate ovulation and menstruation in time. The menstrual cycle app works as an accessible "external memory" that records the date of the last menstruation and is a sort of mirror of what happened with the woman's body over previous weeks and months, at least as far as the information recorded there is concerned. Many women mentioned the advantage of being able to access, by quickly checking the app, the date of their last cycle, which is especially useful during medical consultations.

For menstrual cycle apps, what matters is the history of differences and repetitions the interface is able to process and predict. Menstrual cycle apps seem to demand more frequent engagement and constant input, and they accommodate more oscillations and irregularities from these data, promptly incorporating changes in patterns. As we will see, on the other hand, for pregnancy apps the important data refers to the present (what is happening to the body now), and it is the user's job to compare the information in the app to what she is actually feeling or to information acquired at the medical service.

Only one interlocutor reported using the menstrual cycle app only once a month (sometimes even less); the others used it at least once a week (three interlocutors), twice or three times a week (three interlocutors), or every day (three interlocutors). We have, obviously, a biased sample, since we recruited women who use the apps and were willing to talk about their use. But based on this sample, we can say that using this app demands regular and frequent data input, and if users want the reliable predictions promised by the apps, they have to feed them constantly with accurate data.

Most women mentioned that their main motivations for installing the app were the ability to learn more about their menstrual cycles and to monitor menstruation and fertility, either with the goal of getting pregnant or to avoid pregnancy. The apps are seen as forms of organizing information and rediscovering the signs of one's own body, which tends to happen during the beginning of the app's use.

> MCApp06: When you are a girl, you have no interest in worrying about when you will ovulate or anything like that . . . the volume of your menstruation. . . . I was not interested in those things and I don't remember, really, I have no memory of how my menstruation was before. . . . And when you stop taking contraceptives, it is as if you discovered your body again.

> MCApp07: So, when I first downloaded the app, I didn't understand things very much, I didn't understand the symptoms [sic] my body showed during the whole cycle as well. And then, after [using it], I was able to notice things like: during my fertile period *this* happens in my body. . . . I started noticing the symptoms happening in my body, as the calendar pointed out. . . . Then you understand, you know? So, for me it was fundamental to get to know myself better. When a certain phase was over, the app would let me know about the next phase . . . and I could understand what was going on. So nowadays, sometimes, I don't even have to look at the date in the app, and I know, "Jeez, I am going through the fertile period, because I already feel the symptoms."

Measuring these cyclic repetitions requires a mathematical effort of calendar management that app users promptly delegate to the software, which calculates them and predicts new events. Menstruapps fulfill the job of materializing, through their digital data, these variations and their cyclicity.

Time is an important category, but most of our interlocutors who did not want to become pregnant expected they would be able to measure the cyclicity of their menstruation through this "time management." Six of the ten women migrated from continuous and regular use of hormonal contraceptives to monitoring fertility through these apps, sometimes in combination with other nonhormonal contraceptive methods.

This made us think about the menstruapps as a kind of "digital pill"—something that substitutes the molecular contraceptive coercion carried out by hormones with other techniques, which involve registering information about the perception of fertility, bodily awareness, and the management of sexual relations during the fertile period. The "digital pill" is based on perceiving and monitoring the body and producing digital data.

For Preciado (2008), hormonal contraception is perfectly framed within a pharmaco-pornographic project that turns female bodies temporarily infertile and makes possible heterosexual nonreproductive acts. Science and technology studies and Brazilian feminist studies scholars show how hormonal contraception have helped to produce an alienated form of body modulation, which makes users less likely to interfere with the prescribed use of contraceptive methods (Correa 1994; Roland 1995 and 1998; Citeli, Mello e Souza, and Portela 1998; Cabral, Heilborn, and Brandão 2007; Manica 2012; Sanabria 2016). Policies that promote the use of long-term and low-cost contraception techniques, preferably without the user's control over its discontinuation (such as the IUDs, subdermal implants, injectables, or sterilization procedures), targeted specific populations in Brazil: low-income populations, adolescents, blacks, and marginalized populations in general.

Our interviews indicate that the use of oral hormonal contraception was the standard medical recommendation for all young women, homo/bi/heterosexual, from all classes and races. The convenience of this method was only questioned if the patient explicitly asked for more information and alternative methods or if something unusual occurred while using the pill. That was the case of one of our interlocutors, who found out, due to side effects such as blurred vision, that she had a propensity to thrombosis. As a result, she quit the pill and installed the app.

The continuous use of sex hormones is only intended to be interrupted when these women "plan" to get pregnant (which may involve, for middle-class women, choosing the "ideal" moment, when they have achieved professional and other goals). Unlike the type of relation oral contraceptives create between women and their bodies—daily pill ingestion and temporary interruptions to "technomenstruate" (Preciado 2008)—some of our interlocutors reported an urge to reconnect with their bodies by migrating from the pill to the app and a willingness to start monitoring their fertility and their contraceptive strategies more diligently.

> MCApp09: I think it was only later, when the app arrived, that I became aware, you know, of how much time after menstruation you ovulate, how long after that you menstruate . . . of the phases [the body goes through].

The app demands, and provides, different forms of perceiving and dealing with contraception and with the body:

> MApp10: So, for me, the apps seem to bring women even closer to self-knowledge, you know? And the connection with your own body, the connection with the way things happen within the body. To better understand this process, to learn about how things work by using our calendar. Is it late? Is it not late? I feel this, I feel that. The app tells you, right? You keep inserting information and improving the app's analyses, and then you start to better understand the way your body is functioning.

Based on the empirical material we have gathered and on the theoretical argument we are trying to develop here, we propose thinking about "replacement" in the context of relations between bodies and technologies, where menstrual cycle apps tend to replace the pill regime, thus establishing an informational-communicational form of modulation for cis-female body cycles. As Oudshoorn (1994) showed, in the twentieth century the pill helped to create belief in a regular menstrual cycle of twenty-eight days, by imposing the twenty-eight-day pill pack. This technological framework modulated women's time management (by looking at and following the daily calendar provided by the pharmaceutical industry) and a biochemical/synthetical/hormonal induction that would "biomolecularly" produce infertile, but sexually active, cis-female bodies.

The menstrual cycle apps replace the automatisms the pill provided to deal with time and contraceptive management. Interrupting hormonal contraception involves actively attending to the body, to fertility, and to menstruation. Although it may be seen as a solution for contraception, the effects of monitoring the body surpass the connections between sexuality and reproduction.

> MCApp10: What I observe mostly is that during the fertile period, the libido increases. It is usually when we are looking for, [even] craving for sexual relations. Then I like to observe and get to know these cycles, actively experience these cycles, to really see the thing happening, you know? Not only in the calendar, but in the body, and actions, and everything else.

Although these other forms of dealing with the cycle, fertility, and reproduction/contraception may be less invasive, since they do not employ synthetic hormones, the apps still provide forms of regulation, management, and monitoring the body. Haraway (1991) argued that the "cybernetic turn" was responsible for transforming the world by introducing codification, communication, and information. In this case, hormones (synthetic or endogenous) and informational data both provide the means to control vital and mortal processes. The app is an informational system in which the molecule, formerly the biochemical code-information, is replaced by digital data, in which the cycle and its measurement are enacted by the apps' algorithms, making the user's menstrual cycle more palpable/manageable through the images and graphics produced.

At first, the use of the app may seem more empowering and liberating than a pharmaceutical, freeing the user from synthetic hormones produced by the pharmaceutical industry. Even so, they produce a specific kind of framework in which information and communication technologies become social spaces for data production and accumulation. Users continuously feed databases that may easily work in a regulatory regime for population management, providing sensitive data about menstruation, pregnancy, date and frequency of sexual relations, orgasms, and so on.

Almost no women had read the app's privacy policy, and they were embarrassed that they had not, nervously laughing and commenting, "I know I should have read" or "I know it's important," when asked about this. Still, they took comfort that they did not give away information that they considered sensitive, such as their address or credit card number. Mandatory information solicited by the app, such as name, age, and date of the last period, were not understood as sensitive information that would risk their privacy. There is also the notion that it was impossible to escape the use of technology and data circulation, since "everything is connected." Furthermore, to use any app in Brazil, one has to choose between "accepting" or "denying" the terms of privacy, with no space for negotiation.

Imagining and Monitoring the Not-So-Invisible Fetus: Pregnancy Apps and Expectations

Pregnancy can be seen as a positive period of multiple transformations, but also of surprises, uncertainties, unexpected events, and lack of control. Most of our interlocutors referred to these aspects when asked about the meaning of pregnancy. The "lack of control" had to do with having "another" person inside the body, imposing its own rhythms, demands, and lifestyle changes in terms of bodily care, routine, and diet.

Among the ten women interviewed, four used BabyCenter, four used Pregnancy+, and two used both apps concurrently. They learned about the apps through friends, posts in digital social networks, internet searches on their cell phones, and even through the obstetrician or the obstetrics nurse during prenatal care.

Women generally installed the app right after finding out they were pregnant and accessed it at least once a week (although a few women reported accessing it every day). The frequency of use varied throughout the pregnancy, and the first months were described as the ones of most anxieties and doubts. During this initial period, especially women in the first pregnancy accessed the app more frequently, as a way to reassure themselves about the normality of the gestation and of their feelings (or, in their own words, "symptoms"):

> PgApp02: The other day I had cramps, for example. Then I was: "Am I eating badly?" Then, the app: "No, cramps are normal." So, this is a nice feature of the app, it gives you information: "that is normal, it is common for pregnant women to have these things."[4]

The app is described as a tool that helps women to learn about what is happening "inside them" and what "they should be feeling," but it also allowed them to compare the size and the shape of their belly with other women at the same gestational period. When asked about their motivations to use the app, they replied:

PgApp10: To learn about the progress of gestation, to learn about the size of the embryo, the fetus. . . . Curiosity with what was happening with the gestation, what I should be feeling.

PgApp07: There is a picture there of "how your belly should be at this moment," and then you add the picture you take in front of the mirror, of your own belly. Then you put them side by side to compare. Why should that make people anxious: "Oh, is my belly the right size?" Because people always make comments like this on the streets: "Oh, your belly is very big, are you sure it is just one?" Or even the opposite. I remember when I was seven or eight months many people thought my belly was small, and I said, "No, it's totally acceptable, the doctor has already examined me."

The women interviewed were unanimous in saying that they prefer information about the fetal development week by week, especially in the form of fetal images:

PgApp07: [I prefer] this graphic part. These little images; 3D simulations of how the new little human is growing. . . . It is a way of keeping track of what is happening inside the body, something that I don't control. It is sort of answering the question of what the fetus is doing at that moment. I know it is not what I see, I see an approximate projection. But, still, we are so much alike in this period that even though it is an approximation, it reassures me.

Fetal images, information about the development, and comparisons of the fetus's size every week with fruits and vegetables, for example, helped women to "feel pregnant" and gave a greater sense of concreteness to the gestation, especially at first, when there was no apparent belly yet and fetal movements were imperceptible:

PgApp04: Ah, I think these curiosities are really cute. "Oh, the baby has started to hear," "the baby can blink." . . . It has to do with that, with seeing the photos, learning interesting facts about the baby, imagining how the baby is. We end up having a more real sense of what is going on, you know? Like, "Wow, it already blinks!"; "Wow, the baby is moving, it already has hair." Then I think we start imagining how it really is, it is more palpable.

PgApp05: There was something I liked very much, which was seeing the fetus's size, that was neat, like, keeping up with the size of fruits. These things I liked, because I felt more pregnant when I thought of these baby's developmental milestones.... Then, you know, I felt more pregnant with this app. Because I think the beginning of pregnancy is very ... we still don't feel the baby, we practically don't feel anything. And I, particularly, I feel very nauseated, but besides that I don't feel pregnant, you know? So, for this beginning, it is nice to keep track of things.

As Mitchell and Georges (1998) have noted, the ultrasound is a key technology in the construction of a "cyborg fetus," that is, a fetus whose existence is mediated by a sort of different technologies. Therefore, the ultrasound stimulates the visualization not of a fetus or an embryo, but of an ideal baby, with a distinct appearance, subjectivity, and its own personality. The cyborg fetus emerges as a social actor with an identity of its own. After conducting ethnographic research in obstetric ultrasound clinics in Brazil, Lilian Chazan (2007) observed that the diagnostic technology has increasingly spread throughout the country, becoming an object of consumption that fascinates pregnant women and their families and that induces the "pleasure of seeing the baby." The pregnancy apps take advantage of the fascination that ultrasound fetal images evoke in pregnant women.

If, as Chazan suggests, the obstetric ultrasound is a fundamental element in the process of transformation of fetuses into persons, the apps appear to contribute to the process of transforming these women into "pregnant women" even before the pregnant belly starts to be visible and before fetal movement is detected. They replace the first subjective perceptions of pregnancy by making sense, both in language and through images, of bodily sensations related to pregnancy and the fetus's growth. These apps function as technological mediators in the process of making the "cyborg baby."

In that sense, fetal images available through the app and information about pregnancy weekly development were seen as resources that replace ultrasound. Instead of submitting herself to various and periodic exams, as is common for middle-class women in Brazil, one woman said she would rather look at the app's images weekly to get a visual estimate of the fetus's size and weight. The app also provided a moment of "connection" with the fetus, in the midst of a stressful work routine:

> PgApp07: I remember in old times, the advice from my mother and grandmother was: "Talk to your belly." Looking at the app is like this moment of "talking to your belly" [*laughs*]. I am in a boring meeting, then I discreetly open the app in the cell phone. There it is: my pregnancy is available at any time in my cell phone.

In "materializing," in a digital informational format, the fetus and the pregnancy, these apps configure a "dividual aspect" of their existence

(Deleuze 1992; Rodríguez 2018). And it is in that sense that these images and pieces of information may be put in circulation: as ways of making the fetuses and their pregnant mothers present and shareable. In general, information and images from apps—like estimated fetus size, for instance—were shared by these women with partners and, in a few cases, with friends and other members of the family, extending the existence of the fetus through these technologies of information and communication.

For pregnancy apps, the important and fundamental information is the date of the last menstruation, which allows the app to continuously count the weeks into the pregnancy and to provide general information about what is supposed to happen in each of them. Menstrual cycle apps, on the other hand, demand constant engagement and frequent input of new data. The apps replace previous subjective perceptions and fulfill a few of the many expectations regarding menstrual cycle, pregnancy, and fetal development. They concentrate information about expected bodily events, circumscribing their meanings.

But they are not the only source of information women rely on. Women also looked for information about pregnancy during prenatal care, in support groups for pregnant women, and in books. Unlike apps, though, books are seen as obsolete, since they always bring "the same information." According to some women, the content of books is not updated often enough and so become outdated and repetitive, whereas these apps bring new texts daily, with updated and dynamic information.

Women trusted the information brought by these apps, although they also reported always "checking the sources" through online searches. The information contained in these apps also helped them better "triage" and "decide" what (or not) to ask the obstetricians. Medical professionals were considered the safest and most reliable sources of information and the best experts to talk about pregnancy and labor.

The information brought by the apps is described, on the one hand, as more "meticulous" and hence more reliable. That is why, in cases of controversial recommendations—what kinds of food are harmful during pregnancy, such as some types of teas, for instance—the apps usually have a preventive approach, warning about potential dangers. On the other hand, this same approach could be criticized. According to one of our interviewees, by offering the kind of information that applies to a larger number of people, the app "flattens" the discussions, erasing nuances and controversies:

> PgApp07: This app is too rigid, it presents things only as truths and certainties. It has no subtleties, such as "there are studies affirming that. . . ." Nothing is relativized. It is written in a way to avoid all kinds of ambiguities. I think they try to

do this so that they maintain a minimal common ground. I am a little distrustful. I feel very skeptical and go check [*laughs*]. So, for example, drinking beer during pregnancy, a subject everybody knows there are no sufficient studies about, since no one voluntarily submits to a study that may prove alcohol is bad. Then there is only the observation of a few alcoholic mothers.... There is no safe level for alcohol ingestion because nobody is willing to do this test.

BabyCenter has a forum for debates between pregnant women and recent mothers. Even our interlocutors who only used the app Pregnancy+ were directed to this BabyCenter forum when they searched online for answers to questions regarding their pregnancy. That forum is public and can be accessed through the internet even by people not registered at BabyCenter. In general, most women said they only observe or respond to commentaries, but none reported major interactions in these forums.

Although referred to as useful to answer questions and know of other pregnant women's experiences, the forums were described negatively, as a place that gathered together "clueless people," where there was a lot of "nonsense," "useless information," and questions that should be directed to doctors, not to "untrained people." In that sense, biomedical discourse seems to remain the most legitimate type of knowledge. When these apps do not reaffirm this biomedical discourse and include more personal/individual perspectives and experiences, they are seen as less reliable.

The forums also contain a lot of "horror stories" and "tragedies"—such as cases of complications in pregnancy or in labor—thought to increase the pregnant women's anxieties. Those stories tend to be "avoided," especially in late pregnancy, when labor is approaching. There seemed to be a connection between a major motivation for use (concerns with the normality of pregnancy, healthiness, and development of the fetus) and the constant comparative monitoring of every step of the way, week by week. The fear of miscarriage is always lurking.

Women who experienced miscarriages described the relationship with the apps as "traumatic." The app requires them to delete the "existence" of that pregnancy in its interface, not only to prevent notifications, but also for the database to stop considering the course of that pregnancy. Just deleting the app or canceling the notifications is not enough, since the apps keep a record of all pregnancies and assume they will all follow through the expected course, with the birth of a healthy fetus at approximately forty weeks.

In case of a miscarriage, it is necessary, then, to completely delete the record of that pregnancy in the app—a feature that, apart from being difficult to access, causes great suffering to the women. In those cases, the "cyborg baby," constituted within these technologies, remains "alive" and developing in the app. It is experienced as a second death, happening again in this "dividual" existence through the app. This was reported by three different women, who claimed they were "traumatized" by the app after their miscarriage. Because of this traumatic experience, they preferred to change to a different app when they conceived again.

Remaking the Dilemmas

As Paletta (2019) points out, the rhetoric used to promote these types of apps relies on the higher level of self-acknowledgment women have when they record signs, symptoms, and sensations as "scientific data" (Lupton 2015). Monitoring and measuring the body, which have a quotidian element to them, become relevant practices in a context where people find digital and wearable mobile devices useful, configuring forms of subjectivation that Lupton (2016) calls the "quantified self." In that process, sexual activity is reduced to numbers measuring frequency of occurrence and orgasms reached, a "healthy" menstruation is defined by the (estimated) volume of menstrual blood, and quality of sleep is measured by hours slept. Hence, as Lupton (2016) has pointed out, uncertainties, imprecisions, and unforeseen events of human embodiment are "dominated" through data production.

The side effects of engaging with these techniques may not be so visible, but have to do with feeding huge databases that gather, for the first time in human history, information about menstruation, sexuality, and pregnancy from millions of women around the world. In that sense, we return to the dilemmas pointed out by Sonia Correa when thinking about contraceptive technologies for Brazilian women in the 1990s, which she qualified as a "fetishism of choice" (Correa 1994). It may look like we have more empowering alternatives, since the app seems to be a useful informational tool that helps us remember our periods, check on our baby's development, and improve our body management. But at the same time, we are also testing and proving biomedical models of how cis-female bodily processes are/should be and working "for free" to fill up these systems with our health data. There seems to be a replacement of previous not-so-visible or not-so-sharable perceptions and practices related to the body for new digital, quantified, and self-monitored information, producing highly capitalizable databases that potentialize not-so-new forms of domination and control. Would there be a way out of this dilemma, related to "the will to knowledge" (Foucault [1976] 1988), one that ensures autonomy and safe information?

Daniela Tonelli Manica is a researcher at Labjor, Nudecri, Unicamp. From 2011 to 2018 she was a professor in the Cultural Anthropology Department at the Federal University of Rio de Janeiro (IFCS/UFRJ). She has a master's (2003) and PhD (2009) in social anthropology from Universidade Estadual de Campinas (Unicamp) and held postdoctoral fellowships at the Social Medicine Institute (UERJ, 2010) and the Scientific and Technological Politics Department (Unicamp, 2017). Her research focuses on the anthropology of science and technology, with foci on the following subjects: relationship between nature and culture; gender, technology, and medicine; and hormones, bodily fluids, and techniques.

Marina Fisher Nucci has a master's (2010) and PhD (2015) in collective health from the Social Medicine Institute at the State University of Rio de Janeiro (UERJ). She has experience in gender studies, medicalization, and social studies of science.

Gabriela Cabral Paletta has a master's degree from the Sociology and Anthropology Program at the Federal University of Rio de Janeiro (PPGSA/IFCS/UFRJ). She works with clinical psychology and self-management groups and has been conducting research in the anthropology of science and in technology and feminist studies.

Notes

1. Data collected in May 2018.
2. Data collected in November 2017.
3. None of our interviewees mentioned using these forums.
4. All quotes from interviews were freely translated from Brazilian Portuguese.

References

Cabral, Cristiane, Maria Luiza Heilborn, and Elaine Reis Brandão. 2007. "Teenage Pregnancy and Moral Panic in Brazil." *Culture, Health & Sexuality* 9: 403–14.

Chazan, Lilian. 2007. *"Meio Quilo de Gente": Um Estudo Antropológico Sobre Ultra-Som Obstétrico*. Rio de Janeiro: Editora Fiocruz.

Citeli, Maria Teresa, Cecilia Mello e Souza, and Ana Paula Portela. 1998. "Revezes da Anticoncepção entre Mulheres Pobres." In Luiz Fernando Duarte and Ondina Fachel Leal (eds.), *Doença, Sofrimento, Perturbação: Perspectivas Etnográficas*. Rio de Janeiro: Editora FIOCRUZ, pp. 57–77.

Clarke, Adele, Laura Mamo, Jennifer Fosket, Jennifer Fischman, and Janet Shim, eds. 2010. *Biomedicalization: Technoscience, Health and Illness in the U.S.* Durham, NC: Duke University Press.

Correa, Sonia. 1994. "O Norplant nos Anos 90: Peças que Faltam." *Revista Estudos Feministas* 2: 86–98.
Deleuze, Giles. 1992. "Post-Scriptum Sobre as Sociedades de Controle." In *Conversações: 1972–1990*. Rio de Janeiro: Editora 34, pp. 219–26.
Foucault, Michel. (1976) 1988. *História da Sexualidade I: A Vontade de Saber*. Rio de Janeiro: Edições Graal, 1988.
Haraway, Donna. 1991. "A Cyborg Manifesto: Science, Technology and Socialist-Feminism in the Late Twentieth Century." In *Simians, Cyborgs and Women: The Reinvention of Nature*. New York: Routledge, pp. 149–81.
Lupton, Deborah. 2014. "Beyond Techno-Utopia: Critical Approaches to Digital Health Technologies." *Societies* 4: 706–11.
———. 2015. "Quantified Sex: A Critical Analysis of Sexual and Reproductive Self-Tracking Using Apps." *Culture, Health & Sexuality: An International Journal for Research, Intervention and Care* 17(4): 440–53.
———. 2016. *The Quantified Self*. Malden: Polity.
Manica, Daniela Tonelli. 2012. "Rudimentos da Reconociência Contraceptiva: Experimentações, Biopolítica e a Trajetória de um Cientista." In Claudia Fonseca, Fabíola Rohden, and Paula Sandrine Machado (eds.), *Ciências na Vida: Antropologia da Ciência em Perspectiva*. São Paulo: Terceiro Nome, pp. 185–201.
Mitchell, Lisa, and Eugenia Georges. 1998. "Baby's First Picture: The Cyborg Fetus of Ultrasound Imaging." In Robbie Davis-Floyd and Joseph Dumit (eds.), *Cyborg Babies: From Techno-sex to Techno-tots*. London: Routledge, pp. 105–24.
Oudshoorn, Nelly. 1994. *Beyond the Natural Body: An Archeology of Sex Hormones*. London: Routledge.
Paletta, Gabriela Cabral. 2019. "Menstruapps na Era Farmacopornográfica: Aplicativos de Monitoramento de Ciclo Menstrual e Interseções entre Corpos, Máquinas e Tecnopolíticas de Gênero." Master's thesis, Rio de Janeiro, UFRJ.
Preciado, Paul. 2008. *Testo Yonqui*. Madrid: Editora Espasa Calpe.
Rodríguez, Pablo Esteban. 2018. "Espetáculo do Dividual: Tecnologias do Eu e Vigilância Distribuída nas Redes Sociais." In Fernanda Bruno et al. (eds.), *Tecnopolíticas da Vigilância: Perspectivas da Margem*. São Paulo: Boitempo, pp. 181–98.
Roland, Edna. 1995. "Direitos Reprodutivos e Racismo no Brasil." *Revista Estudos Feministas* 3(2): 506–14.
———. 1998. "Saúde Reprodutiva da População Negra no Brasil: Entre Malthus e Gobineau." In Margareth Arilha and Maria Teresa Citeli (eds.), *Políticas, Mercados, Ética—Demandas e Desafios no Campo da Saúde Reprodutiva*. São Paulo: Editora 34, pp. 97–110.
Sanabria, Emilia. 2016. *Plastic Bodies: Sex Hormones and Menstrual Suppression in Brazil*. Durham, NC: Duke University Press.

CHAPTER 12

Remaking Desires and Femininities
Testosterone "Replacement" for Treating Women's Sexuality in Brazil

FABÍOLA ROHDEN

This chapter investigates the use of the hormone testosterone to improve sexual desire among women.[1] The prescription of testosterone has become common in private clinics in large Brazilian cities. The most common justification for its use has been the supposed need for hormonal "replacement," especially for older women. Doctors, mainly gynecologists, have indicated this treatment based on information presented at congresses and in the medical literature. This study, based on research conducted among male and female doctors and women who use testosterone, discusses the medical indications (or reasons) for issuing this prescription. The analysis considers the contemporary processes of biomedicalization and valorization of self-enhancement, as well as the importance of the dimension of gender relations.

The consumption of hormones by women has a long and polemical history, highlighted by the emergence of the contraceptive pill and hormone replacement therapy (Oudshoorn 1994; Hoberman 2005; Roberts 2007; Rohden 2008; Sanabria 2010, 2016; Faro 2016). Hormones are now indicated for a variety of conditions and are administered and used in a variety of ways, and many of these uses appear to be promising technological innovations that meet the needs of contemporary women. The use of hormone treatments to restore or improve quality of life, especially among older women, can be seen within this context (Manica and Nucci 2017; Sanabria 2016).

Biomedical resources are increasingly common in "enhancing" sexuality. Since the late twentieth century, there has been an increase in the medicalization and pharmaceuticalization of sex and sexuality. Marshall and Katz (2002) have described sexuality and age as fundamental dimensions of the modern individual. These authors highlight the contribution of late twentieth-century lifestyles and cultures, including the emphasis on health, activity and "anti-aging," as part of the process that has given rise to studies and interventions on sexual activity (Marshall and Katz 2002; Marshall 2010).

In the biomedical literature, especially since the 1970s, there was an effort to define female sexual desire as "inhibited" or "hypoactive" and/or to characterize it in terms of passivity, receptivity, responsivity, and complexity (Spurgas 2013; Faro 2016). This contrasts with male desire, which is defined as more spontaneous, focused, initiatory, and constant (Spurgas 2013; Faro 2016). In addition, a growing association between sexuality and organic factors, especially hormonal influences, has also occurred. Efforts to manage "female sexual dysfunction" have ranged from the use of Viagra by women, to the recent US Food and Drug Administration (FDA) approval of Flibanserin, a serotonergic antidepressant, which, if taken regularly, can leave women more relaxed and sexually disposed (Fishman 2004; Tiefer 2006; Moynihan and Minstzes 2010; Fausto-Sterling 2015). More recently, the hormone testosterone has proved to be useful in treating problems related to female sexuality, such as the lack of sexual desire. Thus, we are entering a new chapter in the long and complex history of the so-called "sex" hormones (Oudshoorn 1994).

In Brazil, perspectives on and the treatment of issues related to women's sexuality are largely anchored in biomedicine (Sanabria 2010; Russo et al. 2013). Although testosterone may not legally be prescribed for this purpose, recent medical conferences and articles have promoted testosterone's use for sexual problems, especially among women near menopause (Rohden 2013; Faro 2016; Faro and Russo 2017; Manica and Nucci 2017).

Sanabria's study (2010) on the use of contraceptives and hormones in the city of Salvador in northeastern Brazil is highly relevant. She reports having encountered, especially among middle- and upper-class women, the use of these resources in a context of relatively more autonomous choices and self-improvement. The treatments, including testosterone, were sought for their effects on premenstrual tension, skin, and mood and to improve sexual desire. Although this appears paradoxical to Sanabria's account, women's search for increased desire (which may suggest autonomy) was explained in a context of needing to "keep their husband" and the importance of this for maintaining a certain status for the women.

This helps to illustrate the complex relationship between hormonal "replacement," self-improvement, and gender. Using the material presented here, I will discuss how this logic of testosterone "replacement" can be seen on one hand as an example of the emphasis on enhancement, which characterizes the biomedicalization process, while also corresponding to the reiteration of traditional gender norms. That is, a certain increase of testosterone (a hormone considered the essence of masculinity) is permitted to "recuperate" the capacity to attract or respond to a demand of male sexual desire. Nevertheless, its use is quite restricted, to avoid making the woman "virile."

The data analyzed here come from a study that sought to map the use of biomedical resources and the production of new forms of subjectivity and enhancement. Interviews were conducted with male and female doctors, especially gynecologists, and women who use hormonal treatments to improve their "quality of life" and sexuality, in a large city of southern Brazil.[2] All doctors interviewed were selected because they offer treatments for "sexual problems" and are specialized in and recognized in this field. The women were contacted through a network of interlocutors, mainly healthcare professionals. In addition, the study also included observation at medical congresses, the analysis of scientific articles, and the study of websites of medical associations, pharmaceutical laboratories, social networks, and journalistic materials. This chapter continues with the presentation of the theoretical perspectives used in this analysis, the presentation of statements of a user and of doctors interviewed, and the final discussion of the meanings attributed to the use of testosterone by women.

New Situations of Biomedicalization, Self-Improvement, and Consumption

The use of biomedical resources such as testosterone must be analyzed in the light of discussions around ongoing processes of biomedicalization, consumption, self-improvement, and production of subjectivities, especially in recent decades (Clarke et al. 2010; Rose 2007; Martin 2007; Williams, Martin and Gabe 2011; Dumit 2012). According to Clarke and colleagues (2010), biomedicalization is a complex, multi-situated, and multidirectional process, in which medicalization is redefined as a function of the innovations developed by technoscientific biomedicine. The emphasis given to the prefix "bio" corresponds precisely to the transformations of human and nonhuman elements that are only possible through technoscientific innovations. One consequence of this process is the rise of a new culture or "regime of truth" focused on individual responsibility. A concern for health comes to be a moral attribute of the individual, who should remain informed about new knowledge and practices of caring for oneself, disease prevention, and treatment and be willing to consume the resources now available. In this process, the body is no longer seen as relatively static or immutable and as a focus of control and is converted into something flexible and capable of being transformed and reconfigured. According to the authors, there is a passage from a process of normalization to a process of customization or personalization associated with the institution of technoscientific practices as market niches that sustain a form of "boutique medicine" (Clarke et al. 2010).

Rose (2007) highlighted how contemporary medical technologies are used not only to cure pathologies but to control the vital processes of the body and mind. These technologies for enchancement are associated with the idea of self-improvement as something aimed at the future and with the appearance of individual consumers of these new desires and opportunities to control life. What is new is not the existence of the will for or the practice of enhancement, but the fact of coming to shape the life of subjects. The author also emphasizes a passage from normalization to customization, not only of the body but also of the senses, desires, and emotional and cognitive skills.

In the field of sexuality, Marshall (2009) proposes analyzing the impact of "pharmaceutical imagination." This involves narratives that have in common the supposition of a linear model of scientific progress and the passage from psychological explanations to physiological ones associated with pharmaceutical solutions. These narratives have been quite effective in the promotion of new diagnoses and treatments involving sexuality, because they trigger sensitive values and representations in specific cultural contexts. The pharmaceutical imagination has been quite successful in redefining the paths of sexual life in terms of the effects of the drugs used to treat sexual function.

The (bio)medicalization process has touched women particularly acutely. Due to concern with reproductive and sexual function in specialties such as obstetrics, gynecology, and endocrinology, medicine has focused on the female body as an object of knowledge and intervention. This concern for a supposed specificity of women's bodies gave origin to a unique set of interventions that have been accentuated more recently (Martin 1992; Oudshoorn 1994; Fishman 2004; Roberts 2007; Rohden 2008, 2013).

This finding leads to the need to reflect more critically on the approaches related to biomedicalization and production of the patient-consumer through the dimension of gender. Although Clarke et al. (2010) affirm that biomedicalization tends to accentuate stratifications of gender, race, and social class, other important works have not given deeper attention to this type of analytical mark (Rose 2007; Dumit 2012). It is necessary to incorporate in the analyses how the promotion of the patient-consumer, associated with processes of self-improvement and production of subjectivities, is marked by the contrast of gender, among others. Testosterone "replacement" helps us reflect on the biomedicalization processes underway in Brazilian society through an emphasis on the dimension of gender relations.

"I Went to the Doctor and Asked, 'And Testosterone?'": Patients' Search for Resources

I will now present portions of the statement of a user of testosterone who was interviewed in this study. I consider her experience to be exemplar, in terms of a certain emerging standard of a search for and use of the available pharmaceutical resources in the line that Dumit (2012) expresses in terms of "patient-consumer." I suggest that her case illustrates how the biomedicalization process (Clarke et al. 2010) becomes concrete in individual terms. It also demonstrates in practice a new type of medicalization or pharmaceuticalization of sexuality (Marshall 2009) that is currently developing.

Paula was thirty-six at the time of the interview. She was married, had children, had a degree in administration, and worked in commercial services in the health-care field. When asked about the use of medications and hormones related to sexuality, she said that she had two older family members (one man, one woman) who were using testosterone to decrease fatigue and improve libido. Since she had not been feeling very well after a series of health problems and post-traumatic stress (for which she used antidepressants) after violent episodes at a previous job, she decided to ask her doctor about testosterone. She also took thyroid medication, a formula for losing weight, and oral contraceptives. Her use of and knowledge about various types of medication appears to produce a certain naturalization of the use of one more. She affirmed that she did not "do any research about testosterone" and "simply spoke with her gynecologist," who prescribed a gel form to apply on her skin. In one portion in her interview, she referred to this process in the same tone:

> I was at the doctor and asked, "And testosterone?" And he said, "You can use it; it will help you a lot." And we wound up not speaking about it very much.

The treatment had begun less than a month earlier:

> I'll tell you, in terms of libido and well-being, it's helping a lot. I don't know if it's the action it causes; I don't know anything about testosterone. I know that the

male body produces much more testosterone than the female. They [men] have an easier time losing weight, they feel less irritation, are less sensitive. And from what I have followed, this all has a lot to do with testosterone. It helps, because high levels of testosterone give better equilibrium, I say equilibrium in general. They [men] are less sensitive, have an easier time losing weight. They have a different metabolism than women, and I very much want to lose weight as well.

At another time she also said, "Testosterone may be a bit psychological as well, but it is helping me." Specifically in reference to libido, she added:

I never had a problem, but after I had a son . . . It's not a lack of libido itself, but that thing of having you and your husband at home and at any time it seems the focus is on the child. Today you are tired, another day something else . . . But a man isn't like that! You can talk to ten women and they will all say that for the husbands there is no "I slept badly last night," "I had problems at work." I think that for us women this all interferes with our well-being. I think that as I said, they have high doses of testosterone, they work differently, the body works differently than ours, they have different rhythms, alignments, and completely different conceptions. And it's the same thing: when a man wants to lose weight it's fast; not for us. We have PMS [premenstrual syndrome], I have a headache, in the menstrual cycles. And the doctor thinks that testosterone will help me a lot with this as well.

My husband said to the doctor that he will tell him to prescribe me testosterone forever.

In addition to addressing fatigue and low libido, Paula also expected that testosterone would help her gain "a bit of direction," "clarification of ideas," and "stability":

I get home and have things to do and I don't do them, I don't turn things on. The doctor thinks that testosterone will also help me. He used a specific term . . . that it [the testosterone] will give me a bit of direction, will clarify my ideas, and give me a bit of stability in general.

Paula slips between brief reflection on the possible "psychological effects" of taking a medicine for libido, on the one hand, and an affirmation that men are different because of testosterone, on the other. This difference was always positively qualified by a reference to greater desire and sexual disposition, less sensitivity to "external factors" that interfere with desire, a greater capacity to lose weight (related to a female aesthetic that she desired), and a general state of greater equilibrium and stability. The gap perceived between her sexual disinterest (contextualized with the description of other demands and problems) and her husband's disposition was justified by a supposed hormonal difference and not by means gendered demands, such as caring for children and the home. In addition, she did not report any personal discomfort (or suffering) in perceiving that she had less sexual desire, nor did she refer to the idea that she had any type of hormonal deficit. Although she and the doctor spoke little about this, he immediately prescribed testosterone to "help." The main person to benefit from the treatment appears to be the husband, who was so satisfied that he asked the doctor to prescribe testosterone "forever."

"I Correct the Hormonal Part and the Response Is Fantastic!": Doctors Who Issue the Prescriptions

Statements like that of Paula illustrate the patient-consumer standards that seek and use pharmacological resources in the context of the processes of biomedicalization of society (Dumit 2012; Clarke et al. 2010). However, it is necessary to discuss in greater depth how the use of testosterone is related to the dimension of enchancement and the notion that certain hormones need to be "replaced" or added, seeking better individual performance. It is also necessary to better understand the concepts of gender and sexuality that support this type of "treatment." One way to more deeply examine these issues is to analyze the discourse of the doctors to which she had access. Our interviews with doctors helped to produce some responses (and many questions) that suggest strong harmony between the perspectives of these professionals and the women who use testosterone.

All doctors reported that the main complaint of their patients, in terms of sexuality, was a relative lack of desire or libido. They emphasized that this was usually close to menopause but that this also affect younger women, as experienced by Paula and various others.

Doctors who have been in the field for some time perceived that patient complaints have changed. One doctor, when she began to see patients in the 1990s, noted that "women had other complaints, they said that they did not have orgasms, but over time the population and the profile changed" (Karla, gynecologist). Today "decreased libido" is the main reason why women seek help for sexual problems in Brazil. She also said that when women come to her office, they say that they are "having sex because they are obligated to, that they have not wanted to have sex for more than six months, they can't bear their husbands any more." Lack of desire is seen as a problem due to the demands of the partner, not the woman herself. Male desire—as something to be satisfied and as a reference standard—is constantly present. It is evoked not only as the fundamental parameter of comparison but also as a will or demand to be responded to—a mechanism that reveals the constant re-enacting of traditional gender norms in Brazilian society.

Although there were some differences, nearly all of the doctors interviewed made a direct connection between this complaint of decreased desire and decreased hormones among older women, which is illustrated, for example, by the expression "drop in libido because of hormonal changes" (as Bruna, a gynecologist affirmed). Among the twelve doctors interviewed, ten said that they prescribe testosterone, especially in topical gel form, to increase the desire of their patients. In relation to a legal therapeutic indication for hormonal replacement with testosterone, some doctors interviewed emphasized that this would only be justified when there are proven signs of ovarian insufficiency for production of the hormone. This would only be the case for women in menopause or those who had undergone a total hysterectomy, with the removal of their ovaries as well as their uterus. In this sense, the connection between lack of desire and the possibility of using hormonal treatment, especially with testosterone, is especially associated with women in menopause, although in practice, reference to use by younger women, like Paula, also appears.

Most professionals, when referring to wealthier patients, say that not only is the complaint very common, but that women arrive at the office with a specific demand for a medicine that will solve their problems, as in the case of Paula. A constant reference was also the use of anti-antidepressants by the patients (as Paula reported) and its tendency to decrease sexual desire, which all doctors mentioned as supported by both the scientific literature and clinical practice.

Another common aspect concerns how the doctors conceive the differences between genders and their understanding about what is sexuality or how it can be defined. In general, there is a rhetoric that sexuality would be associated with "multiple factors," a term used to refer to a juxtaposition of organic and cultural aspects. Nevertheless, what prevails is an explanatory logic completely focused on hormones. This would even explain a primordial difference between men and women: while men are governed predominately by the organic, women are much more susceptible to other (social, contextual, and emotional) factors.

The gynecologist Bruna, for example, considers the sexuality of men and women completely different. While a woman must detach from her daily concerns to have desire, "a man is always ready" for biology reasons. The gynecologist Janice agreed:

> Look, it could be because of testosterone itself, that testosterone is the hormone of the libido, and women do have a bit less.... The cycle of a woman's sexual response is much more complex. It depends on if she ate well, if her child is okay, if her partner gave her a proper "good morning," right? A woman's sexual response cycle is not like a man's: he sees a naked woman, gets excited, and ejaculates, right?

Tania, a gynecologist, also affirmed that men deal with sexuality in a "simpler" form. "He is born this way, the path is determined," while women have more difficulties in learning to "permit themselves to have pleasure," requiring "external" stimuli. In organic terms too, female sexuality is more complex than men's:

> Physiologically, female sexuality is more complex. Because we have many more things influencing desire.... A man does not need much stimulus to be excited, to have this erection.... What is studied and perceived is that women need to disconnect their mind a bit from other things to be able to relax and allow themselves to be excited and develop the entire sexual response cycle.

Ivo, an experienced gynecologist who has worked for many decades in this field, expressed an approach that emphasizes the perception of a radical difference between the genders, expressed in terms of a superior, natural, and evolutionary order. He regarded the sexuality of men and women as completely different. He explained the fundamental role of testosterone in terms of the importance of hormones for sexuality:

> Well, testosterone is the sex hormone. And it is the primordial hormone of males. Therefore, males are always ready to have sex as long as they have a testicle. So the daily variability of production of testosterone of males is very little.... Well, females produce testosterone, mammals, whenever they are in heat. This is the period when they are fertile and are ready to reproduce. So they are ready for sex. Then they accept the male. So the level of testosterone is high on those days, they accept the male, the male feels attracted to that female and copulates. A few days after the fertile period, they do not have sex. Everyone knows this: all females accept the male when they are fertile, because sex was made for reproduction, it was not made for something else. So, when women have a high level of testosterone, they have a higher desire to have relations.... What determines this is testosterone.

This doctor made specific reference to the impact of menopause on women's life and sexuality:

> Menopause brings to the female the loss of the elements of femininity, her vagina becomes dryer, it no longer has a scent. Females attract males by the genital scent... and then they go [to seek treatment] with a problem of menopause, because they have difficulty sleeping, hot flashes, emotional instability... and then, they replace the hormone. They replace it for a time, two years, five years, twenty years, depending on what they want. And they live a completely different life.

And, considering the association with sexual desire:

When the capacity to reproduce ceases, sexual desire ceases. Of course, some women persist for years beyond, this is evident, but they are the minority. So, menopause is associated with a series of interferences; they lose the capacity to reproduce and are not interested in sex. So it is up to us to replace these hormones.

Note in these statements not only the firm definition of this period of life of women exclusively in relation to loss, their inexorable dependence on the end of reproductive capacity, but also on the doctor's view to replace lost hormones. Once testosterone is added, the results are guaranteed—that is, sexual desire will increase or return.

However, those interviewed reveal that they do not know precisely if the effect perceived by patients is related to the hormone or to factors such as performance and eagerness about undergoing treatment to improve sexual responsiveness and desire or is the practical result of a recommendation of a topical application of testosterone gel or cream.

Tania, for example, drew attention to the "placebo effect" of using a medication to improve desire:

> You see the placebo effect of the drugs. So you will say [to the patient]: "We will use a drug to get better," to stir things up. So at times this alone unblocks some things and increases desire.

For Janice, testosterone, "the male hormone," clearly increases sexual desire. But she was ambivalent about the specific role of the hormone and the more general effects of treatment to improve sexuality:

> It increases the libido. They are more interested. Just coming to the clinic, a sexology clinic, they think of sex.... But just coming to the clinic, speaking of sex, thinking of sex, helps.

There is also a practical effect involved in the prescription of testosterone, according to the gynecologist Kátia. She reported that at times, she prescribes formulations in cream and gel for topical application to the genitals so that women have to "touch themselves" and "know themselves better"; she says that "masturbation and self-eroticism" are rare among women in their forties and fifties.

These last examples provide an important contrast. On one hand, doctors perceive that "treatments" to "improve" (sexuality) are complex and involve multiple factors. While they reinforce the perception of sexual desire as dependent on levels of testosterone, this is always associated with the male body. A norm that associates desire, testosterone, and masculinity is reinforced and reproduced in the discourses and practices of these professionals.

"Replacing" Testosterone, Why and for Whom?

Both Paula's statements and interviews with doctors raise important points about female sexuality and the possible "treatments" or resources for its enhancement. The first concerns the fact that references are regularly made to other factors that attest to the "complexity" or "multifactoriality" of female sexuality, in contrast to male sexuality, which is presented as more focused, direct, and eminently organic. Paula, like the doctors, reproduces arguments that women are more susceptible to demands, pressure, and constraints related to the life of the couple or the family or even inscribed in a more general plane of "culture." These perceptions are accompanied by comments about the need for women to "disconnect" from these demands and pressures to enjoy a more satisfactory sexual life. In contrast, men are described as more disconnected, which corresponds to the benefit of being "always ready" or available for sex. Nevertheless, this is not accompanied in most statements by the need for more effective guidelines, with the exception of two professionals who revealed that they were opposed to the use of testosterone. For example, they make no comment about the situation of individual patients and do not consider the inequalities of gender in Brazilian society. To the contrary, the prescriptions focus on the indication of the need for hormonal replacement.

Most professionals do not question the meaning of the "complaint" related to the lack of sexual desire presented in their clinics. Many women affirm that they are seeking treatment to improve sexual desire because the demands of their partners are not problematized. Only two professionals thought that testosterone "replacement" was inappropriate, and they argued that sexual dysfunction might reflect suffering by the patient herself. As the gynecologist Karla said, "For hypoactive desire to be a problem, there must be suffering on the part of the woman; it cannot only be a complaint of the husband." This suggests that the characterization of a "problem" (the existence of a woman's suffering) or of something "lacking" would not necessarily be observed in all the cases of treatment to "improve" female sexual desire through testosterone "replacement."

If the search for resources for improving sexual life can be characterized as a phenomenon that indicates freedom and independence, a more traditional framing in terms of gender relations remains quite strong. The search to increase desire appears, in various cases, to respond to demands from partners more than from the women themselves.

The positive effects of the treatment cannot be exclusively attributed to testosterone. Like Paula, who suspected the effects of hormonal treatments were "psychological," the doctors interviewed also referred to the "placebo effect" of the drugs, the direct result of local stimulation with the testosterone gel, or even the effect caused by being engaged in treatment designed to improve sexual life. Little importance is given to these perceptions when compared with the idea that desire depends on the presence or absence of testosterone.

In general terms, what is emphasized is the logic of diagnosis, through the supposition of a lack of a substance, and treatment, by means of its replacement. As doctors indicated (see also Faro 2016; Faro and Russo 2017), testosterone is the treatment most often presented and discussed in the current medical publications and congresses, and consequently it has an important role in doctors' opinions. The presumption of association between testosterone and desire allows that, in practice, it is common for doctors to find that women who have used this hormone have had increased desire and an improved sex life. Although those who mention other effects related to its use do not present this to their patients, because to do so might be counterproductive to the treatment results, the positive results are nearly always attributed to testosterone. The biomedical logic shared by professionals and patients supports their idea that the substance acts with precision and effectiveness. What stands out is that women who use testosterone have more desire. This finding, in turn, reinforces the association between testosterone and sexual desire, characterizing a circular logic.[3]

Both Paula and the professionals presume that there is a deficit in the production of testosterone or, at least, the need for an increase. The term "hormonal replacement" is not always justified, given often no proof of a decrease or lack of testosterone production or no significant mention of a "prior" standard of greater sexual desire, which would thus indicate the need for "recuperation." Therefore, some questions remain: Why and for whom is testosterone "replacement" being promoted? What are the effects of this discourse that reduces female desire to the presence or absence of the hormone, conceived as male?

If we agree with Butler's (1993) affirmation that performativity of gender is defined by the citational and reiterative practice by which discourse produces the effects that it names, we can suppose that also through the recent uses of testosterone in the context of biomedicalization and enhancement of sexuality, the frontiers of gender are being reaffirmed. These uses imply "replacing" or even (re)producing a female desire that responds to the impositions of the traditional norms of gender and sexuality in certain heteronormative and monogamic contexts. However, this treatment with a "male hormone" should respect the binary gender norms, allowing only improved feminity.

All doctors interviewed, when asked about risks in the use of testosterone, referred to the the possible "virilization" of women in association with hormone use: increased body hair, deepening of the voice, and growth of the clitoris. For this reason, great care would be needed with the quantities of testosterone used in the treatment and its duration. The risk of cancer, which appears in the biomedical literature, was rarely cited and always associated with "very high doses," which these professionals would not use. Health risks were given less attention than the risks of masculinization of women who use testosterone. Doctors emphasized that intense control was needed so that any corporal transformations do not extend beyond the frontiers of (conventional) gender.

The two professionals who had transgender patients treated cisgender women very differently. They recognized that the transgender men who sought hormonal treatment are seeking the production of male traits in their bodies, and so testosterone would be legitimate. However, for cisgender women, it is necessary to take maximum care to avoid this. Testosterone should promote the "recovery" of some sexual desire (not excessively) and sustain a marriage, but without any masculinization. While in the era of biomedicalization, the body can be plastic or flexible (Clarke et al. 2010), this is only possible within certain very precise gender limits.[4]

Biomedical resources can be used in innovative contexts and even to the promotion of sexual diversity, as for transgender people. However, in the situation described here, the use of treatments with testosterone helps much more to reproduce traditional binary gender norms. Great care is taken so that the corporal boundaries are not blurred, threatening the characterization considered suitable for female bodies. At the same time, in terms of the "maintenance" or "replacement" of sexual desire, which would keep couples together, an adaptation of female desire is allowed that, as is seen, appears to serve much more the male partners than the women themselves.

Acknowledgments

This chapter presents partial results of the project "Processes of Subjectivation, Corporal Transformations and Productions of Gender via the Promotion and Consumption of Biomedical Resources" supported by the National Council for Scientific and Technological Development–Brazil (CNPq). I would like to thank Chiara Pussetti, Alvaro Jarrin, and Lenore Manderson for their comments on the text. I am also grateful to Glaucia

Maricato, Juliana Loureiro, Eleonora Coelho, and Karine Rodrigues for their collaboration with the fieldwork and to the people who agreed to participate in this study. This chapter was translated by Chris Tunwell.

Fabíola Rohden has a PhD in social anthropology from the Federal University at Rio de Janeiro (2000). She is associate professor and coordinator of the research group Living Sciences: Knowledge Production and Heterogeneous Articulations in the Department of Anthropology at the Federal University at Rio Grande do Sul. She is a researcher at the National Council of Scientific and Technological Development (CNPq).

Notes

1. This chapter focuses exclusively on cisgender women and does not address the use of hormones by transgender women. The term "trans/transgender" refers to people who do not recognize themselves in the sex to which they were assigned at birth. The term "cis/cisgender" refers to people who identify with the sex they were assigned at birth. The discussion around these terms is relevant here particularly because it calls attention to how all the different forms of expression and materialization of bodies, behaviors, and identities are arduously elaborated.
2. In respect for ethical determinations, the name of the city as well as the real names of the people interviewed remain classified.
3. This argument is developed in greater depth in Rohden (2019), based on the concept of ontonorms proposed by Mol (2012).
4. These cases of some doctors who disagree with prescribing testosterone to cisgender women, as well as the contrast with doctors who treat transgender people, were analyzed in another article in which I discuss particularly the controversies around the effects, or "risks," of "virilization" due to the use of this hormone (Rohden 2018).

References

Butler, Judith. 1993. *Bodies That Matter*. New York: Routledge.
Clarke, Adele E., Janet Shim, Laura Mamo, Jennifer Fosket, and Jennifer Fishman. 2010. *Biomedicalization: Technoscience and Transformations of Health and Illness in the U.S.* Durham, NC: Duke University Press.
Dumit, Joseph. 2012. *Drugs for Life: How Pharmaceutical Companies Define Our Health*. Durham, NC: Duke University Press.
Faro, Livi. 2016. "Mulher com Bigode nem o Diabo Pode: um Estudo sobre Testosterona, Sexualidade Feminina e Biomedicalização." PhD dissertation. Rio de Janeiro: Federal University of Rio de Janeiro.
Faro, Livi, and Jane Russo. 2017. "Testosterona, desejo sexual e conflito de interesse: periódicos biomédicos como espaços privilegiados de expansão do mercado de medicamentos." *Horizontes Antropológicos* 23(47): 61–92.

Fausto-Sterling, Anne. 2015. "'Female Viagra' Is No Feminist Triumph." *Boston Review*, 23 November.
Fishman, Jennifer. 2004. "Manufacturing Desire: The Commodification of Female Sexual Dysfunction." *Social Studies of Science* 34(2): 187–218.
Hoberman, John. 2005. *Testosterone Dreams. Rejuvenation, Aphrodisia, Doping*. Berkeley: University of California Press.
Manica, Daniela, and Marina Nucci. 2017. "Sob a pele: implantes subcutâneos, hormônios e gênero." *Horizontes Antropológicos* 23(47): 93–129.
Marshall, Barbara. 2009. "Sexual Medicine, Sexual Bodies and the 'Pharmaceutical Imagination.'" *Science as Culture* 18(2): 133–49.
———. 2010. "Science, Medicine and Virility Surveillance: 'Sexy Senior' in the Pharmaceutical Imagination." *Sociology of Health & Illness* 32(2): 211–24.
Marshall, Barbara, and Stephen Katz. 2002. "Forever Functional: Sexual Fitness and the Ageing Male Body." *Body & Society* 8(4): 43–70.
Martin, Emily. 2007. *Bipolar Expeditions: Mania and Depression in American Culture*. Princeton, NJ: Princeton University Press.
———. 1992. *The Woman in the Body: A Cultural Analysis on Reproduction*. Boston: Beacon Press.
Mol, Annemarie. 2012. "Mind Your Plate! The Ontonorms of Dutch Dieting." *Social Studies of Science* 43(3): 379–96.
Moynihan, Roy, and Barbara Minstzes. 2010. *Sex, Lies + Pharmaceuticals: How Drug Companies Plan to Profit from Female Sexual Dysfunction*. Vancouver: Reystone.
Oudshoorn, Nelly. 1994. *Beyond the Natural Body: An Archeology of Sex Hormones*. London: Routledge.
Roberts, Celia. 2007. *Messengers of Sex: Hormones, Biomedicine and Feminism*. New York: Cambridge University Press.
Rohden, Fabíola. 2008. "The Reign of Hormones and the Construction of Gender Differences." *História, Ciências, Saúde—Manguinhos* 15: 133–52.
———. 2013. "Gender Differences and the Medicalization of Sexuality in the Diagnosis of Sexual Dysfunctions." In Horacio Sivori, Sergio Carrara, Jane Russo, Maria Luiza Heilborn, Ana Paula Uziel, and Bruno Zilli (eds.), *Sexuality, Culture and Politics: A South American Reader*. Rio de Janeiro: CEPESC/CLAM, pp. 620–38.
———. 2018. "Sexual Desire, Testosterone and Biomedical Interventions: Managing Female Sexuality in 'Ethical Doses.'" *Vibrant* 4(3): 1–12.
———. 2019. "Adjusting Hormones and Constructing Desires: New Materialisations of Female Sexuality in Brazil." *Culture, Health & Sexuality* 21(9): 1045–58.
Rose, Nikolas. 2007. *The Politics of Life Itself: Biomedicine, Power, Subjectivity in the Twenty-First Century*. Princeton, NJ: Princeton University Press.
Russo, Jane, Fabíola Rohden, Livi Faro, Marina Nucci, and Alaim Giami. 2013. "Clinical Sexology in Contemporary Brazil: The Professional Dispute among Divergent Medical Views on Gender and Sexuality." *International Journal of Sexual Health* 25: 59–74.
Sanabria, Emilia. 2010. "From Sub—to Super—Citizenship: Sex Hormones and the Body Politic in Brazil." *Ethnos Journal of Anthropology* 75(4): 377–401.
———. 2016. *Plastic Bodies: Sex Hormones and Menstrual Suppression in Brazil*. Durham, NC: Duke University Press.

Spurgas, Alyson. 2013. "Interest, Arousal, and Shifting Diagnoses of Female Sexual Dysfunction, or: How Women Learn about Desire." *Studies in Gender and Sexuality* 14(13): 187–205.

Tiefer, Leonor. 2006. "Female Sexual Dysfunction: A Case Study of Disease Mongering and Activist Resistance." *Public Library of Science Medicine* 3(4): 1–5.

Williams, Simon J., Paul Martin, and Jonathan Gabe. 2011. "The Pharmaceuticalisation of Society? A Framework for Analysis." *Sociology of Health & Illness* 33(5): 710–25.

AFTERWORD

Beyond the Flesh

LENORE MANDERSON

The concrete poles of street lamps and traffic lights are the perfect places to post advertisements and capture the attention of pedestrians. In Johannesburg, from where I write, one kind of advertisement is predictably present, even when communication content and other details change. These are advertisements for body enhancements—for larger buttocks, breasts, thighs, and penises—with the first point of contact via SMS or WhatsApp. Sometimes other bodily and other services are offered—the recovery of lost keys and lost lovers, the availability of abortions, successes in exams and fertility journeys. But services to change the contours of the body are most frequently promoted; those who offer such services do so at the low cost of printing and pasting the posters, with little risk of state surveillance and apprehension. Together with tattoo parlors, hair salons, body piercing studios, and nail salons, body modification is big business, and how bodies are modified moves within and outside of the boundaries of the law.

Meanwhile, globally, each week changes in biomedical technology, medicine, and surgery offer alternatives to people living with chronic health problems, the long-term effects of infection and injury, physical differences, and functional difficulties. These same technologies, and the foundational research that have made them possible, can—for some people—make independent living possible or make life simpler, less confronting, and less tiring. Those at the forefront of medical technology offer to restore that which is lost—sight and hearing, for example—notwithstanding the contradictions of such promises with a growing awareness of the limits of these technologies and those whom they might help and the social imperative to break down attitudes and practices that discriminate on the basis of difference. South Africa's largest cities—Cape Town and Johannesburg—compete with other major cities worldwide in pursuit of research and its translation; the country continues to build on the legacy of Christiaan Barnard's pioneer heart transplant surgeries over fifty years ago (McKellar 2017).

Globally, these technologies of treatment, repair, and restoration find their way, too, into experimental and commercial, nontherapeutic domains. The menu of common cosmetic techniques derives from the methods, procedures, and materials of highly skilled plastic surgery. The skills of cranio-maxillofacial surgery for clefts, head and neck cancers, and facial injuries translate into cosmetic dentistry and various reshaping surgeries of the jaw and nose; dermatological lasers remove age spots and unwanted hair. Rods implanted to stabilize fractures in long bones, and so assist in healing, and to limit fractures and allow mobility in people with conditions such as osteogenesis imperfecta (brittle bones) are inserted in limb-lengthening surgery. Liposuction and augmentation surgery with fat from other parts of the body and injections of silicon and hydrogel are part of the stock in trade of cosmetic surgeons, as much as techniques for repair after serious injuries and following cancer surgery.

The profits of cosmetic surgery sustain the practices of many surgeons, and the vanities and anxieties that create a market for aesthetic practices become part of a virtuous cycle as surgeons give time to perform corrective surgeries in resource-poor settings. The Mercy Ship and other surgical missions, with global north surgeons and nurses volunteering their time to undertake cleft lip and palate repair and benign tumor interventions, are almost always presented as benevolent correctives given the lack of services in low-income countries (Campbell, Sherman, and Magee 2010; Laub 2015). At the same time, people from high-income settings seek affordable care and cheaper cosmetic procedures in hospitals and clinics in middle-income countries (Ackerman 2010; Whittaker, Manderson, and Cartwright 2010). The infrastructure of tourism facilitates such medical and health travel, and local tourism economies share the benefits.

Medical Remaking

In this section, I expand on the ways in which biotechnology, pharmaceuticals, and medical and surgical practices have taken the lead beyond the body and pushed the boundaries of what a body is and what it might do. I then return to the specific examples of body remaking, reshaping, reclaiming, and expanding, as the authors explore in this volume.

When life is a market matter and aging is apparently obsolete, what of its beginnings and its middles? In understanding how governments, established medical technological and pharmaceutical companies, start-ups, physicians, and surgeons are approaching health, disease, and dysfunction, I turn first to medical interventions and, in doing so, raise questions about access and equity. I work here with an extended understanding of technology, its employment in preventing and managing disease, and its various impacts on well-being, social identity, and everyday life. Technologies are not limited to material artifacts, but include all kinds of objects, products, and systems. Although the availability of such body technologies presumes specific skills, resources, services, and affordances, I take for granted here that these are in place in cosmopolitan (biomedical) settings. Such technologies include, diversely, contraceptive devices, rapid test kits for pregnancy and HIV, pharmaceuticals, ultrasound and MRI, pacemakers and prostheses, and emerging technologies such as the menstruation app that Daniela Tonelli Manica, Marina Fisher Nucci, and Gabriela Cabral Paletta discussed in their contribution to this volume. I include, too, items like medical diagnostics and monitors that extend into increasingly globalized clinical environments and beyond—basic primary health-care clinics in rural areas, primary school classrooms, and the private homes of those who can afford them.

While I use the term "technology" to refer to hardware—physical items linked to the clinical tasks of preventive health actions, diagnosis, surveillance, and treatment—I also include procedures and processes in which such products might feature. Institutions and regulations, protocol and cognitive instrumentation, are all technologies. These are also globally available and used, as reflected in the processes of validating protocols and screening tools. So too are classification systems, including various definitions of disability, globalized (Schneider 2016; 2009; Warren and Manderson 2013), with contexts and local biologies subsumed by the universal. The encodings of such systems reflect norms and shape and sanction social actions, relationships, and procedures of care.

These diverse technologies are promoted worldwide to meet the needs of people in particular local settings and in exploring this relationship, technologies exercise, produce, control, and reflect flows of power. Understanding technologies' uses requires that we attend to the ideological and ideational structures that give value to specific objects or forms and shape how these are used in different cultural, institutional, and personal environments. This is particularly significant when we examine how technologies travel, as the authors of this volume explore. Low libido and erectile dysfunction, for example, are not absolute states; these are not necessarily recognized as medical conditions warranting treatment even by those who seek medical advice, as Emily Wentzell, Raffaella Ferrero Camoletto, and Fabíola Rohden have illustrated in this volume.

Techno-repair

Depending on diagnosis, prognosis, and technical availability, a range of extra- and intracorporeal technologies are used to redress, mitigate, and manage different conditions. Most extracorporeal technologies—even mundane items like false teeth, hearing aids, and glasses—are increasingly treated as temporary. Internally sited technologies and procedures obviate them, rendering the use of technology invisible in the present or as anticipated to be available in an imagined yet feasible, even probable, future (Adams, Murphy, and Clarke 2009). False teeth are displaced by implants, and through the processes of osseointegration, the metal implant and bone merge. Glasses and contact lenses are replaced by intraocular lenses, corneal grafts, whole eye transplants, electronic vision enhancement systems of increasing sophistication, and at an accelerating pace, high-performing bionic eyes that can "see" with increasing acuity. Svetlana Borodina's account of retinal implants in Russia, in this volume, again draws attention to the ambivalence with which such technology is received.

Body system functions have long been replaceable. The use of a cardiac pacemaker or an implantable cardioverter defibrillator to regulate heartbeat and dialysis to take over from nonfunctioning kidneys are commonplace instances of intracorporeal and extracorporeal technologies, respectively. These technologies have long been used. A pacemaker, for instance, is a device (a generator) with wires (or leads) leading into the heart, through which electrical pulses are delivered to prompt the heart to beat at a normal rate and so control abnormal health-threatening rhythms. Pacemakers were developed as external devices in the 1920s (Bains et al. 2017; Ward, Henderson, and Metcalfe 2013); over one hundred years they have become increasingly small and light, operating with a lithium battery and now implanted, usually with a local anaesthetic. The electrodes in the leads are both conductors and sensors, which identify changes in the electrical activity from the heart, send this information to the microprocessor in the generator, record the heart's electric activity and rhythm, and if needed, create a small current that travels through the leads into the heart to slow or regulate beat. Contemporary pacemakers can adjust heart rate and timing in response to changes in activity, monitor blood temperature and respiratory rate, and can be adjusted using wireless technology via a cell phone or radiofrequency signals. The heart's activity can be recorded, pacemaker functions and battery status checked, and the signaling rate reprogrammed if need be. This sounds like simple magic.

Although infection from the leads is far less common because the node (device, pacemaker) is internal, there is a high risk of infection when placing (or resiting) the leads of the node or when replacing the battery (after five to seven years). The possibility to replace lithium-battery-powered devices with new infinite-duration cardio-powered pacemakers, around 2012, has not eventuated. Current research includes work on micro-implants, wireless power, advanced microsurgery (on "sutureless bioprostheses" for instance), and the use of "biologicals" (genes and cells) (Albertini et al. 2015; Boink et al. 2015; Ho et al. 2014). For many people, continuing life rests on the fact that the heart is a beyond-human organ.

My second example is of dialysis, developed as an extracorporeal technology in the 1920s in response to kidney failure (Benedum 2003; McAlister 2005; Peitzman 1997). As I have described elsewhere (see chapter 6 in Manderson 2011), dialysis takes place around three times a week if hemodialysis is used. With hemodialysis, blood is transported from the large artery, usually at the person's wrist, via a cannula through a disposable tube to the dialysis machine. Waste products and excess water diffuse across the membrane; clean blood is returned to the body through the vein. Alternatively, patients can opt for daily peritoneal dialysis. In this case a permanent catheter is inserted into the abdomen to allow fluid to flow into and from the peritoneal cavity to filter out waste products and to drain used fluid into a waste bag, via a catheter. This may occur overnight or intermittently through the day. Again, we rely on the beyond-human for life support.

In summary: A pacemaker keeps the heart working. It is not a "mechanical heart," but part of a heart, although mechanical hearts were developed as research progressed toward heart transplants. Dialysis does the work of kidneys, preventing salt and other waste products accumulating to toxic levels. While dialysis is seen as a temporary intervention and a kidney transplant the ultimate solution, the lack of available body organs makes this next step speculative but uncertain. Even with a transplant, medical surveillance and expensive medication must continue (Manderson 2011); organs may be rejected and may need to be replaced. Hence the ongoing costs of managing kidney disease are inevitably accessible primarily to people with sizable realizable wealth.

So, mechanics can do the work of hearts and kidneys. Lungs too—again, extracorporeal artificial "lungs" is an old technology used to manage polio (Emerson 1985; Ott 2016), as illustrated in their peculiarity in the film *Breathe* (2017). In these machines, negative pressure ventilation continually displaces and replaces the air inside of the machine and compresses and depresses the chest to simulate respiration for the duration of paralysis. The iron lung is no longer used, not because polio has been nearly eliminated, but because—as we might expect—other technologies have replaced it. ECMO—extracorporeal membrane oxygenation—functions as an external lung, either for a temporary condition or as a temporary intensive-care measure prior to finding a donor for a lung transplant.

Contemporary medicine is characterized by pre-emptive practice, the present shaped by prescience via our emerging knowledge and imagination of the possibilities of molecular, nanoparticulate, and genetic structures, as well as by various already available mechanical, pharmaceutical, surgical, and other technologies. The growing capacity through blood tests, genetic testing, and molecular profiling to diagnose, differentiate, and so transpose people—from a state of wellness, to being "at risk," to being pre-diseased—has influenced how we plan our own health and that of future generations. It has reshaped imagined health systems and financing, provided the scripts for investment in medical technology (on banking and investment in global public health [Erikson 2015]), and tempered anxieties about the limits to medicine.

In this context, medical technological interventions, presented as preventive medical strategies with the potential to benefit populations at large, provide a way forward. But this approach does other things too: it marginalizes people with particular bodies, health status, class, and gender; diverts scarce resources from other grossly underfunded parts of the health system; ignores the structural factors that influence health status; and creates new risks of drug-resistant infection that threaten to undermine medicine's great wins of the past century.

Techno-appropriation

Understanding and thinking about what might unfold, over decades and across generations, opens up questions of an ethics of practice: for pre-emptive or anticipatory medicine, personalized medicine, personal investment in uncertain experiments, and stalling or heading off what might once have been seen as the inevitability of death. Developments in medical science are (always) unevenly distributed; so too are the losses and gains in health within and between nation-states. I have suggested that technologies frame life's beginnings and ends, and I have noted that access to these and the implications of their use are quite different in different health and economic systems. But the uneven application and uncertain outcomes of technologies also draw attention to the friability of a universal ethics. These practices of optimism build on a twentieth and twenty-first century distribution of resources that dismisses as irrelevant a public health, one that has already been eroded, globally and locally, through poverty and inequality.

Many of the developments and technologies that I have discussed above are used for people whose life depends on them, but this is not always so.

In this volume, the focus is on how technology comes to be appropriated and democratized, both through the mediating role of doctors and surgeons and through their travel into less regulated settings. Technology is extended, simplified, devolved, and repurposed to reach multiple markets, and its uptake, in such contexts, highlights further inequalities, vulnerabilities, and values.

I start here not by tracking the order of the chapters, but by moving from surgery to medication to resistance, in ways that illustrate the power of what is seen as normative or, conversely, discrepant, at the implicit promises of engaging with modifying technologies, processes, and procedures, at acts of care in both compliance with and resistance to body practices characteristic of normative behavior, and at pushback, interrogation, and experimentation. In the chapters in this volume, as I reflect below, ethnography has the power to highlight the complex ways by which human bodies are stretched in meaning and material practice.

I turn first to surgical interventions to people's ears and faces. Marcelle Schimitt describes the role of surgeons in correcting protruding ears in Brazilian children. Her ethnography begins with a program, announced by the mayor of Rio de Janiero, for otoplasties for children "as an essential ally in the fight against bullying"; this was not the first time that outer ears were targeted for nonconformity (Jarrín 2015). Schimitt sets this program against the eugenic concerns of plastic surgeons and others for over a century and notions of nation that have long been aligned with ideal body types. While elsewhere eugenic sentiment has been tethered to race, not aberrant or unruly body parts, race and the body are imbricated, and while nonconforming outer ears might seem an extraordinary reason for state-sanctioned surgery, social uneasiness and embarrassment cohere with ideas of national improvement.

Alejandro Arango-Londoño turns to plastic surgery provided for men in Colombia. Arango-Londoño illustrates the economic role of biomedicine and heath and beauty industries in building an economy apart from drug trafficking—cosmetic clinics, gyms, spas, public parks, medical clinics, medical schools, wellness services, and supplement shops all operate to enhance women's and men's social value and biocapital. In this social and political context, men invest in their bodies as a way of investing in well-being and a future, tying self-esteem, self-confidence, and self-trust, and ultimately social success, to appearance. The men who Arango-Londoño worked with aspired to muscular athleticism, leanness, healthy (and preferably lighter) skin, good teeth and hair. Height was least mutable, but men worked to increase core strength and supplemented gym workouts with liposuctions, nose jobs, chest fat reductions, chest implants, and fat removal from their cheeks. Perhaps not ironically, one reason that men gave for turning to cosmetic surgery was "pressure" from their partners. I return to this below, in reference to women seeking testosterone to reverse loss of libido.

Eva Carpigo, in discussing hair salons in Mexico City, and Chiara Pussetti, on the use of skin-lightening products in Portugal, highlight how the body is read in social space and how body modification can reassure individuals, allow expressions of care, and promise social inclusion. The Beauty Brigade in Mexico City, as Carpigo describes it, offers those who are in need haircuts free of charge, and the acts of care and intimacy during this grooming nurture individuals while providing them with their bodies remade, as capital in everyday social interactions of appearance. Pussetti presents the obverse; the use of skin-lightening products by Afro-Portuguese women highlights their own understandings and experiences of a persistent racial hierarchy. Beauty, as defined in Portugal (as elsewhere) is defined by class, age, sexuality, gender, race, and not least, skin color, even when this is overtly rejected for social and political reasons.

Body appearance matters. Begonya Enguix Grau illustrates how communities of men and women resist dominant norms. She describes the "bear" subculture of gay men and how a globalized aesthetic that values fat and hairy bodies is realized in Catalunya. Her second example is of feminist activists working for Catalan independence, who counter gender norms by dressing and acting in ways that confront local conventions of the feminine. These are bodies, Enguix Grau argues, that go beyond the skin: in her words, they are "embedded and entangled in complex assemblages of emotions, affects, ideologies, mobilizations, corporations, activisms, and other expressions of (for) social and political action." Through their presentation against local stereotypes, these men and women resist the social and political constraints placed on normative bodies.

Enguix Grau's bodies are sexual and gendered, and here I return to questions of sex, gender, and sexual function. As noted earlier, Wentzell and Camoletto are concerned with erectile dysfunction and the drive to "repair" masculinity in Mexico, the United States, and Italy. Rohden attends to Brazilian women's sexual function and the prescription of testosterone to redress loss of libido, a need, as foreshadowed above, that derives from complaints from partners rather than their own concerns about appropriate levels of desire. In these three cases, men and women are ambivalent and often reject medical discourses that medicalize changes to body function; they do not universally embrace the idea of a timeless youthful sexual body and ageless active sexuality.

Daniela Tonelli Manica, Marina Fisher Nucci, and Gabriela Cabral Paletta provide the one example of how fertility and reproduction have been subject to technology, although this is a domain where investment in technology has been heavy and beyond-human reproduction has been normalized (Inhorn and Patrizio 2015) and further imagined (Lewis 2018). Manica, Nucci, and Paletta describe the use of apps to monitor pregnancies and the menstrual cycle in Brazil, in ways that medicalize and monitor women's bodies, generating data external to their bodies and, one might argue, alienating them from quotidian body functions. David Howe and Carla Filomena Silva likewise explore how technologies add to the body, in this case by examining the use of prosthetic technologies in the Paralympics. They draw attention to the status that accrues with the use of such technologies and, correlating with this, the marginalization of people who cannot afford high-level prosthetic technology or do not require their use. While some of the instances above illustrate how technology, including cosmetic surgery, is oriented to disguise or absorb difference, such that normalization is a means of "passing," in this example the more sophisticated the technology, the higher the status.

How Bodies Bite Back

Art has long provided a vehicle for resistance to the stereotypes of gendered bodies and beauty that feed bodily insecurities and a demand for various body-altering practices. Performance art in particular has provided a means by which artists have confronted audiences with bodies that divert from expectations by gender, race, size, shape, and ability. Consider the work of artist-activist Ju Gosling (2020), working from the United Kingdom, and her use of an external corset-brace to support her torso and insert her disability into social interactions; or German choreographer and dancer Raimund Hoghe (2020), arguing the importance of nonconforming bodies on stage to resist what he sees as the shift from bodies in action to bodies with the "status of design objects."

I began with Johannesburg and the informal market in body modification, and I return here now. South Africa provides a very particular space in which bodies are always on show, precisely because under apartheid most bodies were out of place by law; apartheid's aftermath means that bodies in any place are always remarkable. But at the same time, race, shape, sexuality, and gender offer multiple opportunities of transgressive performance art, experiment, and resistance, including by artists working with their own bodies (Pather and Boulle 2019; Shefer 2019). Dean Hatton's genderqueer performances, including in street settings and shopfronts, are perhaps best known: viewers are confronted by the ampleness and full-breasted masculinity of Hatton's near-naked body (Hatton 2020).

Beaudoin's chapter on bioart in Australia and Canada tacks from an artist's use of their body as a whole to artists' use of body components (tissue, fat, bodily exudence, for instance) (Bagnolini and Stellino 2019). In laboratories at the University of Western Australia, artists like Stelarc create tissue cultures and other artworks from mammals or from their own bodies. Stelarc has used both the interior and exterior of his body as matters of art since the 1970s, pushing the limits of being human and pursuing the constaints and liberation of working beyond-human (Dixon 2019; Elsenaar and Scha 2002). In the laboratory, Beaudoin describes how Stelarc and collaborator Nina Sellars extract and blend together their own fat and biomaterials. Stelarc, Sellars, and other bioartists in Australia, Canada, and beyond challenge the practices and norms associated with biological systems and biotechnology and play with conventional notions of bodies, body materials, and biology to rethink what is and is not human.

As Jarrín and Pussetti suggest in their introduction to this volume, "hacking" the human—as reflected in bioart practice and in the resistant noncomformity of the bears and feminist activists—transforms our understandings of bodies and human potentiality. In these chapters, and all contributions to this volume, we are confronted with ways in which people both embrace and conform, and challenge and resist, dominant norms of what it means to be human and in what ways being human is prescribed and constrained. As the authors illustrate, being human means that we can step beyond the constraints of our physical bodies and the normative roles that often contain them. The materiality of being human becomes the material of moving beyond the human body, to embrace the opportunities of being fully human.

Lenore Manderson is distinguished professor of public health and medical anthropology in the School of Public Health, University of the Witwatersrand, South Africa, and holds appointments also with Brown University, United States, and Monash University, Australia. She is known internationally for her work on inequality and the social context of infectious and chronic diseases and disability in Australia, Southeast and East Asia, and Africa. Her publications include *Surface Tensions: Surgery, Bodily Boundaries and the Social Self* (2011); most recently she coauthored and edited *Connected Lives: Households, Families, Health and Care in Contemporary South Africa* (2020).

References

Ackerman, Sara L. 2010. "Plastic Paradise: Transforming Bodies and Selves in Costa Rica's Cosmetic Surgery Tourism Industry." *Medical Anthropology* 29(4): 403–23.

Adams, Vincanne, Michelle Murphy, and Adele E. Clarke. 2009. "Anticipation: Technoscience, Life, Affect, Temporality." *Subjectivity* 28: 246–65.

Albertini, Alberto, Elisa Mikus, Marica Sabarese, Luca Caprili, Mauro Del Giglio, and Mauro Lamarra. 2015. "New Cardiac Bioprostheses: The Case of 'Sutureless' Valves." *European Heart Journal Supplements* 17: 34–37.

Bagnolini, Guillaume, and Paolo Stellino. 2019. "Bioart: Definition(s) and Ethical Issues; Introductory Essay." *Philosophical Readings* 11(1): 1–5.

Bains, Perminder, Safia Chatur, Maya Ignaszewski, Simroop Ladhar, and Matthew Bennett. 2017. "John Hopps and the Pacemaker: A History and Detailed Overview of Devices, Indications, and Complications." *British Columbia Medical Journal* 59: 29–37.

Benedum, J. 2003. "The Early History of the Artificial Kidney." *Anasthesiologie Intensivmedizin Notfallmedizin Schmerztherapie* 38(11): 681–88.

Boink, Gerard J., Vincent M. Christoffels, Richard B. Robinson, and Hanno L. Tan. 2015. "The Past, Present, and Future of Pacemaker Therapies." *Trends in Cardiovascular Medicine* 25(8): 661–73.

Campbell, Alex, Randy Sherman, and William P. Magee. 2010. "The Role of Humanitarian Missions in Modern Surgical Training." *Plastic and Reconstructive Surgery* 126(1): 295–302.

Dixon, Steve. 2019. "Cybernetic-Existentialism in Performance Art." *Leonardo* 52(3): 247–54.

Elsenaar, Arthur, and Remko Scha. 2002. "Electric Body Manipulation as Performance Art: A Historical Perspective." *Leonardo Music Journal* 12: 17–28.

Emerson, J. H. 1985. "Some Reflections on Iron Lungs and Other Inventions." *Respiratory Care* 43(7): 577.

Erikson, Susan L. 2015. "Secrets from Whom? Following the Money in Global Health Finance." *Current Anthropology* 56(S12): S306–16.

Gosling, Ju. 2020. Ju Gosling website. Retrieved 1 March 2020 from http://www.ju90.co.uk/.

Hatton, Dean (aka goldendean). 2020. Goldendean website. Retrieved 2 March 2020 from http://2point8.co.za.

Ho, John S., Alexander J. Yeh, Evgenios Neofytou, Sanghoek Kim, Yuji Tanabe, Bhagat Patlolla, Ramin E. Beygui, and Ada S. Y. Poon. 2014. "Wireless Power Transfer to Deep-Tissue Microimplants." *Proceedings of the National Academy of Sciences of the United States of America* 111(22): 7974–79.

Hoghe, Raimund. 2020. Raimund Hoghe website. Retrieved 1 March 2020 from http://www.raimundhoghe.com/english.php. .

Inhorn, Marcia C., and Pasquale Patrizio. 2015. "Infertility around the Globe: New Thinking on Gender, Reproductive Technologies and Global Movements in the 21st Century." *Human Reproduction Update* 21(4): 411–26.

Jarrín, Alvaro. 2015. "Towards a Biopolitics of Beauty: Eugenics, Aesthetic Hierarchies and Plastic Surgery in Brazil." *Journal of Latin American Cultural Studies* 24: 535–52.

Laub, Donald R. 2015. "Globalization of Craniofacial Plastic Surgery: Foreign Mission Programs for Cleft Lip and Palate." *Journal of Craniofacial Surgery* 26(4): 1015–31.

Lewis, Sophie. 2018. "Cyborg Uterine Geography: Complicating 'Care' and Social Reproduction." *Dialogues in Human Geography* 8(3): 300–16.

Manderson, Lenore. 2011. *Surface Tensions: Surgery, Bodily Boundaries, and the Social Self*. Walnut Creek, CA: Left Coast Press.

McAlister, Vivian C. 2005. "Clinical Kidney Transplantation: A 50th Anniversary Review of the First Reported Series." *American Journal of Surgery* 190(3): 485–88.

McKellar, Shelley. 2017. "Clinical Firsts—Christiaan Barnard's Heart Transplantations." *New England Journal of Medicine* 377(23): 2211–13.

Ott, Katherine. 2016. "The Iron Lung in History and Cultural Memory." In M. J. Arnoldi (ed.), *Engaging Smithsonian Objects through Science, History, and the Arts*. Washington, DC: Smithsonian Institution Press, pp. 192–205.

Pather, Jay, and Catherine Boulle, eds. 2019. *Acts of Transgression: Contemporary Live Art in South Africa*. Johannesburg, South Africa: Wits University Press.

Peitzman, Steven J. 1997. "Origins and Early Reception of Clinical Dialysis." *American Journal of Nephrology* 17(3–4): 299–303.

Schneider, Margueritte. 2016. "Cross-National Issues in Disability Data Collection." In B. M. Altman (ed.), *International Measurement of Disability: Purpose, Method and Application: The Work of the Washington Group*. Social Indicators Research Series 61. Dordrecht, The Netherlands, and New York: Springer, pp. 15–28.

———. 2009. "The Difference a Word Makes: Responding to Questions on 'Disability' and 'Difficulty' in South Africa." *Disability and Rehabilitation* 31(1): 42–50.

Shefer, Tamara. 2019. "Activist Performance and Performative Activism towards Intersectional Gender and Sexual Justice in Contemporary South Africa." *International Sociology* 34(4): 418–34.

Ward, Catherine, Susannah Henderson, and Neil H. Metcalfe. 2013. "A Short History on Pacemakers." *International Journal of Cardiology* 169(4): 244–48.

Warren, Narelle, and Lenore Manderson, eds. 2013. *Reframing Disability and Quality of Life: A Global Perspective*. Dordrecht, The Netherlands, and New York: Springer.

Whittaker, Andrea, Lenore Manderson, and Elizabeth Cartwright. 2010. "Patients without Borders: Understanding Medical Travel." *Medical Anthropology* 29(4): 336–43.

INDEX

Note: Page numbers in italics refer to figures.

age: bodies, 2, 4, 8, 12, 93, 152, 160; bodies and technologies, 3, 37; colonialism, 145; erectile dysfunction (ED), 9, 18–19, 22–23; fitness, 36; gender, 25, 36; hormones, 240; masculinities, 21, 25; men, 35–38, 132, 152, 263; neoliberalism, 36–37; pharmaceuticals, 36–38, 44, 45, 46; race, 8; repair, 8, 35–46; sexualities, 9, 11, 20–23, 31, 35–46, 241, 246–47, 248–49, 263; whiteness, 95; women, 263
Agier, Michel, 68–69
Anthropocene, the, 11, 165, 166, 171, 172, 178–82
anthropo-plassein and *anthropo-poiesis*, 5–6, 84
Appadurai, Arjun, 135
apps, 73, 224–37. *See also* menstruation apps (Brazil); pregnancy apps (Brazil); *individual apps*
Arango, Luz Gabriela, 81, 84
Arango-Londoño, Alejandro, 10, 262
Argentina, 148–49
Argus II (prosthetic device), 209–10
Arran (militant group), 141–42, 144, 153, 155–58, 160
Australia, 10–11, 165, 169, 177, 264–65

BabyCenter (app), 225–26, 232, 236. *See also* pregnancy apps (Brazil)

Bakkum, Douglas, 173
Bates, Tarsh, 172, 174–76, 177
Bears subculture, 10, 142, 144, 146–53, 159, 160, 263, 265. *See also* queerness
Beaudoin, Christine, 10–11, 264–65
beauty: age, 263; bioart, 264; biocapitalism, 126–27, 134, 262; biomedicine/medical technologies, 126, 127, 134, 137; biopolitics, 2–3, 115; bodies, 60, 93, 96, 100, 114, 115, 127, 134, 137, 158; class, 10, 98–100, 106, 115, 123–24, 128–29, 133, 134, 135–36, 137, 138, 263; Colombia, 123–38; colonialism, 96; culture, 124; *A Cura da Fealdade* (The cure for ugliness), 56; disabilities, 110; economics, 3, 124–29, 130, 132–33, 134–38; ethnicities, 95, 101–3; eugenics, 67; Europe, 96–97, 99, 100–101, 111, 114; femininities, 94, 95, 130; feminists, 110; gender, 98, 106, 115, 123–24, 128, 134, 138, 263; Gilman, Sander L., 60, 85; globalization, 2–3, 115, 127, 128, 137; health risks, 135–36, 137, 138; masculinities/men, 123–38; Mexico, 71, 88n20; morality, 118n22, 128–29; nationalities, 98, 106, 115; neoliberalism, 134, 138; pharmaceuticals, 127, 135; plastic surgeries, 1, 126; Portugal, 93–101, 102, 115n1, 263; race, 7–8, 10, 67, 94–115, 117n16, 128, 134, 263;

Remotti, Francesco, 84; sexualities, 98, 127, 263; skin lighteners, 117n16, 263; social value, 123, 127–29, 132, 134–36, 137–38, 262; technologies/United States, 3; whiteness, 94–96, 98, 103, 106–7, 111–15; women, 110, 114, 115, 117n14, 130, 134, 148, 158. *See also* European bodies

Beauty Brigade (Mexico), 9–10, 67–85; *apapacho estético*, 79–83, 84, 85; biopolitics, 67; bodies, 67, 80–81, 86n2, 87n10; catharsis, 78–79, 82, 84; class, 70, 84; description of, 68, 70–72; disabilities, 71, 76–77, 81, 82–83, 85, 89n36; empathy, 75–77, 84; as family, 73–75, 84, 88n23; inhibitions, 77–78, 85; recovery, 70–73, 83, 263; recreation, 72–73, 84; repair, 9–10, 67–85; social value, 68–70, 74–75, 83–85, 263; volunteers, 70–71, 72, 73–85, 87nn12–13, 88n31, 88n34. *See also* elderly sex workers; Sexto, Diego

Beauty Without Borders (Afghanistan), 67

Ben-Ary, Guy, 169, 172, 173–74, 177, 180

Berlant, Lauren, 2

bioart, 165–82, 264–65; the Anthropocene, 166, 171, 172, 178–82; beauty, 264; *Bennu/Blender*, 177; biohacks, 10–11, 167–68, 171, 172, 181–82, 265; biotechnologies, 165–71, 172, 181–82, 265; bodies, 10–11, 165–67, 171–78, 180–82, 264–65; *CellF* (project), 173–74, 180; definition of, 167; DIYbio (Do-it-yourself biology), 167–68, 171; the environment, 165, 166, 174–75, 178; gender, 176, 264; post-humanism, 165–66, 171, 176, 178, 180–82; race, 264. *See also individuals; individual laboratories*

biocapitalism, 7, 10, 126–27, 134, 262

bioethics, 12, 261

biohacks: bioart, 10–11, 167–68, 171, 172, 181–82, 265; biotechnologies, 144, 167–68; bodies, 3, 144, 146, 159–60, 177, 265; gender, 10, 142, 160; skin lighteners/lightness, 144

biomedicine: beauty, 126, 134, 137; blindness, 208, 210, 219, 256; bodies, 252; bodies and technologies, 256–57, 258, 261; Brazil, 228, 236, 237, 243–44; class, 243–44; disabilities, 219; economics, 262; gender, 242, 243–44, 251–52; health tourism, 257; limits of, 256–57, 261; men, 45, 130, 134, 263; menstruation and pregnancy apps (Brazil), 228, 236, 237; neoliberalism, 134; pharmaceuticals, 246, 261; plastic surgeries, 130, 257; race, 243–44; repair, 36, 257; retinal implants (Russia), 207, 215, 219; sexualities, 36, 241, 243, 252; testosterone, 240, 242–44, 251; women, 243, 263

biopolitics: Bears subculture, 142; beauty, 2–3, 115; Beauty Brigade (Mexico), 67; biocapitalism, 7; bodies, 2–3, 8, 45, 67, 141–46, 158–61; Catalan militants, 10, 141–42; feminists, 159; fertilities/reproduction, 224; gender, 142–43; hormones, 3; menstruation and pregnancy apps (Brazil), 224–25; pharmaceuticals, 3, 224; plastic surgeries, 3, 54; prosthetics, 3, 202; repair, 45; Russia, 219; skin lighteners, 3, 7. *See also* politics

biotechnologies, 3, 144, 165–71, 172, 177, 178–82, 257–58, 261–62, 265. *See also* bodies and technologies; menstruation apps (Brazil); pregnancy apps (Brazil)

Black Atlantic, 7–8

blindness, 11, 83, 85, 207–20, 221n1, 256. *See also* retinal implants (Russia)

bodies: age, 2, 4, 8, 12, 93, 152, 160; the Anthropocene, 165; Arango, Luz Gabriela, 81; assemblages, 145–46, 153–61; Bears subculture, 10, 142, 146–53, 159, 160, 263, 265; beauty, 60, 93, 96, 100, 114, 115,

127, 134, 137, 158; Beauty Brigade (Mexico), 67, 80–81, 86n2, 87n10; becoming, 145–46; bioart, 10–11, 165–67, 171–78, 180–82, 264–65; biohacks, 3, 144, 146, 159–60, 177, 265; biomedicine, 243, 252; bio/politics, 2–3, 8, 10, 45, 67, 141–46, 158–61, 263; biotechnologies, 166, 177, 180–82, 257–58; Brazil, 53, 62, 224–32; Catalan militants, 141–42, 144, 155–59; class, 4, 12, 93, 138, 146; disabilities, 2, 4, 189; economics, 2, 127, 137; Enguix Grau, Begonya, 3, 10–11, 263; the environment, 175, 180, 181; ethnographies, 12, 143, 148–49, 262; femininities, 161; feminists, 141–43, 153–59, 160, 230, 265; fitness, 2, 106, 128; Foucault, Michel, 128; gender, 4, 10, 12, 93, 141–46, 148–49, 153–61, 263; globalization, 2–3; health, 53; masculinities, 133, 138, 146–53, 161; men, 123, 125–26, 127–28, 130, 132–35, 138, 146–53, 263; menstruation and pregnancy apps (Brazil), 224–32; Mexico, 88n27; nationalities, 12; nations, 2–3, 9, 10, 52, 60, 153–59, 160, 220; neoliberalism, 3, 45; overflown/protest bodies, 143, 146, 153, 156–58, 159–60; parasports, 190, 192–93, 195–202; pharmaceuticals, 257–58; plastic surgeries, 52–54, 59, 60, 138, 144, 257–58; post-humanism, 181; queerness, 2, 3, 147, 149–53; race, 2, 4, 7–8, 12, 93, 96, 110–11, 114, 262; repair, 4, 8, 46, 52–54, 60, 62–63; reshaping, 4, 129–38, 160, 166, 172, 180, 257–58; retinal implants (Russia), 209, 220; sexualities, 2, 4, 93, 143–46, 148–49, 229–30, 263; South Africa, 256–57, 264; whiteness, 110–11; women, 130, 132–33, 141–42, 144, 158, 229–30, 237, 243, 263–64. *See also* European bodies

bodies and technologies, 3–7; access and equity, 261–62; age, 3, 37; bioart, 10–11, 166, 167, 174, 177, 180; bioethics, 12, 261; biohacks, 144, 167–68; biomedicine, 256–57, 258, 261; biopolitics, 3; Catalan militants, 158–59; class, 8, 138, 261; dialysis, 260; economics, 261; erectile dysfunction (ED), 258; gender, 8, 11–12, 261; globalization, 258, 261; lungs, 260–61; masculinities, 153; men, 134, 138; pacemakers, 259–60; parasports, 190, 193–96, 198–202, 264; repair, 12, 37, 259–61; replacement, 4, 8, 9, 12; Rose, Nikolas, 243; sexualities, 8, 37, 229–30, 258. *See also* biotechnologies; menstruation apps (Brazil); pregnancy apps (Brazil); reshaping

Bonnett, Alastair, 111
Borodina, Svetlana, 11, 259
Braidotti, Rosi, 142
Brazil, 52–63, 224–37, 240–52; biomedicine, 228, 236, 237, 243–44; bodies, 53, 62, 224–32; contraception, 11, 230, 237, 241; ear surgeries, 9, 52–63, 63n4, 262; eugenics, 9, 56–57, 61–63, 63n5, 64n6, 67, 262; fitness, 62; gender, 224–25, 243–44, 246, 250; hormones, 7, 11–12, 240–52; neoliberalism, 54; plastic surgeries, 7, 9, 52–54, 57, 58–59, 62–63, 63n1; repair, 9, 52–63; reproduction, 224–25; sexualities, 240–52, 263; testosterone, 240–52; whiteness, 67; women, 11–12, 224–37, 240–52. *See also individuals*; menstruation apps (Brazil); pregnancy apps (Brazil)
Brazilian Ministry of Health, 52
Bunt, Stuart, 169
Butler, Judith, 251
Butryn, Ted, 195, 200

Cali (Columbia), 123–38
Camoletto, Raffaella Ferrero, 9, 258, 263
Campbell, Fiona Kumari, 211
Canada, 10–11, 167–68, 264–65
Canguilhem, George, 215

Carpigo, Eva, 9–10, 263
Carrigan, Tim, 147–48
Casa Xochiquetzal, 72, 74, 75, 76, 82–83
Castañeda, Luzia Aurelia, 56
Catalan militants, 10, 141–42, 144, 153–59, 160, 263. *See also individual groups*
Catalunya, 10, 155, *156*, 158, 263
Catts, Oron, 169, 172, 174, 179, 180
CellF (project), 173–74, 180
Chapelle, Gauthier, 68
Charles, John, 195
Chazan, Lilian, 234
children. *See* ear surgeries (Brazil)
cisgender, 24, 25. *See also* gender; men; menstruation apps (Brazil); pregnancy apps (Brazil); women
Clare, Eli, 216
Clarke, Adele E., 242, 243–44
class: beauty, 10, 98–100, 106, 115, 123–24, 128–29, 133, 134, 135–36, 137, 138, 263; Beauty Brigade (Mexico), 70, 84; biomedicine, 243–44; bodies, 4, 12, 93, 138, 146; bodies and technologies, 8, 261; Colombia, 123–24, 128–29; colonialism, 145; contraception, 230; erectile dysfunction (ED), 9, 22–23, 31; Europe, 96, 99, 111; European bodies, 98–100, 111; gender, 8, 143; hormones, 7, 241; human malleability limits, 7; intersectionalities, 8; masculinities, 134; men, 146; men's health medicine, 24, 28, 30–32; Mexico, 68–69, 70, 76, 83, 84; plastic surgeries, 53, 55–56; Portugal, 99, 103; race, 96, 98; skin lightness, 96, 99, 111; whiteness, 95, 96, 98–99, 111–12, 115
Clue (Calendario do ciclo menstrual e ovulacao) (app), 226
Cochennec, Morgan, 71–72
Colombia, 10, 123–38, 262
colonialism: age/class/disabilities/gender/nationalities, 145; beauty, 96; ethnicities, 102–3, 116n5, 117n11; human malleability limits, 7; Portugal, 10, 95–98, 102–3; race, 98, 116n5, 117n11, 145; sexualities, 95–96, 116n2, 116n5, 145; skin lighteners/lightness, 102–3, 106, 111; whiteness, 10, 95–98, 100, 102–3, 106, 116n3. *See also* European bodies
Connell, Bob, 147–48
Connell, Raewyn, 133, 148
contraception, 11, 166, 228, 229–31, 237, 240, 241, 258
Cooper, Melinda, 126–27, 134
Correa, Sonia, 237
COS (Coordinadora Obrera Sindical), 153
cosmetic surgeries. *See* plastic surgeries
Crime: Its Causes and Remedies (Lombroso), 56–57
Crivella, Marcelo, 54–55, 57, 60
Csordas, Thomas, 196
CUP (Candidatura d'Unitat Popular), 141–42, 144, 153, 158, 160
Cura da Fealdade, A (The cure for ugliness) (Kehl), 56
cyborg athletes, 11, 189, 190, 193–202. *See also* parasports
cyborg babies, 234, 236–37. *See also* fetuses
cyborgs, 3, 4, 8, 189, 197, 200–202, 224, 231

de Barbieri, Teresa, 143
deafness, 58, 83, 208, 209, 211, 256
Deleuze, Gilles, 145
dialysis, 260
Dijsselbloem, Jeroen, 111
disabilities: beauty, 110; Beauty Brigade (Mexico), 71, 76–77, 81, 82–83, 85, 89n36; biomedicine, 219; blindness as, 208–9, 214–15, 216–19, 221n1; bodies, 2, 4, 189; colonialism, 145; cure ideologies, 216–17; eugenics, 6; globalization, 258; Gosling, Ju, 264; IBYCIM (Instituto de Belleza y Cultura Incluyente México), 82–83; intersectionalities, 8; IOSD (International Organisations of Sport for the Disabled), 190–91;

men's health medicine, 28; *The Normal and the Pathological* (Canguilhem), 215; parasports, 190–91, 193, 197–98, 201–2; replacement, 9, 11, 189–202; Russia, 208, 219, 220, 221n1; sexualities, 8, 197; technologies, 11, 189–90, 191–92, 195, 201–2, 220. *See also* cyborg athletes

DIYbio (Do-it-yourself biology), 167–68, 171, 181–82

Dumit, Joseph, 244

Dyer, Richard, 95

ear surgeries (Brazil), 9, 52–63, 63n4, 262

economics: beauty, 3, 124–29, 130, 132–33, 134–38; bioart, 171; biomedicine, 262; bodies, 2, 127, 137; bodies and technologies, 261; Colombia, 123–29, 137, 138; plastic surgeries, 10, 126, 128, 129, 133, 135–37, 257; prosthetics, 264

Ecuador, 6

Edel, Mike, 173

Edmonds, Alexander, 136, 137

EI (Esquerra Independentista), 141–42, 144, 153–59, 160

elderly sex workers, 71, *72, 74,* 75

Enguix Grau, Begonya, 3, 10–11, 263

environment, the, 5, 11, 165, 166, 174–75, 178–81. *See also* Anthropocene, the

Equatorial Guinea, 148–49

erectile dysfunction (ED), 17–32; age, 9, 18–19, 22–23; bodies and technologies, 258; class, 9, 22–23, 31; gender/race, 9; Italy, 9, 43, 263; masculinities, 9, 18–23, 37–38, 263; men, 18–19; men's health medicine, 9, 18, 26–28; Mexico, 9, 18, 19–23, 31, 37–38, 263; pharmaceuticals, 37–38; repair, 9, 17–32, 263; United States, 9, 263. *See also* Viagra

ethnicities: beauty, 95, 101–3; colonialism, 102–3, 116n5, 117n11; ear surgeries, 60; gender, 143; men's health medicine, 25–26, 30, 31;

plastic surgeries, 100, 101–2, 116n8; Portugal, 103; sexualities, 94–96; skin lighteners/lightness, 67, 101–3, 108–9, 111. *See also* race

ethnographies: Beauty Brigade (Mexico), 67; bioart, 165; bodies, 12, 143, 148–49, 262; Colombia, 123–24; menstruation and pregnancy apps, 226–27, 234; methodologies, 4, 67, 115n1, 117n14, 226–27, 242; Pussetti, Chiara, 88n28; testosterone, 242; whiteness, 101, 103

eugenics, 6, 9, 56–57, 61–63, 63n5, 64n6, 67, 262. *See also* Kehl, Renato

Europe, 7–8, 38–39, 96–97, 98, 99, 100–101, 111–12, 114. *See also* colonialism; *individual countries*

European bodies, 93–115; class, 98–100, 111; colonialism, 10, 116n5; Portugal, 10, 93–101; race, 110–11; skin lighteners, 10, 101–10; social value, 10, 93, 100–101, 105–6, 116n5. *See also* whiteness

femininities: beauty, 94, 95, 130; bodies, 161; face slimmers, 1; feminists, 10, 263; gender, 143, 144, 151; masculinities, 148, 149; menstruation apps (Brazil), 228; plastic surgeries, 138; race, 10, 94–96; testosterone, 242, 251–52; whiteness, 10, 95, 96, 111, 115

feminists: beauty, 110; biopolitics, 159; bodies, 141–43, 153–59, 160, 230, 265; Catalan militants, 141–42, 153–59, 160, 263; contraception, 230; femininities, 10, 263; gender, 141–42, 263; masculinities, 142; menstruation and pregnancy apps (Brazil), 224–25. *See also* EI (Esquerra Independentista)

Ferguson, James, 104

Ferrando, Francesca, 166

fertilities, 224–32, 263–64. *See also* pregnancy apps (Brazil); reproduction

fetuses, 232–37. *See also* pregnancy apps (Brazil)

Fitch, Andrew, 173
fitness: age, 36; bodies, 2, 106, 128; Brazil, 62; Colombia, 125–26, 128, 131–32, 133; plastic surgeries, 131–32, 133; queerness, 147, 150, 151–52, 160; spornosexualities, 147
Foucault, Michel, 52, 61, 67, 128
France, 38–39, 111, 155

gayness. *See* queerness
gender: age, 25, 36; assemblages, 153–59; Bears subculture, 144; beauty, 98, 106, 115, 123–24, 128, 134, 138, 263; bioart, 176, 264; biohacks, 10, 142, 160; biomedicine, 242, 243–44, 251–52; biopolitics, 142–43; bodies, 4, 10, 12, 93, 141–46, 148–49, 153–61, 263; bodies and technologies, 8, 11–12, 261; Brazil, 224–25, 243–44, 246, 250; Catalan militants, 10, 141–42, 155–56, 158, 160; class, 8, 143; Colombia, 123; colonialism, 145; erectile dysfunction (ED), 9; ethnicities, 143; face slimmers, 1; femininities, 143, 144, 151; feminists, 141–42, 263; hormones, 242, 245–48; human malleability limits, 7; intersectionalities/race/repair, 8; masculinities, 143, 144; medical technologies, 11–12, 17–18; medicine, 43; men's health medicine, 23–32; menstruation and pregnancy apps (Brazil), 224–25; Mexico, 20; nations, 153–59; pharmaceuticals, 224, 250; plastic surgeries, 10, 53, 130–33, 134; Portugal, 103; queerness, 25; sexes, 143–45; sexualities, 8, 36, 43, 46, 143–46, 148, 149–51, 246–48, 250–52; technologies, 224; testosterone, 240, 242, 245, 251–52; whiteness, 95. *See also* men; women
Georges, Eugenia, 234
Germany, 111, 226
Giami, Alain, 39
Gill, Rosalind, 100
Gillespie, Marcia Ann, 94, 95
Gilman, Sander L., 53, 60, 85

Gilmore, David, 147
Gilroy, Paul, 7
Glenn, Evelynn Nakano, 100
globalization, 2–3, 100, 115, 126–27, 128, 137, 258, 261
Gosling, Ju, 264
Gott, Merryn, 46
Gould, Stephen J., 56
GPs (general practitioners). *See* Italy
Grounds, Miranda, 169
Guattari, Félix, 145

Haraway, Donna: the Anthropocene, 179, 181; cyborgs, 4, 190, 197, 200, 202, 231; hybrid bodies, 192; overflown bodies, 146
Hardon, Anita, 135
Hastings, Jaden J. A., 172, 177
Hatton, Dean, 264
Hayles, Katherine, 4, 5
health risks, 7, 100, 108, 116n9, 117n12, 117n18, 135–37, 138, 252
health tourism, 126, 129–30, 137, 138, 257, 262
Hearn, Jeff, 147
Hennen, Peter, 151
Hodgetts, Stuart, 173
Hoghe, Raimund, 264
Holland, Sharon Patricia, 8
hormones, 240–52; biopolitics, 3; Brazil, 7, 11–12, 240–52; class, 7, 241; contraception, 229–30, 231; gender, 242, 245–48; masculinities, 153; men's health medicine, 23, 27; transgender men, 252. *See also* testosterone
Howe, David, 11, 264
human malleability limits, 4–7
Hunter, Margaret, 100

IBYCIM (Instituto de Belleza y Cultura Incluyente México), 82–83
ICT (information and communication technologies), 224–25, 227–29, 231–32, 235, 237, 264. *See also* menstruation apps (Brazil); pregnancy apps (Brazil); technologies

Ihde, Don, 6
immigrants, 7, 10, 85, 93, 100–101, 103, 116n5
in vitro fertilization, 6. *See also* reproduction
IOSD (International Organisations of Sport for the Disabled), 190–91
IPC (International Paralympic Committee), 189, 190–91, 193, 194, 199, 202
IPC World Athletics Championships (paralympic sports), 190, 194, 198, 199, 202
Italy, 9, 35–46, 100–101, 111, 263
Iwakuma, Miho, 196
IWAS (International Wheelchair and Amputee Sport Association), 191, 196, 197

Jarrín, Alvaro, 54, 55, 67, 103, 265

Kac, Eduardo, 167
Kafer, Alison, 216
Kalra, Pryanka, 101
Kama, Amit, 202
Katz, Stephen, 241
Kaufman, Sharon, 220
Kehl, Renato, 56–57, 59, 60, 61, 62, 63n5, 64n6
Keinz, Anika, 100
Kropotkin, Peter, 68
Kurenkov, Vyacheslav, 214
Kurzweil, Ray, 4–5

Laivina, Evija, 1–2
Lapworth, Andrew, 171
LeCain, Timothy J., 179
Lee, John, 147–48
Levine, Martin, 149–51
Lewicki, Pawel, 100
LGBTQ communities, 25, 70, 153. *See also* Bears subculture; queerness
libido. *See* sexualities
Liebelt, Claudia, 3
Lisbon. *See* Portugal
Lobato, Monteiro, 56
Lombroso, Cesare, 56–57
Luckett, William H., 60

lungs, 260–61
Lupton, Deborah, 237

machismo, 9, 19–22, 31, 123, 131. *See also* masculinities
MacIntyre, Alasdair, 201
Making the Body Beautiful (Gilman), 60
Malafouris, Lambros, 6
Manderson, Lenore, 3
Manica, Daniela Tonelli, 11, 258, 263–64
Markowitz, Sally, 95
Marshall, Barbara L., 45, 241, 243
Martin, Wendy, 36
masculinities, 123–38, 147–53; age, 21, 25; Bears subculture, 146–53, 160; beauty, 123–38; bodies, 133, 138, 146–53, 161; class, 134; Colombia, 10, 123–38; concepts of, 147–48; Connell, Raewyn, 133; erectile dysfunction (ED), 9, 18–23, 37–38, 263; femininities, 148, 149; feminists, 142; gender, 143, 144; Hatton, Dean, 264; hegemonic masculinities, 147–48; men's health medicine, 23, 25–27, 29, 30–32; Mexico, 19–23, 263; neoliberalism, 123, 134, 138, 148; plastic surgeries, 10, 133, 138; queerness, 148–53; race, 25–26, 134; repair, 9, 18, 19, 35, 263; reshaping, 129–38; sexualities, 11–12, 20–23, 31, 37, 153; testosterone, 242; women, 147–48. *See also* machismo; men
Mauss, Marcel, 82
medical technologies: beauty, 127, 137; gender, 11–12, 17–18; men, 18, 127, 130, 134; sexualities, 11–12, 17–18; women, 3–4, 7. *See also individual medical technologies*
men, 123–38; age, 35–38, 132, 152, 263; beauty, 123–38; biomedicine, 45, 130, 134, 263; bodies, 123, 125–26, 127–28, 130, 132–35, 138, 146–53, 263; bodies and technologies, 134; Catalan militants, 156, 158; class, 146; gender, 23; medical technologies, 18, 127, 130,

134; nations, 155; pharmaceuticals, 35; plastic surgeries, 10, 123, 125–26, 129–38, 262–63; repair, 18–19, 23–32; sexualities, 18–19, 20–23, 26–28, 30–31, 35–38, 40–46, 133–34, 144, 146–47, 241–42, 246–52; skin lightness, 127, 262; social value, 262; testosterone, 244–45, 249–52; transgender men, 24, 25, 29, 252. *See also* Bears subculture; erectile dysfunction (ED)

men's health medicine, 17–32; class, 24, 28, 30–32; disabilities, 28; erectile dysfunction (ED), 9, 18, 26–28; ethnicities, 25–26, 30, 31; gender, 23–32; masculinities, 23, 25–27, 29, 30–32; nationalities, 25–26, 32; race, 24, 25–26, 30–32; repair, 23–32; reproduction, 29–30; sexualities, 26–28, 30, 31, 35; testosterone, 23, 27; United States, 18, 23–24, 30–31

Menstrual Calendar (Calendario Menstrual) (app), 226

menstruation apps (Brazil), 11, 224–32, 235, 258, 264

Merleau-Ponty, Maurice, 196

Mexico: *apapacho*, 79–80, 88n29; beauty, 71, 88n20; bodies, 88n27; brigades, 69–70, 87n9; class, 68–69, 70, 76, 83, 84; criminality, 68–69, 76, 86n3, 86n6, 87nn7–8; erectile dysfunction (ED), 9, 18, 19–23, 31, 37–38, 263; gender, 20; machismo, 19–22, 31; masculinities, 19–23, 263; natural disasters, 69, 86n4, 88n22; race, 19–20; sexualities, 31, 37–38. *See also* Beauty Brigade (Mexico)

Mexico City, 9–10, 68–70, 71, 75, 76, 83, 86n6, 87n7, 263. *See also* Beauty Brigade (Mexico); Casa Xochiquetzal

"Mirror Mirror" (Gillespie) (essay), 94

miscarriages, 11, 236–37
Mitchell, Lisa, 234
Moore, Darren, 173
Mori, Masahiro, 2
Murphy, Robert, 197

nationalities, 8, 12, 25–26, 32, 95, 98, 106, 115, 145

nations, 2–3, 9, 10, 52, 54–57, 60–63, 153–59, 160, 220. *See also individual nations*

neoliberalism: age, 36–37; beauty, 134, 138; biocapitalism, 126–27, 134; bodies, 3, 45; Brazil/plastic surgeries, 54; Colombia, 10, 125–26; masculinities, 123, 134, 138, 148; queerness, 148

Nguyen, Mimi Thi, 3, 67

Normal and the Pathological, The (Canguilhem), 215

Nucci, Marina Fisher, 11, 258, 263–64

Ochoa, Marcia, 3
Orelhinha Bonitinha (Beautiful little ears) (program), 54–55, 57. *See also* ear surgeries (Brazil)
otoplasties. *See* ear surgeries (Brazil)
Oudshoorn, Nelly, 231

pacemakers, 3, 259–60
El País (newspaper), 129, 130–31, 133, 136
Paletta, Gabriela, 11, 237, 258, 263–64
Paralympics, 11, 189–94, 196–202, 264
parasports, 11, 189–202, 264. *See also* cyborg athletes; *individuals*; *individual paralympic organizations*
Pelling, Andrew, 168, 169
Pelling Lab for Augmented Biology, 167–71
Perry, Imani, 100
pharmaceuticals: age, 36–38, 44, 45, 46; beauty, 127, 135; biomedicine, 246, 261; biopolitics, 3, 224; biotechnologies/bodies, 257–58; contraception, 229–30, 231; erectile dysfunction (ED), 37–38; gender, 224, 250; Italy, 40; men, 35; reshaping, 8–9, 257; sexualities, 35, 36–38, 40, 44, 45–46, 241, 243–44; skin lighteners, 108, 111, 112–14, 117n18. *See also* hormones; Viagra
Pico della Mirandola, Giovanni, 5–6
Pistorius, Oscar, 189, 198, 200

Pitanguy, Ivo, 55–56, 57, 59, 60
plastic surgeries: beauty, 1, 126; biomedicine, 130, 257; biopolitics, 3, 54; bodies, 52–54, 59, 60, 138, 144, 257–58; Brazil, 7, 9, 52–54, 57, 58–59, 62–63, 63n1; class, 53, 55–56; Colombia, 10, 123, 124–26, 128, 129–37, 262; economics, 10, 126, 128, 129, 133, 135–37, 257; ethnicities, 100, 101–2, 116n8; eugenics, 9, 262; Europe, 100; femininities, 138; fitness, 131–32, 133; gender, 10, 53, 130–33, 134; health risks, 7, 135–37, 138; health tourism, 129–30, 257; masculinities, 10, 133, 138; men, 10, 123, 125–26, 129–38, 262–63; Portugal, 101–2, 103, 117n15; queerness, 131; race, 53, 101–2, 103; repair, 52–54, 257; reshaping, 8–9, 138, 257; sexualities, 133–34; social value, 9, 59–60, 85; technologies, 127; United States, 62, 64n15, 85, 116n8; women, 7, 130–33, 134. *See also* ear surgeries (Brazil); *individuals*
Plastic Surgery in School (Brazil), 55, 57. *See also* ear surgeries (Brazil)
Plastic Surgery League (Brazil), 57
Polikanov, Dmitriy, 213
politics, 10, 263. *See also* biopolitics
Portugal, 93–115; beauty, 93–101, 102, 115n1, 263; class, 99, 103; colonialism, 10, 95–98, 102–3; ethnicities/gender, 103; European bodies, 10, 93–101; health risks, 117n18; plastic surgeries, 101–2, 103, 117n15; race, 103–4, 114–15, 263; Russian women, 99; sexualities, 38, 93–96, 98; skin lighteners/lightness, 7, 10, 93–96, 99, 101–10, 111, 112–15, 117n18, 263; social value, 10, 93, 100–101, 103, 105–6; whiteness, 93–99, 105–10, 114–15
post-humanism, 4, 5, 11, 165–66, 171, 176, 178, 180–82
Potts, Anne, 37
Preciado, Paul B., 144, 229–30

pregnancy apps (Brazil), 11, 224–27, 232–37, 264
Pregnancy+ (Gravidez+) (app), 225–26, 232, 236
prosthetics: biopolitics, 3, 202; biotechnologies, 3, 258; ear surgeries, 57–58, 61; economics, 264; human malleability limits, 4–5; parasports, 11, 190–96, 198–202, 264; retinal implants (Russia), 207, 209–13, 219; technologies, 191–92, 195–96, 198–202. *See also* cyborg athletes
Puar, Jasbir, 8, 159
Pussetti, Chiara, 10, 88n28, 263, 265

queerness: Beauty Brigade (Mexico), 70; bodies, 2, 3, 147, 149–53; fitness, 147, 150, 151–52, 160; gender, 25; Hatton, Dean, 264; masculinities, 148–53; men's health medicine, 23; neoliberalism, 148; plastic surgeries, 131; sexualities, 148. *See also* Bears subculture

race: age/gender/intersectionalities, 8; beauty, 7–8, 10, 67, 94–115, 117n16, 128, 134, 263; bioart, 264; biomedicine, 243–44; Black Atlantic, 7–8; bodies, 2, 4, 7–8, 12, 93, 96, 110–11, 114, 262; class, 96, 98; colonialism, 98, 116n5, 117n11, 145; contraception, 230; erectile dysfunction (ED), 9; eugenics, 262; Europe, 7–8, 96, 98; European bodies, 96–101, 110–11; femininities, 10, 94–96; human malleability limits, 7; masculinities, 25–26, 134; men's health medicine, 24, 25–26, 30–32; menstruation and pregnancy apps (Brazil), 227; Mexico, 19–20; plastic surgeries, 53, 101–2, 103; Portugal, 103–4, 114–15, 263; reproduction, 6; sexualities, 8, 10, 94–96, 110, 116n2, 116nn4–5; skin lighteners, 101–10, 117n16, 263; whiteness, 110; women, 110–11. *See also* ethnicities

Remotti, Francesco, 5, 84
repair, 8–10, 17–86; age, 8, 35–46; Beauty Brigade (Mexico), 9–10, 67–85; biomedicine, 36, 257; biopolitics, 45; bodies, 4, 8, 46, 52–54, 60, 62–63; bodies and technologies, 12, 37, 259–61; Brazil, 9, 52–63; ear surgeries, 52–63; gender, 8; masculinities, 9, 18, 19, 35, 263; men, 18–19, 23–32; men's health medicine, 23–32; plastic surgeries, 52–54, 257; replacement, 19; sexualities, 35–46. *See also* erectile dysfunction (ED)
replacement, 8–9, 11–12, 189–265; bodies and technologies, 4, 8, 9, 12; disabilities, 9, 11, 189–202; hormones, 240–52; parasports, 189–202; reproduction apps, 224–37; retinal implants (Russia), 207–20; technologies, 9, 193–94
reproduction, 3–4, 5, 6, 26, 29–30, 224–37, 248, 263–64. *See also* pregnancy apps (Brazil)
reshaping, 10–12, 93–182; Bears subculture, 141–61; bioart, 165–82; bodies, 4, 129–38, 160, 166, 172, 180, 257–58; Catalan militants, 141–42, 153–59, 160, 263; Colombia, 129–38; gender, 141–61; masculinities, 129–38; pharmaceuticals/plastic surgeries, 8–9, 257; Portugal, 93–95; whiteness, 93–115
retinal implants (Russia), 11, 207–20, 259. *See also individuals; individual organizations*
Revista Imagen (magazine), 129–30, 132, 134
Reynolds White, Susan, 135
Rhee, Jennifer, 2
Roberts, Elizabeth, 6
robotics, 2, 174, 177, 180
Rohden, Fabíola, 11, 258, 263
Rose, Nikolas, 6, 243
Rubin, Gayle, 143
Russia, 99, 207–20, 221n1. *See also* retinal implants (Russia)

Sanabria, Emilia, 7, 241
Sandberg, Linne, 38
Santo, Espírito, 61
Scharff, Christina, 100
Schimitt, Marcelle, 9–10, 262
Scott, James C., 86n2
SecondSight, 212
Sellars, Nina, 172, 177, 180, 265
SEPC (Sindicat d'Estudiants dels Països Catalans), 153
Servigne, Pablo, 68
sexes, 17–18, 158. *See also* gender; men; women
Sexto, Diego, 70, 73, 75, 76, 87n11. *See also* Beauty Brigade (Mexico)
sexualities: age, 9, 11, 20–23, 31, 35–46, 241, 246–47, 248–49, 263; Bears subculture, 144; beauty, 98, 127, 263; biomedicine, 36, 241, 243, 252; bodies, 2, 4, 93, 143–46, 148–49, 229–30, 263; bodies and technologies, 8, 37, 229–30, 258; Braidotti, Rosi, 142; Brazil, 240–52, 263; colonialism, 95–96, 116n2, 116n5, 145; contraception, 229–31; disabilities, 8, 197; ethnicities, 94–96; Europe, 38–39, 111; gender, 8, 36, 43, 46, 143–46, 148, 149–51, 246–48, 250–52; intersectionalities/nationalities, 8; Italy, 35–46; masculinities, 11–12, 20–23, 31, 37, 153; medical technologies, 11–12, 17–18; men, 18–19, 20–23, 26–28, 30–31, 35–38, 40–46, 133–34, 144, 146–47, 241–42, 246–52; men's health medicine, 26–28, 30, 31, 35; menstruation and pregnancy apps (Brazil), 224–25, 228, 229–30, 231–32, 237; metro/sporno sexualities, 146–47, 148; Mexico, 31, 37–38; pharmaceuticals, 35, 36–38, 40, 44, 45–46, 241, 243–44; plastic surgeries, 133–34; Portugal, 93–96, 98; queerness, 148; race, 8, 10, 94–96, 110, 116n2, 116nn4–5; repair, 19, 35–46; skin lightness, 93–96; testosterone, 11, 240–52,

263; whiteness, 10, 93–96. *See also* erectile dysfunction (ED); women and sexualities
Seymour, Wendy, 197–98
Shogan, Debra, 199
Silva, Carla Filomena, 11, 264
Simay, Philippe, 71
Simmel, Georg, 71, 87n17
Simpson, Mark, 146–47
skin lighteners, 101–15; beauty, 117n16, 263; biohacks, 144; biopolitics, 3, 7; colonialism, 102–3, 106; ethnicities, 101–3, 108–9; Europe, 101, 111; European bodies, 10, 101–10; health risks, 100, 108, 116n9, 117n12; immigrants, 100–101; Italy, 100–101, 111; pharmaceuticals, 108, 111, 112–14, 117n18; Portugal, 7, 10, 101–10, 111, 112–15, 117n18, 263; as practice, 4; race, 101–10, 117n16, 263; social value, 3, 10, 263
skin lightness: biohacks, 144; class, 96, 99, 111; colonialism, 111; Ecuador, 6; ethnicities, 67, 111; Europe, 101, 111; immigrants, 100–101; men, 127, 262; morality, 114, 118n22; Portugal, 93–96, 99; sexualities, 93–96; social value, 101. *See also* whiteness
Slovenia, 158
So-Edinenie (foundation), 209, 211, 213
sound, 211. *See also* deafness
South Africa, 256–57, 264
Spain, 111, 148–49, 153–58
Spanish Legion, 155
Stelarc (performance artist), 172, 177, 180, 265
Stevenson, Lisa, 220
Sunder Rajan, Kaushik, 126
supercrips, 11, 193–94, 199–200, 201, 202. *See also* cyborg athletes
Surface Dynamics of Adhesion (Bates), 174–76
Sweden, 38, 174
SymbioticA Centre of Excellence in Biological Art, 165, 169–70, 172, 173–78, 179, 180

Takhchidi, Khristo, 210, 213
technologies: beauty, 3, 127; biocapitalism, 262; blindness, 215, 218–19, 220; disabilities, 11, 189–90, 191–92, 195, 201–2, 220; gender, 224; globalization, 258; humanity, 6; parasports, 190–202; plastic surgeries, 127; prosthetics, 191–92, 195–96, 198–202; replacement, 9, 193–94; reproduction, 224–25, 263–64; Russia, 207, 213–14, 219–20. *See also* bodies and technologies; medical technologies; menstruation apps (Brazil); pregnancy apps (Brazil)
testosterone, 11–12, 23, 27, 240–52, 263. *See also* hormones
Thompson, Nathan, 173
El Tiempo (newspaper), 133–34, 136
Tórtima, Pedro, 56
transatlantic slave trade, 7–8
transgender people, 24, 25, 29, 85, 252
Twigg, Julia, 36

Uliyanov, Grigoriy, 207–8
uncanny aesthetics and uncanny valley, 2, 4
United Kingdom, 24, 38–39, 111, 264
United States: beauty, 3; Beauty Without Borders (Afghanistan), 67; Colombia, 124–25; ear surgeries, 60; erectile dysfunction (ED), 9, 263; men's health medicine, 18, 23–24, 30–31; pharmaceuticals, 241; plastic surgeries, 62, 64n15, 85, 116n8; pregnancy and menstruation apps, 225; recovery, 87n18; Russia, 209, 214

van der Geest, Sjaak, 135
Viagra, 9, 18–23, 26, 35, 37, 38–39, 40, 46, 241
vision impairments, 199. *See also* blindness; retinal implants (Russia)
VOS (All-Russia Society for the Blind), 217–18

Wentzell, Emily, 9, 258, 263
White (Dyer), 95
whiteness, 93–115; age, 95; beauty, 94–96, 98, 103, 106–7, 111–15; bodies, 110–11; Brazil, 67; class, 95, 96, 98–99, 111–12, 115; colonialism, 10, 95–98, 100, 102–3, 106, 116n3; Europe, 96, 100–101, 111–12; European bodies, 96–101; femininities, 10, 95, 96, 111, 115; gender, 95; globalization, 100; nationalities, 95; Portugal, 93–99, 105–10, 114–15; race, 96–99, 110; sexualities, 10, 93–96. *See also* skin lightness
whitening products. *See* skin lighteners
Who Embodies Europe? (Keinz and Lewicki), 100
Wilmut, Ian, 5
Wissinger, Elizabeth, 115
women: age, 263; beauty, 110, 114, 115, 117n14, 130, 134, 148, 158; biomedicine, 243, 263; bodies, 130, 132–33, 141–42, 144, 158, 229–30, 237, 243, 263–64; Brazil, 11–12, 224–37, 240–52; Catalan militants, 156, 158, 160; Colombia, 130; gender, 23, 25, 143, 158; masculinities, 147–48; medical technologies, 3–4, 7; nations, 155; plastic surgeries, 7, 130–33, 134; race, 110–11; reproduction, 3–4, 26, 231, 248; social value, 262; testosterone, 11–12, 240–52; women's health, 23, 24. *See also* CUP (Candidatura d'Unitat Popular); European bodies; femininities; feminists; gender; menstruation apps (Brazil); pregnancy apps (Brazil)
women and sexualities: age, 11, 36, 41–42, 44–45, 46; beauty, 130; Brazil, 224–25, 228, 229–32, 237, 240–52, 263; CUP (Candidatura d'Unitat Popular), 158, 160; femininities, 130; Italy, 36, 41–42, 44–45, 46; testosterone, 11, 240–52. *See also* contraception; menstruation apps (Brazil); pregnancy apps (Brazil); reproduction
World Athletics Championships (paralympic sports). *See* IPC World Athletics Championships (paralympic sports)
World Health Organization, 53, 64n14

youth. *See* age
Yuval-Davis, Nira, 155

Zakharchenko, Antonina, 207–8
Zurr, Ionat, 169, 172, 178, 179, 180

www.ingramcontent.com/pod-product-compliance
Lightning Source LLC
Chambersburg PA
CBHW051531020426
42333CB00016B/1872